MW00463531

Basic Principles of Ophthalmic Surgery

Third Edition

Ayman Naseri, MD
Executive Editor

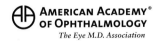

AMERICAN ACADEMY®
OF OPHTHALMOLOGY
The Eye M.D. Association

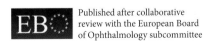

Published after collaborative
review with the European Board
of Ophthalmology subcommittee

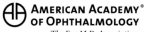
AMERICAN ACADEMY®
OF OPHTHALMOLOGY
The Eye M.D. Association

Box 7424
San Francisco, CA 94120-7424

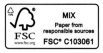
MIX
Paper from
responsible sources
FSC
www.fsc.org   FSC® C103061

The Academy provides this material for educational purposes only. It is not intended to represent the only or best method or procedure in every case, nor to replace a physician's own judgment or give specific advice for case management. Including all indications, contraindications, side effects, and alternative agents for each drug or treatment is beyond the scope of this material. All information and recommendations should be verified, prior to use, with current information included in the manufacturers' package inserts or other independent sources, and considered in light of the patient's condition and history. Reference to certain drugs, instruments, and other products in this publication is made for illustrative purposes only and is not intended to constitute an endorsement of such. Some materials may include information on applications that are not considered community standard, that reflect indications not included in approved FDA labeling, or that are approved for use only in restricted research settings. **The FDA has stated that it is the responsibility of the physician to determine the FDA status of each drug or device he or she wishes to use, and to use them with appropriate patient consent in compliance with applicable law.** The Academy specifically disclaims any and all liability for injury or other damages of any kind, from negligence or otherwise, for any and all claims that may arise from the use of any recommendations or other information contained herein.

Financial Disclosures

Academy staff members who contributed to the development of this product state that within the past 12 months, they have had no financial interest in or other relationship with any entity discussed in this book that produces, markets, resells, or distributes ophthalmic health care goods or services consumed by or used in patients, or with any competing commercial product or service.

The authors and reviewers state that within the past 12 months, they have had the following financial relationships:*

Dr Bandello: Alcon Laboratories (C), Alimera Sciences (C), Allergan (C), Bausch & Lomb (C), Bayer Schering Pharma (C), Farmila-Thea Farmaceutici S.p.A. (C), Genentech (C), F. Hoffmann-La Roche AG (C), Novagali Pharma SA (C), Novartis Pharmaceuticals (C), Pfizer (C), Sanofi S.A. (C), ThromboGenics (C)

Dr Creuzot-Garcher: Alcon Laboratories (C, S), Allergan (C, L, S), Bausch & Lomb (C), Bayer, Novartis Pharmaceuticals (C, L, S), Laboratoires Théa (C)

Dr Gedde: Alcon Laboratories (C), Allergan (C)

Dr Grupcheva: Johnson & Johnson (L), Théa (L)

Dr Andrew G. Lee: Credential Protection (O)

Dr Lustbader: LCA Vision (E), Novartis Pharmaceuticals (O)

Dr Winn: US Patent application: P5224US00 (P)

Dr Wladis: Lions Eye Foundation (S)

The other authors and reviewers state that within the past 12 months, they have had no financial interest in or other relationship with any entity discussed in this book that produces, markets, resells, or distributes ophthalmic health care goods or services consumed by or used in patients, or with any competing commercial product or service.

*C = consultant fees, paid advisory boards, or fees for attending a meeting; L = lecture fees (honoraria), travel fees, or reimbursements when speaking at the invitation of a commercial sponsor; O = equity ownership/stock options of publicly or privately traded firms (excluding mutual funds) with manufacturers of commercial ophthalmic products or commercial ophthalmic services; P = patents and/or royalties that might be viewed as creating a potential conflict of interest; S = grant support for the past year (all sources) and all sources used for a specific talk or manuscript with no time limitation

Contributors

Maria M. Aaron, MD
Professor of Ophthalmology
Director, Section of Comprehensive Ophthalmology
Emory University
Atlanta, Georgia

Daniel I. Bettis, MD
Glaucoma Fellow
John A. Moran Eye Center
University of Utah
Salt Lake City, Utah

Keith D. Carter, MD
Lillian C. O'Brien and Dr C. S. O'Brien Chair in
    Ophthalmology
Chair and Head, Department of Ophthalmology
University of Iowa Carver College of Medicine
Iowa City, Iowa

Jack A. Cohen, MD
Associate Professor of Ophthalmology
Associate Chair for Education
Resident Program Director
Rush University Medical Center
Chicago, Illinois

Sarah W. DeParis, MD
Resident Physician
Department of Ophthalmology
University of California, San Francisco
San Francisco, California

J. Paul Dieckert, MD, MBA
Medical Director for Member Education
Director, Division of Vitreoretinal Disease and Surgery
Baylor Scott & White Healthcare
Temple, Texas

Robert B. Dinn, MD
Eye Physicians, Inc.
Kokomo, Indiana

James P. Dunn, MD
Professor of Ophthalmology
Director, Uveitis Unit
Wills Eye Hospital Retina Service
Philadelphia, Pennsylvania

Kian Eftekhari, MD
Salt Lake Regional Medical Center
Salt Lake City, Utah

Steven J. Gedde, MD
John G. Clarkson Chair in Ophthalmology
Vice Chair of Education
Professor of Ophthalmology
Bascom Palmer Eye Institute
Miami, Florida

William G. Gensheimer, MD
Instructor/Fellow
Department of Ophthalmology
University of Colorado School of Medicine
Aurora, Colorado

Eric R. Holz, MD
Clinical Associate Professor of Ophthalmology
Baylor College of Medicine
Houston, Texas
Retina and Vitreous Associates of Texas
Houston, Texas

Yousuf M. Khalifa, MD
Chief of Service
Department of Ophthalmology
Grady Memorial Hospital
Associate Professor of Ophthalmology
Cornea and External Diseases
Emory Eye Center
Atlanta, Georgia

Anna S. Kitzmann, MD
Department of Ophthalmology
Mayo Clinic Health System
Fairmont, Minnesota

Alla Kukuyev, MD
Robert Cizik Eye Clinic
Clinical Assistant Professor
Department of Ophthalmology & Visual Science
The University of Texas
Houston, Texas

Paul D. Langer, MD
Associate Professor of Ophthalmology
Director, Division of Ophthalmic Plastic,
    Reconstructive, and Orbital Surgery
Department of Ophthalmology, New Jersey Medical
    School
Newark, New Jersey

Andrew G. Lee, MD
Professor of Ophthalmology, Neurology, and
    Neurological Surgery, Weill Cornell Medical
    College
Chair, Department of Ophthalmology, Houston
    Methodist Hospital
Clinical Professor of Ophthalmology, UTMB Galveston
Clinical Professor of Head and Neck Surgery, UT MD
    Anderson Cancer Center
Adjunct Professor of Ophthalmology, The University of
    Iowa and Baylor College of Medicine

Jennifer Lee, MD
Washington Pacific Eye Associates
Kirkland, Washington
Clinical Assistant Professor of Ophthalmology
University of Washington
Seattle, Washington

Yunhee Lee, MD, MPH
Assistant Professor of Clinical Ophthalmology
Bascom Palmer Eye Institute
Miami, Florida

Jay M. Lustbader, MD
Chair, Departments of Ophthalmology, MedStar
    Georgetown University Hospital and MedStar
    Washington Hospital Center
Professor of Ophthalmology, Georgetown University
    School of Medicine
President, Washington National Eye Center

Casey Mickler, MD
Storm Eye Institute
Medical University of South Carolina
Charleston, South Carolina

Frank Moya, MD
Assistant Professor of Ophthalmology, Glaucoma
    Section
Duke Eye Center
Winston-Salem, North Carolina

Hreem Patel, MD
Rush University Medical Center
Chicago, Illinois

Ensa K. Pillow, MD
Attending Physician, Ophthalmology
Oklahoma City Veterans Affairs Medical Center
Oklahoma City, Oklahoma
Clinical Assistant Professor, Department of
    Ophthalmology
University of Oklahoma

Dmitry Pyatetsky, MD
Assistant Professor
Ophthalmology Residency Program Director
Northwestern University Feinberg School of Medicine
Chief, Ophthalmology, Jesse Brown VA Medical Center
Chicago, Illinois

Peter A. Quiros, MD
Assistant Professor, Department of Ophthalmology
University of Southern California
Doheny Eye Institute
Los Angeles, California

Anvesh C. Reddy, MD
Department of Ophthalmology
University of Missouri–Kansas City School of Medicine
Kansas City, Missouri

Mahendra K. Rupani, MD
Assistant Professor, Ophthalmology
University of Missouri–Kansas City School of Medicine
Kansas City, Missouri

Paul J. Tapino, MD
Associate Professor of Clinical Ophthalmology
Director, Ophthalmology Residency Program
The Scheie Eye Institute
Philadelphia, Pennsylvania

M. Reza Vagefi, MD
Associate Clinical Professor of Ophthalmology
Associate Residency Program Director
University of California, San Francisco
San Francisco, California

Nicholas J. Volpe, MD
Chair, Department of Ophthalmology
George and Edwina Tarry Professor of Ophthalmology
Northwestern University Feinberg School of Medicine
Chicago, Illinois

Jonathan D. Walker, MD
Assistant Clinical Professor
Indiana University School of Medicine
Fort Wayne, Indiana
Allen County Retinal Surgeons
Fort Wayne, Indiana

David K. Wallace, MD, MPH
Professor of Ophthalmology & Pediatrics
Director of Clinical Research
Duke Eye Center
Durham, North Carolina

Andrew A. Wilson, MD
Dean McGee Eye Institute
Oklahoma City, Oklahoma

Bryan J. Winn, MD
Assistant Professor of Ophthalmology at
Columbia University Medical Center
Residency Program Director
Columbia University
New York, New York

Edward J. Wladis, MD
Associate Professor, Ophthalmic Plastic Surgery
Department of Ophthalmology
Lions Eye Institute
Albany Medical College
Albany, New York

Sandra M. Woolley, PhD, CPE
Ergonomist, Occupational Safety
Mayo Clinic
Rochester, Minnesota

Norman A. Zabriskie, MD
Vice-Chair Clinical, Medical Director
Department of Ophthalmology/Visual Sciences
John A. Moran Eye Center
University of Utah
Salt Lake City, Utah

Contents

Foreword   ix
Preface   xi

Part I
Evaluation and Preparation   1

Chapter 1
Patient Selection   3
Maria M. Aaron, MD

Criteria for Surgical Intervention   3
Factors Affecting Surgical Risk   4
Ethical Considerations   7
Implications of the Surgeon's
   Experience   8

Chapter 2
Preparation of the Patient   11
Hreem Patel, MD
Jack A. Cohen, MD

Preparations in the Office   11
Process in the Operating Room   13

Chapter 3
Preparation of the Surgeon   17
Eric R. Holz, MD
Alla Kukuyev, MD

Familiarization   17
Understanding the Planned
   Procedure   18
Knowing the Tools   18
Physical Factors Affecting the
   Surgeon   18
Hand Preparation   20
Operating Room Environment   20

Chapter 4
Informed Consent   25
Kian Eftekhari, MD
Paul J. Tapino, MD

Importance of Informed Consent   25
Elements of Informed Consent   26

Challenges for Residents Obtaining
   Informed Consent   28
Summary   31

Chapter 5
Simulation in Surgical Training   35
William G. Gensheimer, MD
Yousuf M. Khalifa, MD

Wet Laboratory   35
Intraocular Simulation   36
Virtual Reality   39

Part II
Surgical Logistics   43

Chapter 6
The Importance of Ergonomics for
Ophthalmologists   45
Sandra M. Woolley, PhD, CPE
Anna S. Kitzmann, MD

Ergonomics and Ergonomic Risk
   Factors   45
Adopting Ergonomically Friendly
   Practices   46
Reducing the Risk of Developing
   Musculoskeletal Disorders   58

Chapter 7
The Operating Microscope and
Surgical Loupes   63
Norman A. Zabriskie, MD
Daniel I. Bettis, MD

Advantages and Disadvantages of
   Magnification   63
Patient Positioning   64
Surgeon Positioning   68
Positioning the Bed   70
Stabilizing the Hands   72
Microscope Function   76
Surgical Loupes   81

Chapter 8
Surgical Instruments and
Blades 85
Jay M. Lustbader, MD
Robert B. Dinn, MD

Surgical Instruments 85
Other Specialized Surgical
   Instruments 105
Surgical Blades 107

Chapter 9
Suture Materials and Needles 111
Jennifer Lee, MD
Keith D. Carter, MD

Characteristics of Sutures 111
Classification of Sutures 111
Needles 115

Chapter 10
Lasers 119
Jonathan D. Walker, MD

Laser Physics 119
Laser/Tissue Interactions 120
Wavelength 123
Controlling the Energy 124
Putting the Variables Together 125
Laser Safety 127
Patient Issues 127
New Directions 129

Chapter 11
ACGME Requirements for Surgical
Training 133
Bryan J. Winn, MD

ACGME Case Logs 133
Common Pitfalls 135
Tips on Maintaining an Accurate Surgical
   Log 136
Beyond Residency and the ACGME 137
Milestones 137

Part III
Intraoperative Considerations 141

Chapter 12
Aseptic Technique and the Sterile
Field in the Operating Room 143
Ensa K. Pillow, MD
Andrew A. Wilson, MD

Skin Preparation 143
Application of Antiseptic Agents 144
Hand Scrubbing 144
Gowning and Gloving 146
Draping 147
Sterile Field 150

Chapter 13
Ophthalmic Anesthesia 153
Steven J. Gedde, MD
Yunhee Lee, MD, MPH

Sedation 153
Local Anesthetic Agents 154
Regional Anesthetic Agents 155
Local Anesthesia 157
Regional Anesthesia 158
General Anesthesia 163
Facial Nerve Blocks 164
Complications of Ophthalmic
   Anesthesia 165

Chapter 14
Hemostasis 171
J. Paul Dieckert, MD, MBA

Prevention 171
Heating 171
Vasoconstriction 173
Biochemical Enhancement of
   Hemostasis 173
Mechanical Tamponade 174
Embolization 174

Chapter 15
Suturing and Knot Tying 177
Edward J. Wladis, MD
Paul D. Langer, MD

Simple Square Knot (Instrument
   Tie) 177
Basic Suturing Principles 179
Common Suturing Techniques 180

Chapter 16
Intraocular Fluids 187
James P. Dunn, MD

Ophthalmic Viscosurgical Devices 187
Irrigating Fluids 191
Mydriatics and Miotics 192
Anesthetics 193
Corticosteroids, Antibiotics, and
   Antifungals 194

Capsular Staining Agents 194
Vascular Endothelial Growth Factor
  Antagonists 195
Compounding Intraocular Drugs 195

Chapter 17
Patient Safety Issues 199
Andrew G. Lee, MD

Infection Prophylaxis 199
Surgery on the Incorrect Eye 199
Incorrect Intraocular Lens
  Placement 201
Minimizing Medication Errors:
  Communication about Drug
  Orders 202
Preventing Surgeon-Related Fire in the
  Operating Room 204

Part IV
Postoperative Considerations 211

Chapter 18
Postoperative Management 213
Nicholas J. Volpe, MD
Dmitry Pyatetsky, MD

Postoperative Instructions 213
Timing of Postoperative Care 215
Focus of the Examination 217
Pain Management 219
Management of Complications 219

Chapter 19
The Healing Process 225
Frank Moya, MD
Peter A. Quiros, MD
Casey Mickler, MD

Healing by Intention 225
The Process of Healing 226
Wound Healing in Dermal/Conjunctival
  Tissue 229
Corneal Wound Healing 233
Scleral Wound Healing 235
Uveal Wound Healing 236
Modifying Wound Healing 237
Wound Healing Enhancers 238
The Ultimate Goal 240

Chapter 20
Dressings 243
David K. Wallace, MD, MPH

Advantages and Disadvantages of
  Postoperative Dressings 243
Indications 244
Supplies 244
Technique for Dressing Placement 246
Postoperative Instructions 248
Dressing Removal 248

Chapter 21
**Handling of Ocular Tissues for
Pathology 251**
Mahendra K. Rupani, MD
Anvesh C. Reddy, MD

Preoperative Planning, Frozen and
  Routine Specimens 251
Supplies and Equipment,
  Requisitions 252
Labeling of Specimen Containers 254
Specimen Requisitions 254
Transportation 256
Frozen Sections 256
Pearls for Handling of Routine
  Specimens 256
Special Procedures 260
Gross Specimens Only 260

Chapter 22
**Complications and Their
Consequences 263**
Sarah W. DeParis, MD
M. Reza Vagefi, MD

Care of the Patient 263
Medicolegal Implications of an
  Error 265
Care of the Surgeon in the Event of an
  Error 267

Appendix A
**Preferred Responses, Chapter
Self-Assessment Tests 271**

Index 273

Foreword

How do you teach surgery? How do you learn surgery? We surgeons have vivid memories of events in our surgical learning path—the first time we scrubbed in as medical students, the first time we sutured a laceration, or the first time we touched a beating heart—and many, many more.

As ophthalmologists, we remember the first successful cataract surgery and the patient's vision the next day—and we remember our first serious intraoperative complication and the steps we took to manage it. We likely all shared a similar surgical learning process in residency training as we built on our general medical and surgical experience, sequentially adding knowledge, specific manual maneuvers, and procedural components through a combination of didactics, surgical "wet laboratories," observation, and supervised patient experience. Then, under supervision, we assembled it all into the complete package as primary surgeon.

Is that the best way to learn surgery? Ultimately, no. In an ideal system, ophthalmic surgical simulation technology will soon allow us to gain not only technical proficiency but also experience in intraoperative decision-making and complication management. When surgeons in training then perform their "first case" as a primary surgeon, they will do so having had important near-real-life experience. The process will benefit surgeons in training and patients alike.

But surgery is much, much more than the technical performance of a set of skill components. A well-constructed set of surgical learning objectives must involve many subjects, including the biomechanics of wound construction and healing, instrument design, surgical materials (such as sutures and irrigation fluids), and sterility and infection control. It should include patient selection, the informed consent processes, medical ethics, postoperative management, and complication avoidance and management, among other topics.

For ophthalmology, surgery is a core and a complex competency, and education in this complex subject remains a process equally daunting for teacher and student alike. Anything that can facilitate the process benefits future patients. *Basic Principles of Ophthalmic Surgery,* together with the Academy's companion volume, *Basic Techniques of Ophthalmic Surgery,* packages many of the key elements of the surgical process and environment into an invaluable adjunct to the learning program for residents.

Simulators, texts, and videos are only imperfect tools in this educational process. But they can better prepare us to meet the challenges. There is one other critical component to surgical education—the experienced operative teacher and mentor who sits (or stands) at our side and guides us through the exciting, exacting, and at times stressful process of altering living human tissue. This volume, both text and video, reflects the commitment and talents of some of those incredible ophthalmic educators who have shepherded the earlier editions.

As surgeons we have a profound obligation to our patients. They honor us by trusting to us their sight and sometimes their lives. This text acknowledges the scope and complexity of that obligation.

David W. Parke II, MD
Chief Executive Officer
American Academy of Ophthalmology

Preface

Many years ago when the American Academy of Ophthalmology began development of *Basic Principles of Ophthalmic Surgery,* respected educators immediately recognized the need for a comprehensive resource to aid in navigating the surgical learning curve experienced by all ophthalmology residents. Led by Dr Anthony Arnold in its inaugural edition and by Dr Thomas Oetting in the second edition, this book shares the collective knowledge and experience of passionate surgical educators accumulated over thousands of hours of professional dedication. The hope is that residents and educators from around the corner and around the world can benefit from this text in traversing among the most challenging aspects of residency training: the interface between the patient and the novice surgeon.

This edition is divided into 4 major sections: Evaluation and Preparation, Surgical Logistics, Intraoperative Considerations, and Postoperative Considerations. All of the previous chapters has been updated where appropriate, and several new chapters have been added to further expand on specific topics in greater depth. New chapters include "Informed Consent" (by Kian Eftekhari, MD, and Paul J. Tapino, MD), "Simulation in Surgical Training" (by William G. Gensheimer, MD, and Yousuf M. Khalifa, MD), "ACGME Requirements for Surgical Training" (by Bryan J. Winn, MD), and "Complications and Their Consequences" (by Sarah DeParis, MD, and M. Reza Vagefi, MD).

For all of the authors in this book, we are grateful for their generous contributions of time, effort, and expertise, offered on behalf of many future generations of ophthalmologists. I am also personally grateful for the support of Kim Torgerson and for her patience and guidance in creating this edition.

Ayman Naseri, MD
Ophthalmology Residency Program Director, University of California
Chief of Ophthalmology at the San Francisco Veterans Affairs Medical Center
San Francisco, California

Acknowledgments

The Academy wishes to acknowledge the following people who reviewed the second edition and suggested changes for the third edition. For the Committee on Resident Education: Christopher B. Chambers, MD; Laura K. Green, MD; Jean R. Hausheer, MD; Andrew G. Lee, MD; Alison R. Loh, MD; Laura L. Wayman, MD; Jennifer S. Weizer, MD; and Evan L. Waxman, MD, PhD. For the European Board of Ophthalmology: Wagih Aclimandos, London, UK; Christina Grupcheva, MD, Varna, Bulgaria; Catherine Creuzot-Garcher, MD, PhD, Dijon, France; Hanne Olsen Julian, Copenhagen, Denmark; Francesco Bandello, MD, FEBO, Milan, Italy. For peer review of new chapters: Michele M. Bloomer, MD;

Laura K. Green, MD; Jean R. Hausheer, MD; Andrew G. Lee, MD; Nick Mamelis, MD; Anne Menke (OMIC); Todd J. Mondzelewski, MD; Jennifer S. Weizer, MD; and Evan L. Waxman, MD.

A special thanks to Richard Caesar, MBBS, FRCOphth, and Bryn M. Burkholder, MD, for providing videos.

The Academy thanks the following for supplying photographs for the instruments chapter, including Anthony Kroboth, Ambler Surgical; Anne Bohsack, FCI Ophthalmics; Gordon Dahl, Katena Products; Larry Laks, MicroSurgical Technology; Scott Heck, Wilson Ophthalmic; and Amy Wang, ASICO, LLC. Photo credits: figures for this chapter are courtesy of Ambler Surgical unless otherwise noted. Figures 8-18, 8-39, and 8-46 are courtesy of FCI Ophthalmics; Figures 8-37, 8-38, 8-53, 8-66, 8-67, 8-75, 8-76, and 8-86 are courtesy of Katena Products; Figures 8-40, 8-41, 8-45, and 8-71 are courtesy of Micro-Surgical Technology; Figure 8-72, part 2, is courtesy of ASICO, LLC; and Figures 8-74 and 8-91 are courtesy of Wilson Ophthalmic.

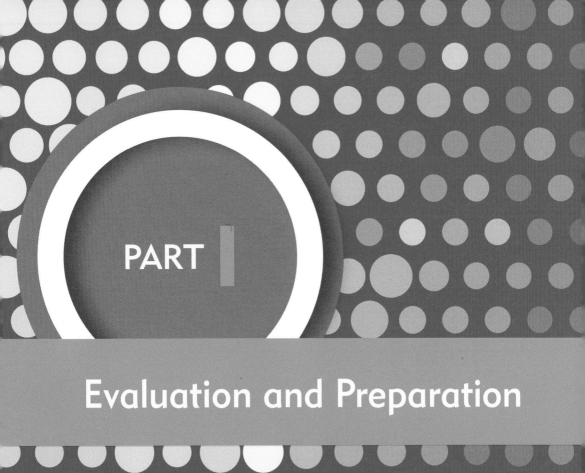

PART I

Evaluation and Preparation

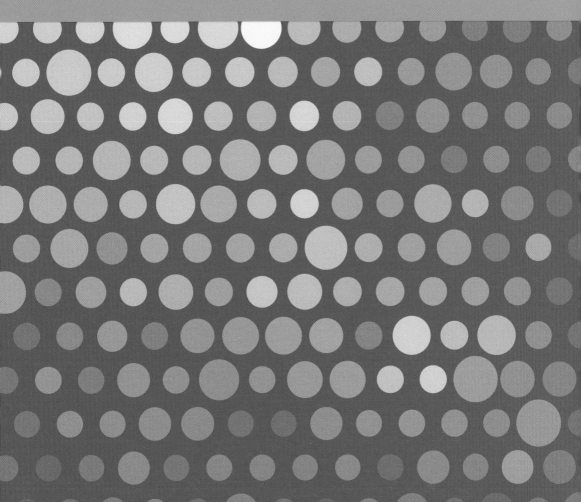

CHAPTER 1

Patient Selection

Maria M. Aaron, MD

The performance of surgery involves much more than the procedure itself. The beginning surgeon often focuses on the successful completion of the technical procedure—merely getting from point A to point B—without complications. Successful surgery, however, also requires careful patient selection, preoperative evaluation, and postoperative care. This chapter focuses on issues of patient selection, including criteria for surgical intervention, factors affecting surgical risk, ethical considerations including informed consent and advertising, and the implications of the surgeon's experience.

Criteria for Surgical Intervention

The surgeon must carefully assess the patient's complaints and expectations for surgery. Upon reviewing the clinical pathology, he or she must determine if the surgical procedure will accomplish the desired outcome. For example, the patient with mild to moderate macular degeneration undergoing cataract extraction might be expecting a 20/20 result similar to that of others who have had the procedure; consequently, the surgeon must communicate a reasonable expectation of more limited visual acuity in this situation. Moreover, a patient with severe macular degeneration and a dense posterior capsular opacity may not benefit at all from a YAG capsulotomy, and therefore the laser procedure is not justified.

In addition to understanding the patient's expectations, the surgeon must carefully review the clinical findings in order to accurately assess risk, evaluate whether surgery is justified, and communicate the risk-benefit ratio clearly to the patient. Careful clinical evaluation may reveal coexisting disease that might increase the potential risks of surgery. For example, a patient who has a moderate degree of corneal endothelial guttata who is undergoing phacoemulsification for a dense brunescent lens has the added risk of corneal decompensation. Table 1-1 lists common coexisting findings to consider when evaluating patients for cataract surgery, which is the type of surgery in which the beginning surgeon is most likely to be involved. While the implications of such abnormalities may vary depending upon the clinical situation and the experience of the surgeon, preoperative examination should include their consideration in every case. Many first-year residents may be involved in eyelid and laser procedures.

Table 1-1 Common Concerns to Consider Before Cataract Surgery

Condition	Risk
History	
Previous trauma	Zonular or capsular weakness
General physical condition	
Dementia	Altered response to anesthesia, movement during procedure
Severe spine/neck disease	Inability to lie supine
Congestive heart failure	Inability to lie supine
Prior use of an alpha blocker	Intraoperative floppy iris syndrome
Anterior segment	
Abnormally shallow anterior chamber	Reduction of working space
Abnormally deep anterior chamber	Difficulty with maneuvers
Exposure keratopathy	Corneal decompensation
Endothelial guttata	Corneal decompensation
History of iritis or inflammatory condition	Severe postoperative inflammation
Poor pupillary dilation	Challenging nuclear removal, iris prolapse
Pseudoexfoliation	Poor dilation and zonular weakness
Advanced glaucoma	Spike in intraocular pressure
Prior trabeculectomy	Failure of shunt
Corneal scars	Poor visualization
Phacodonesis	Zonular weakness
Mature cataract or poor red reflex	Poor visualization of capsulorrhexis
Posterior segment	
Previous pars plana vitrectomy	Loss of vitreous support
High myopia	Retinal detachment
Diabetic retinopathy	Progression of disease
Macular degeneration	Possible progression of disease
Other macular pathology	Limited visual outcome

Factors Affecting Surgical Risk

Ophthalmic surgical procedures are often performed on elderly patients who require careful medical evaluation to avoid surgical or systemic complications. While a patient's age does not necessarily correlate with his or her physical and mental status, older patients often have concomitant medical conditions requiring multiple medications. Proper preoperative medical assessment allows for selection of proper surgical candidates and helps ensure a smooth operative procedure and course in those who proceed to surgery.

Preoperative medical evaluation, either a brief survey by the surgeon or a detailed assessment by a medical specialist, depending on the clinical situation, allows for selection of those patients who can safely undergo surgery and identification of those who either require medical care before surgery or cannot safely proceed. The examiner should take a thorough history—including questions about medications, allergies, bleeding disorders and prior surgical procedures—during the preoperative assessment. The surgeon should detect the past use of alpha-blocking agents such as tamsulosin, as a history of these agents increases the risk of the intraoperative floppy iris syndrome. He or she should also pay careful attention to a patient's use of aspirin-containing products and additional medications that may cause bleeding, including warfarin sodium (Coumadin), heparin, nonsteroidal anti-inflammatory drugs (NSAIDs), and herbal therapies such as Ginkgo biloba, garlic, and ginger. Many patients are unaware that aspirin and NSAIDs may cause bleeding and therefore do not report them unless specifically questioned.

Anticoagulants are of particular concerns when considering eyelid, periorbital, or orbital procedures. In patients requiring oral anticoagulants for prevention of stroke and transient ischemic attack, suspension of these agents carries risks, and alternative anesthesia or consultation with the patient's physician should be considered. Systemic situations that may require special evaluation or therapy before surgery include cardiac disease, hypertension, pulmonary disease, and diabetes. Issues of anesthesia may be a concern with children and people with altered mental status.

Cardiac Disease

Patients with cardiac disease should be evaluated for any recent ischemic events, arrhythmias, or congestive heart failure (CHF). Patients with severe CHF may have difficulty lying supine for the duration of the procedure and may require intensive therapy to optimize cardiac status before surgery. (See Chapter 2 for discussion of positioning the patient.) If the patient is unstable or if the surgeon has any degree of uncertainty about the cardiac stability, the cardiologist or primary care provider should clear the patient before the performance of the ophthalmic procedure.

Hypertension

Arterial blood pressure control is essential in patients undergoing ophthalmic surgery, as uncontrolled pressure increases risk of cardiovascular complications. Patients with a systolic blood pressure over 180 mmHg and a diastolic blood pressure over 100 mmHg should be evaluated and treated before the performance of an elective procedure.

Postural Limitations

Proper positioning of the patient for surgical or laser procedures is essential for uncomplicated, successful surgery. The majority of intraoperative procedures require the patient to be in the supine position; however, patients with severe kyphosis, cerebral palsy, myotonic dystrophy, or obesity may present challenges. These patients may also be difficult to position for office procedures at the slit lamp. Adjusting the operating table and/or chair, rotating the surgical microscope or laser apparatus, altering the surgical/laser approach, and using pillows, sheets, foam, and so on are effective techniques for minimizing discomfort for patients and surgeons.

Pulmonary Disease

The patient with severe chronic obstructive pulmonary disease or asthma will need clearance by his or her pulmonary or primary care physician before elective surgery.

Optimization of pulmonary function reduces cardiopulmonary risks of anesthesia. Uncontrolled cough increases risk of complications in intraocular surgery, in both intraoperative and postoperative periods; patients with this condition require careful screening and management before consideration for surgery.

Diabetes

Optimal control of diabetes may reduce risks of general anesthesia and postoperative infection. Patients with uncontrolled diabetes should be evaluated and managed by a medical specialist before elective ophthalmic surgery.

Children

Children who have a family history of unexplained morbidity with anesthesia should be suspected of having a predisposition to malignant hyperthermia, a rare genetic disorder of skeletal muscle metabolism. Any such question should be addressed by the patient's medical and anesthesia team before surgery. Chapter 13 reviews symptoms of malignant hyperthermia; early recognition and action may be life-saving.

Altered Mental Status

Patients with altered mental function present specific problems in understanding the surgical procedure and postoperative conditions and may be unable to cooperate for surgery under local anesthesia. These patients require the participation of a family member in the preoperative, operative, and postoperative states. They also need additional consideration with regard to the choice of anesthesia (eg, general or local).

Ocular Conditions

Specific ocular conditions should also be considered to ensure proper preparation for surgery. While Table 1-1 lists many of these, some require special consideration. In particular, patients will severe dry eye require careful consideration, especially when contemplating lid procedures, refractive surgery, or other corneal or intraocular surgeries. Most commonly, dry eye worsens following surgery from damage to the epithelial cells, cutting of corneal nerves, or use of drops after surgery. Ideally, the dry eye symptoms should be treated preoperatively and continued in the postoperative period for several months.

Corneal diseases

Epithelial, stromal, or endothelial disease can all complicate cataract surgery either by obscuring proper visualization during the procedure or by contributing to postoperative corneal edema following the surgery. If possible, such concerns should be addressed prior to or during cataract surgery to provide the best possible surgical outcomes.

Iris abnormalities

Any conditions causing poor pupillary dilation (eg, pseudoexfoliation, posterior synechiae, or medications causing intraoperative floppy iris syndrome [IFIS]) should be noted preoperatively so that they may be addressed, helping to avoid difficulty with nucleus removal or iris prolapse. Specifically, surgeons should inquire about the use of systemic α-1 blockers for the treatment of urinary symptoms associated with benign prostate hypertrophy. Treatment options to consider include iris retractors, pupil expansion rings, or viscoelastic agents that mechanically hold the pupil in position.

Lens concerns

Extremely dense nuclei, subluxed lens, or phacodonesis can create challenges during cataract surgery. Proper planning regarding technique (ie, conversion to extracapsular cataract surgery, posterior approach to cataract removal, placement of capsular tension ring) can prevent intraoperative complications.

Ethical Considerations

Informed Consent

Chapters 2 and 4 review details of the informed consent process. With regard to patient selection, however, 3 primary issues apply to the discussion of informed consent:

1. The surgeon has the responsibility to determine whether a patient is able to understand the nature of the procedure and potential risks, and then to make an autonomous decision whether to proceed. If the patient is unable to do so, or if uncertainty exists about his or her competence to make this decision, elective surgery should be deferred pending clarification of the issue (possibly with legal consultation). In some circumstances, a chosen surrogate may make the decision.
2. The patient has the right to make his or her own decisions regarding medical treatment, and he or she may contribute to the process of selection for surgery. For example, a moderate nuclear cataract in a patient with 20/50 vision may or may not require surgery. An airline pilot might desire that his or her cataract be removed, whereas an elderly person may feel comfortable continuing daily life with 20/50 vision.
3. The patient has the right to know if a resident in training, supervised by an experienced faculty, will be the primary surgeon for a portion or all of the procedure. This must be explicitly explained during the consent process. Patient selection must take into account those who are uncomfortable with this situation, so that alternate planning for surgical care can be made.

Advertising

The fundamental principle in medical advertising is that communications to the public must be accurate. Individuals who engage in false advertising may be subject to punishment under state and federal laws, but physicians must also be aware of the rules outlined by state medical boards as well as the American Medical Association's Code of Ethics. Before the twentieth century, advertising for patient recruitment was prohibited because it was considered "derogatory to the dignity of the profession to resort to public advertisements." However, in 1977, it became unlawful for physicians to restrict advertising. With the recent explosion of refractive surgical procedures, the ethical concepts of advertising must be carefully considered. Care must be taken to portray all aspects of surgery accurately, without misleading the public, and to avoid claims of superiority or exclusivity that promote the physician's business rather than the patient's best interest. Similarly, one must avoid any patient education program or referral process that utilizes coercion to encourage surgery or limit patient options for surgical referral.

Implications of the Surgeon's Experience

The surgeon is responsible for assessing whether he or she has attained the level of experience required to perform specific surgical procedures. In residency training, the attending faculty generally sets guidelines and monitors them, with increasingly complex or difficult cases being assigned to senior residents with greater surgical experience. Thus, the patient selection process includes assigning certain categories of surgical candidates to residents at the appropriate level of training. For example, in cataract surgery, cases that might be expected to present challenges at surgery (eg, patients who are monocular, have poor pupil dilation, poor visualization due to corneal disease, phacodonesis, or high myopia) are reserved for experienced surgeons. Similarly, patients who require surgery to be completed in the shortest time (eg, those who have limited cooperation due to altered mental status or those with severe medical problems limiting tolerance for prolonged procedures) are assigned to the most experienced surgeons.

This principle also holds after the completion of residency training, as surgical technology advances and new techniques become available. Patients who are candidates for new techniques must be selected according to the expertise of the surgeon.

Key Points

- A thorough preoperative medical evaluation is essential in appropriate patient selection.
- Patients with cardiac disease, hypertension, postural limitations, pulmonary disease, or diabetes may require special evaluation or therapy before surgery. Issues of anesthesia may be a concern with children and people with altered mental status.
- Appropriate patient selection includes
  - ensuring that indications for surgical intervention are appropriate and that the risk-benefit ratio is satisfactory
  - carefully assessing medical risk factors and ensuring that the patient's general medical status is optimized prior to surgery
  - ascertaining that the patient understands and agrees to the indications, risks, benefits, and alternatives for surgery
  - avoidance of coercion in proceeding with surgery
  - ensuring that the proposed surgical procedure is one for which the surgeon has adequate training and experience

American Academy of Ophthalmology. *Communications to the Public* [Advisory Opinion of the Code of Ethics]. San Francisco: American Academy of Ophthalmology; 2012.

American Academy of Ophthalmology. *Ethical Ophthalmologist Series* [online courses]. San Francisco: American Academy of Ophthalmology; 2010.

American Academy of Ophthalmology. *Informed Consent* [Advisory Opinion of the Code of Ethics]. San Francisco: American Academy of Ophthalmology; 2013.

Berdahl JP and Vann RR. Cataract surgery: preoperative evaluation. In: Henderson BA, Rineda R, Chen, SH, eds. *Essentials of Cataract Surgery.* 2nd ed. Thorofare, NJ: Slack; 2014.

Durfee DA, ed. Ethics and the American Academy of Ophthalmology. In: *The Profession of Ophthalmology: Practice Management, Ethics, and Advocacy.* San Francisco: American Academy of Ophthalmology; 2010:186–197.

Rowe S. Appropriateness of cataract surgery. In: Henderson BA, Rineda R, Chen, SH, eds. *Essentials of Cataract Surgery.* 2nd ed. Thorofare, NJ: Slack; 2014.

Self-Assessment Test

1. Medications that may increase the risk of bleeding include which of the following? (Choose all that apply.)
   a. Ginkgo biloba
   b. nonsteroidal anti-inflammatory drugs
   c. Coumadin
   d. all of the above
2. List at least 3 features that a preoperative medical evaluation should address.
3. The decision to recommend cataract surgery includes consideration of which of the following factors? (Choose all that apply.)
   a. coexistent macular disease
   b. patient's visual requirements
   c. coexistent corneal disease
   d. family history of macular degeneration

For preferred responses to these questions, see Appendix A.

CHAPTER 2

Preparation of the Patient

Hreem Patel, MD
Jack A. Cohen, MD

Appropriate preparation of a patient for surgery greatly impacts both the surgeon's and the patient's entire surgical experience. Recognition of the importance of this process early in residency encourages the development of good habits seen in successful surgeons who maintain good rapport with their patients and effectively manage expectations. Patient preparation begins in the office and continues preoperatively in the operating room.

Preparations in the Office

After the surgeon has assessed the patient and decided that surgery is a viable option, the next steps involve obtaining informed consent and scheduling the surgery. The essence of the informed decision-making process lies in effective physician–patient communication. The physician empowers the patient with the knowledge required to make an educated decision regarding medical care. At all times, the patient should feel in control of the decision-making process and able to decide what happens to his or her body.

Informed Consent

Chapters 1 and 4 include discussion of concepts of informed consent that should be considered in selecting patients for surgery. Informed consent in preparing the patient for surgery develops from the patient's understanding of several elements.

These elements include

- the nature of the procedure
- reasonable alternatives to the proposed intervention
- explanation of the risks, benefits, and uncertainties related to each alternative
- assessment of the patient's understanding
- acceptance of the intervention by the patient

Procedure, alternatives, and risks

The depth of the discussion depends on the nature of the procedure and the number of risks, benefits, and alternatives. The American Academy of Ophthalmology suggests that the content of this discussion should include what a "reasonable" patient would want to know. However, the difficulty in implementing a reasonable patient standard is also recognized because it involves determining what information is relevant for a particular patient. In most ophthalmic surgeries, the ultimate goals are to improve vision, preserve vision, or enhance appearance. The most common risks include infection, bleeding, loss of vision, scarring, and possible need for repeat surgery.

Discussion of alternatives should incorporate all options including medical management and observation even if these choices are not ideal. Allow the patient to ask as many questions as necessary to facilitate comprehension of the intervention. This also enables the physician to assess the patient's understanding of the procedure. Encourage patients to have family members present during the preoperative discussion so that they can provide support for the patient not only for the surgery itself, but during the decision-making process as well. Clearly outline any rehabilitation that will be needed after surgery and the average number of postoperative visits needed so the patient has an understanding of the postoperative course as well. Attention to these types of details helps ensure that adequate informed consent is obtained.

Discussion of the procedure should also include a description of anesthesia options. In ophthalmology, surgery may be performed with a variety of anesthetic techniques including topical, local, intravenous sedation, and general anesthesia. (See Chapter 13.) The physician should explain the preferred anesthetic option for the procedure so that the patient knows what to expect and the physician can anticipate potential problems. A review of the medical history and physical examination results will determine indications or contraindications for specific anesthesia techniques. The anesthesia service determines the choice of anesthesia technique and informed consent process for anesthesia.

Assessment and acceptance

Special situations to consider in the consent process include surgery for minors, incompetent individuals, and emergencies. With minors and incompetent individuals, the consent process occurs with the legal guardian. If there is no legal guardian, state laws provide guidance for the hierarchy of appropriate decision makers. If no surrogate decision maker exists or if the situation is emergent, the physician acts in the best interests of the patient until a surrogate is found. Legal standards in these situations may vary by state, and in any questionable case, counsel should be consulted before proceeding with surgery.

Medical Clearance

Medical clearance should be obtained from the patient's internist or family practitioner before surgery. Although routine preoperative laboratory testing has not been proven to increase the safety of cataract surgery, consideration may be given to such testing on the recommendation of the patient's physician or for specific requirements of the medical facility involved. Basic tests in this workup include a complete metabolic profile, a complete blood count (CBC), and an electrocardiogram (EKG). For patients undergoing general anesthesia, a chest x-ray is also recommended. The surgeon must ensure that all diagnostic test results are reviewed before surgery.

Additional common preoperative issues (eg, prophylaxis against endocarditis, managing anticoagulation, and medication interaction with herbal supplements) should be discussed and managed in conjunction with the patient's physician. The American Heart

Association guidelines for prophylactic management of patients with cardiac valvular disease must be followed. Guidelines and quantification of risks for discontinuing anticoagulation have been published; typically anticoagulation is continued in patients at high risk for thromboembolism. Certain herbal supplements, such as Ginkgo biloba and vitamin E, increase the risk of bleeding in patients taking warfarin sodium (Coumadin) and must be considered.

Process in the Operating Room

Various chapters in this book discuss aspects of the surgical process. The following overview summarizes operative considerations with the focus on ensuring the patient's comfort. (Chapter 17 reviews specific precautions that are necessary to ensure the safety of the patient during ophthalmic surgery.)

Meeting the Patient

In the preoperative holding area, it is important that the patient see the surgeon. He or she may be the only familiar face among the many people that the patient will see during the surgical experience. This contact reassures the patient and provides an opportunity for any last-minute questions.

Marking the Surgical Eye

Many surgeons mark surgical eye in the holding area before any sedation is given. This confirms the surgical eye with the patient and avoids any confusion in the operating room. (In the operating room, the surgeon marks the site of the incision as well.) Surgery on the incorrect eye is the most feared but fortunately preventable medical error in the ophthalmic operating room. (See Chapter 17.)

Administering Medications

Review the history and physical report to ascertain any changes in the patient's health status. In cataract surgery and many retinal procedures, dilating drops will be administered in the preoperative holding area. Many surgeons also use preoperative topical antibiotic on the day of surgery or several days before surgery, although there is no consensus on which antibiotics to use and no studies show that this course prevents endophthalmitis. Some cataract surgeons apply topical anesthetic such as nonpreserved lidocaine jelly in the holding area with or without a device such as a Honan balloon to lower intraocular pressure.

Consider communicating any concerns or special requirements to the anesthesia service as soon as possible. For example, if the patient had problems with anesthesia during a prior surgical procedure, make sure the service is aware of this. If a local anesthetic block is needed, notify the anesthetist so the patient receives adequate sedation. Bear in mind that in many institutions, anesthesiology administers local anesthetic blocks so they need to be scheduled preoperatively.

Communicating With the Staff

Before the patient is brought back to the operating room, speak with operating room staff members to see whether they have any questions. If any special materials were ordered, verify that they are available. When doing cataract surgery, check that the correct intraocular lens has been set out for the procedure.

When the patient is brought into the operating room, the circulating nurse verifies the patient's name, surgical procedure, surgical site, and medical allergies with the patient. In addition, a time out is taken to identify all members of the operating room, verify the patient's name, verify the correct procedure, and identify any special precautions that maybe needed. Then, the bed is positioned in the most ideal location near the microscope to maximize viewing of the surgical eye (often the floor is marked to help guide the placement of the bed). If general anesthesia is required, positioning of the bed occurs after the patient is intubated. Positioning the patient's head on the bed and relative to the microscope is the foundation upon which the remainder of the surgery is built. When this is done incorrectly, every subsequent step of the procedure may become a challenge. When working under the microscope, the eye should be positioned so that it is parallel to the ground. The height of the bed should be adjusted to optimize surgeon comfort when looking under the microscope. When first learning to operate, check the positioning of the microscope by turning it on and looking through the oculars to assess whether the patient's placement is correct. This also serves to check if the microscope is functioning properly. (Chapter 7 discusses in detail the positioning of the microscope, patient, and surgeon.)

Ensuring the Patient's Comfort

Make sure the patient is comfortable. Operating rooms are often cold, and the patient may prefer an extra blanket. The nurse can provide support for the patient's back as needed by placing a blanket roll or foam log under the knees. Since many surgeries are done with topical anesthesia with or without intravenous sedation, wrist bracelets that attach to the bed rails are sometimes employed to ensure that the patient does not attempt to touch his or her face during the surgery. Taping down the patient's head is helpful in preventing head movement during surgery.

If a local anesthetic block is needed, it is best to do it after positioning the patient. After adequate intravenous sedation, the planned block can be administered. Typically, the nurse or the anesthetist holds the patient's head so it does not move during the block due to the noxious stimulus. Taping of the head should occur after the block so the head can be placed in the most comfortable position for the block. The surgical prep and draping follow final positioning of the patient. (See Chapter 2 for information about surgical prep and draping.)

Key Points

- In providing informed consent to the patient, the surgeon must explain the nature of the procedure, reasonable alternatives to the proposed intervention, and the risks, benefits, and uncertainties related to each alternative.

- Medical clearance for surgery includes assessment of cardiopulmonary status, anticoagulants, and antiplatelet agents. Clearance should be coordinated with the patient's primary care physician.
- In the operating room, the surgeon is responsible for meeting and reassuring the patient, supervising preoperative ophthalmic medications, coordinating with anesthesia and nursing staff, and ensuring proper positioning and comfort of the patient.

American Academy of Ophthalmology, Ophthalmic Mutual Insurance Company. *Practice Guidelines for Informed Consent.* San Francisco: American Academy of Ophthalmology; 2010; revised Dec 2011.

Douketis JD, Berger PB, Dunn AS, et al. The perioperative management of antithrombotic therapy: American College of Chest Physicians Evidence Based Clinical Practice Guildelines (8th Edition). *Chest.* 2008;133(6 Suppl):299S–339S.

Durfee DA, ed. Ethics in ophthalmology. In: *The Profession of Ophthalmology.* 2nd ed. San Francisco: American Academy of Ophthalmology; 2010.

Gower EW, Lindsey K, Nanji AA, Leyngold I, McDonnel PJ. Perioperative antibiotics for prevention of acute endophthalmitis after cataract surgery. *Cochrane Database Syst Rev.* 2013 Jul 15;7:CD006364.

Kearon C, Hirsh J. Management of anticoagulation before and after elective surgery. *N Engl J Med.* 1997;336(21):1506–1511.

Venugopalan P, Ganesh A, Rafay AM, Dio N. Low frequency of bacteraemia during eye surgery obviates the need for endocarditis prophylaxis. *Eye (Lond).* 2001; 15(Pt 6):753–755.

Self-Assessment Test

1. Which of the following is involved in the informed consent process? (Choose all that apply.)
   a. providing preoperative counseling alone
   b. discussing the risks, benefits, and alternatives of surgery
   c. delegating this responsibility to the surgical nurse
   d. discouraging consideration of alternatives to surgery that the surgeon feels are less appropriate

2. Which of the following is involved with the preoperative medical preparation of the patient? (Choose all that apply.)
   a. abstaining from any involvement in the preoperative preparation
   b. obtaining chest x-ray, electrocardiogram, urinalysis, and complete blood count
   c. discontinuing anticoagulants
   d. communicating with patient's primary physician if medical conditions coexist

3. When preparing the patient in the operating room, attention must be given to which of the following? (Choose all that apply.)
   a. communicating with the patient
   b. proper positioning of the head

    c. providing support for the back and knee
    d. stabilizing the patient (control of hands and head)
    e. ensuring a comfortable temperature
    f. all of the above

For preferred responses to these questions, see Appendix A.

CHAPTER 3

Preparation of the Surgeon

Eric R. Holz, MD
Alla Kukuyev, MD

A great body of literature addresses ophthalmic surgical management, including details of surgical techniques, preparation of the patient, management of the operating theater, and postoperative care (aspects of these topics are discussed elsewhere in this book). Very little, however, has been written about preparation of the surgeon. The surgeon's ability to attain peak performance is clearly a key element in obtaining optimal surgical outcomes. Thorough familiarity with the patient, procedure, and operating room environment are the foundation of preparation. Other considerations include physical factors affecting the surgeon, hand washing, and control of the operating room environment. This chapter serves as a guide to creating a personalized routine for your own preparation as a surgeon. The development of good habits through repetition limits stress and anxiety and prepares the physician to perform to optimum potential.

Familiarization

Chapters 1 and 2 discussed aspects of becoming familiar with the patient, deciding that surgery is the best option, and preparing the patient for surgery. In summary, several elements are important in the physician's interaction with his or her patient:

1. The surgeon should fully examine the patient preoperatively. This evaluation consists of a complete examination, including best-corrected visual acuity measurement, a review of pertinent ancillary testing, and directed systemic evaluation. Review of ancillary testing may include intraocular lens calculation data, fluorescein angiography, or neuroimaging such as magnetic resonance imaging films.
2. A discussion ensues in order to understand the patient (especially reactions and concerns), educate the patient, answer questions, and obtain informed consent.
3. A surgical plan evolves during the preoperative examination. Clearly, first meeting a patient on a gurney in the operating room is ill advised. Delegating preoperative evaluation and management to technicians, optometrists, and colleagues is another practice to avoid if you are to be optimally prepared. The exception to this might be an emergently added surgery, in which case it may be appropriate for the surgeon to examine the patient in the preoperative area if logistics preclude an examination in the office.

Understanding the Planned Procedure

Knowledge of the anticipated surgical procedure is an essential part of the familiarization process. As noted in Chapter 1, the surgeon is responsible for assessing whether he or she has attained the level of experience required to perform specific surgical procedures. Ideally, the beginning surgeon is prepared through the mentored experiences provided during ophthalmology residency training. Established techniques continue to evolve and new techniques are employed, and these developments require the surgeon's continuing education.

On an ongoing basis, long after the completion of residency training, the surgeon must ensure that he or she is facile in all aspects of a proposed procedure; if knowledge gaps or uncertainties exist, the surgeon has the responsibility to arrange for consultation with and possible intraoperative assistance from an expert in the field.

Knowing the Tools

Familiarity with the overall operating room environment is also crucial to preparation of the surgeon. Ophthalmic surgical instrumentation and machinery, including the phacoemulsification and vitrectomy units, are increasingly complex, and the surgeon needs to understand their inner workings in detail. Detailed discussion of surgical instrumentation and machinery is beyond the scope of this book. Equipment company representatives and other experienced surgeons are valuable sources of information in this area. (See Chapter 8 for an introduction to surgical instruments and blades.)

Consider performing a "dry run," including opening up surgical packs, setting up the machine, running through machine settings, and becoming familiar with the foot pedals and handpieces. The properly prepared surgeon knows the equipment better than the nursing staff! In cases of equipment malfunction or requirement for special measures, the surgeon's ultimate responsibility is to manage the situation correctly. In addition, an important, but frequently overlooked, area involves the location of items in the room. The physician is advised to go to the operating room during downtime and go through each drawer and cabinet with the nursing staff. The location of suture material, intraocular lenses, non-set surgical instruments, and so on should be identified so that the surgeon is prepared to give instructions when the primary nurse is unavailable, particularly during after-hours cases.

Physical Factors Affecting the Surgeon

A multitude of factors affects a physician's preparedness to perform surgery. Two of the commonly discussed physical factors are exercise and sleep deprivation. Physical exertion before surgery, involving as few as 20 knee bends, has been shown to significantly increase hand tremor when performing microsurgical tasks. This supports widely held beliefs that strenuous exercise, particularly upper-body weight lifting, should be avoided the day before and the day of surgery.

The relationship between sleep deprivation and physician performance has been studied superficially. Conclusions have been reached that "patient care may be compromised if a fatigued, sleep-deprived clinician is allowed to operate, administer an anesthetic, manage a medical crisis, or deal with an unusual or cognitively demanding clinical presentation" (Weigner, Ancoli-Israel, 2002). There is controversy regarding performance of particular activities but in general, there is more degradation on tasks of longer duration requiring vigilance. Performance of longer, repetitive surgery may be more severely affected by sleep deprivation. Avoidance of physical exertion and a good night's sleep are important components in the preparation of the surgeon.

Substance Use or Abuse

Both legal and illicit drug use can affect surgical performance and the prepared surgeon understands their impact. It is obvious that physicians impaired by alcohol or illicit drugs should never operate; however, the use of caffeine and β-blockers has been an area of controversy.

Many doctors routinely drink coffee or tea before performing surgery, yet studies involving hand steadiness support the assertion that caffeine increases hand tremor. One study noted that after ingestion of 200 mg of caffeine, tremor was significantly increased when measured with a handheld laser pointer model. Another study, employing a high-resolution, noncontact position tracking system, found that ingestion of 200 mg of caffeine caused a 31% increase in tremor from baseline. Based on these data, caffeine should be avoided to minimize tremor during ocular surgery.

Performance artists and surgeons have employed β-adrenergic blocking drugs to improve their performance. Several studies assess the effect of β-blockers on ocular surgery, or hand tremor. Using the same high-resolution, noncontact position tracking system as employed for the caffeine study, subjects who ingested 10 mg of propranolol (a nonselective β-blocking agent) were found to have 22% less tremor than at baseline. No adverse effects or side effects were reported. Ophthalmology residents given 40 mg of propranolol 1 hour before performing ophthalmic microsurgery experienced a significant reduction in tremor and perceived anxiety. However, there was no difference in complication rates or difficulties during surgery. Similarly, no negative effects or side effects were encountered in study participants. A study involving ingestion of timolol 12.5 mg as well as a postural orthotic concluded that neither "accorded a significant benefit in allaying hand tremor." In summary, β-blocker use, particularly oral propranolol, may diminish hand tremor, but this difference has not been proven to affect surgical outcomes.

Illness

Short-term illness such as the flu or an injury can temporarily impair the surgeon to varying degrees. It is the surgeon's responsibility to adequately assess any conditions that may affect surgical judgment and performance. It is reasonable to arrange for a qualified colleague to take over an emergency surgery and to postpone elective cases until such a time that the surgeon is no longer affected by his or her condition. Most ophthalmologic surgeries are elective, and with good communication with the patient can be rescheduled in the interest of patient safety.

Hand Preparation

Hand washing or scrubbing is a time-honored routine in surgery. Without question, hand washing decreases the surgeon's skin flora counts, which may in turn lower postoperative infection rates, especially in the event of glove failure. Several areas of controversy surround the surgical scrub, however. The duration of hand washing has been studied, with results indicating that a 2-minute period of chlorhexidine use is equivalent to 4- and 6-minute periods. Improved alcohol solutions for hand rubbing have become popular and are present in most institutions. A study reported that the use of a 75% aqueous alcoholic solution containing propanol-1, propanol-2, and mecetronium etilsulfate caused no difference in postoperative infection rates compared with use of 4% povidone-iodine or 4% chlorhexidine gluconate. Additionally, hand rubbing with an alcohol-based solution has been shown to result in a significantly lower skin flora count than hand washing with antiseptic soap during routine patient care.

In light of these findings, preparation of the hands for surgery should consist of a 2-minute scrubbing with chlorhexidine or povidone-iodine or simple hand washing with soap followed by hand rubbing with an appropriate alcohol-based solution. Generally accepted practice for the first scrub of the day includes a total duration of 5 minutes. Chapter 12 reviews the steps in the surgical hand scrub as well as the steps for gowning and gloving after the wash is complete.

Operating Room Environment

The surgeon must be able to give his or her full attention and concentration to the patient and the procedure. Preparation of the environment before surgery is an important step in minimizing distractions. Ideally, the physician should clear his or her schedule a bit before and after surgery to avoid potential conflicts. Having to run to clinic or to another hospital creates significant stress and is suboptimal. Likewise, during surgery, minimize interruptions by telephone calls and pages or avoid them altogether.

Giving forethought to ergonomic issues is a simple, but often overlooked, element. A few minutes spent before the procedure to adjust the bed height, microscope (eyepiece pupillary distance, power, and centration), and wrist rest result in greater comfort and less stress for the surgeon. (Chapter 7 reviews these adjustments in detail. See also Chapter 6.) Additionally, speaking with the scrub nurse and circulating nurse before the case allows them to anticipate your needs and to have readily available the necessary equipment and instruments. Simple communication before the surgery makes the team in the room more involved, understanding, and efficient. As a result, the case runs more smoothly.

Time Out

Wrong site surgery (including wrong eye surgery and incorrect intraocular lens implantation) can be prevented. The American Academy of Ophthalmology endorses a preoperative checklist based on the JCAHO universal protocol (Joint Commission of Accreditation of Healthcare Organizations, 2003). Many surgery centers and hospitals have their own protocols also adapted from the universal protocol. In an American Ophthalmological Society thesis, a thorough analysis of surgical errors made in ophthalmology was performed. The study found that 77% of the errors were preventable by use of the universal protocol. The typical time-out checklist introduces everyone present in the operating room, addresses any concerns from all members of the team, and reviews relevant equipment and choice of implants.

The Surgeon's Voice

Conversations and verbal orders are both common and necessary in the operating theater. The surgeon should attempt to give clear, audible instructions to the surgical staff in order to avoid any confusion with the surgeon's request. It should be kept in mind that the vast majority of ophthalmic patients are awake during surgery, so great care should be taken with conversations. Both the tenor and content should be professional. In addition, the conversations in the room should not distract in any way from the critical task at hand.

What About Music?

A frequent component of the operating room environment is music. Although music may relax the surgeon, staff, and patient, it should not be allowed to become a distraction. The musical selection, choice of playlist, or radio station should be prepared before the surgical scrub. Volume and static should be checked and refined before surgery in order to avoid distractions while changing volume, playlists, or stations.

Several studies have tried to measure how distracting the music itself is to the surgeon and how it might affect the surgeon's performance. One study investigated auditory processing in the presence of various levels of noise typical of an operating room with and without a task to perform. The authors suggested that operating room noise, including music, might be the most important contributing factor to breakdown of communication between operating room teams (Way et al, 2013). In another simulated surgical task, residents were asked to perform a laparoscopic cholecystectomy in the presence of typical operating room distractions and demonstrated poorer task performance with noise than without (Pluyter et al, 2010). Researchers at Oregon State reported that less experienced general surgeons were more susceptible to making errors when distracted by typical operating room noise than their more experienced colleagues (Feuerbacher et al, 2012).

Key Points

- Preparation of the surgeon includes detailed review of the patient's ophthalmologic and general medical status along with the planned surgical procedure.
- The operating surgeon should become familiar with the complex equipment to be used in the procedure, including setup, positioning, and common malfunction remedies.
- Sleep deprivation, physical exertion, caffeine ingestion, illness, and medication use may all have a detrimental effect on a surgeon's performance.

Arnold RW, Springer DT, Engel WK, Helveston EM. The effect of wrist rest, caffeine, and oral timolol on the hand steadiness of ophthalmologists. *Ann Ophthalmol.* 1993;25(7):250–253.

Durfee DA, ed. Ethics in ophthalmology. In: *The Profession of Ophthalmology.* 2nd ed. San Francisco: American Academy of Ophthalmology; 2010:174–252.

Elman MJ, Sugar J, Fiscella R, et al. The effect of propranolol versus placebo on resident surgical performance. *Trans Am Ophthalmol Soc.* 1998;96:283–294.

Feuerbacher RL, Funk KH, Spight DH, Diggs BS, Hunter JG. Realistic distractions and interruptions that impair simulated surgical performance by novice surgeons. *Arch Surg.* 2012;147(11):1026–1030.

Girou E, Loyeau S, Legrand P, Oppein F, Brun-Buisoon C. Efficacy of handrubbing with alcohol based solution versus standard handwashing with antiseptic soap: randomized clinical trial. *BMJ.* 2002;325(7360):362–367.

Holmes JM, Toleikis SC, Jay WM. The effect of arm exercise and ocular massage on postural hand tremor. *Ann Ophthalmol.* 1992;24(4):156–158.

Humayun MU, Rader RS, Pieramici DJ, Awh CC, de Juan E Jr. Quantitative measurement of the effects of caffeine and propranolol on surgeon hand tremor. *Arch Ophthalmol.* 1997; 115(3):371–374.

Joint Commission on Accreditation of Healthcare Organizations (JCAHO). JCAHO Universal Protocol for preventing wrong site, wrong procedure. *JCAHO Perspectives on Patient Safety.* 2003;3:1–11.

Lubahn JD, Dickson BG, Cooney TE. Effect of timolol versus a postural orthotic on hand tremor during microsurgery. *Microsurgery.* 2002;22(6):273–276.

Mürbe D, Hüttenbrink KB, Zahnert T, et al. Tremor in otosurgery: influence of physical strain on hand steadiness. *Otol Neurotol.* 2001;22(5):672–677.

O'Shaughnessy M, O'Malley VP, Corbett G, Given HF. Optimum duration of surgical scrub-time. *Br J Surg.* 1991;78(6):685–686.

Parienti JJ, Thibon P, Heller R, et al. Hand-rubbing with an aqueous alcoholic solution vs traditional surgical hand-scrubbing and 30-day surgical site infection rates: a randomized equivalence study. *JAMA.* 2002;288(6):722–727.

Pluyter JR, Buzink SN, Rutkowski AF, Jakimowicz JJ. Do absorption and realistic distraction influence performance of component task surgical procedure? *Surg Endosc.* 2010; 24(4): 902–907.

Samkoff JS, Jacques CH. A review of studies concerning effects of sleep deprivation and fatigue on residents' performance. *Acad Med.* 1991;66(11):687–693.

Way, TJ, Long A, Weihing J, et al. Effect of noise on auditory processing in the operating room. *J Am Coll Surg.* 2013;216(5):933–938.

Weinger MB, Ancoli-Israel S. Sleep deprivation and clinical performance. *JAMA.* 2002; 287(8):955–957.

Self-Assessment Test

1. In the surgeon's preparation for surgery, which statements apply? (Choose all that apply.)
   a. need not necessarily examine the patient personally
   b. must be facile with all steps of the planned procedure

    c. should be familiar with all major equipment involved, including common causes of malfunction and their correction

    d. should review all pertinent ancillary tests personally

2. List 2 physical factors that may negatively affect surgical performance.

3. The caffeine contained in 1 cup of coffee may induce detrimental hand tremor. Is this statement true, or false?

4. The controversy in surgical hand preparation includes which of the following? (Choose all that apply.)

    a. duration of scrub

    b. composition of the antibacterial agent

    c. necessity to scrub

    d. requirement for gloves

For preferred responses to these questions, see Appendix A.

CHAPTER 4

Informed Consent

Kian Eftekhari, MD
Paul J. Tapino, MD

Informed consent is a critical component of the physician–patient relationship in surgical specialties. Simply stated, informed consent includes discussion of risks, benefits, and alternatives when medical or surgical treatments are proposed. Establishing a goal of educating patients about their diseases, treatment alternatives, and the risks of various treatment options is a basic mandate by the Accreditation Council for Graduate Medical Education (ACGME) to ensure core competencies among residents.

During the process of informed consent, 5 of the 6 ACGME core competencies are involved (systems-based practice being the sixth):

- patient care
- medical knowledge
- practice-based learning and improvement
- interpersonal and communication skills
- professionalism

Importance of Informed Consent

Ophthalmologists have a unique role within medicine in the process of caring for patients. Often, treatments are being recommended for conditions that neither the patients nor other healthcare providers can readily diagnose or observe themselves. Therefore, patients and providers are left to take the ophthalmologist's word regarding the presence of cataracts, high intraocular pressure, or diabetic retinopathy. Informed consent is a necessary step in the medicolegal process of treating patients but should be viewed in the larger context of educating patients about their diseases and possible treatments.

Informed consent has obvious medicolegal implications. Malpractice litigation is, unfortunately, a common occurrence in ophthalmology, and most malpractice suits involve cataract surgery. There are extensive findings in the literature that despite the most conscientious efforts, patients may not remember the salient elements of the informed consent discussion after surgery. This may be due to an elderly patient population or low

---

This chapter includes related videos, which can be accessed by scanning the QR codes provided in the text or going to www.aao.org/bposvideo.

health literacy among certain patient populations. Other reports find that providers do not always do an adequate job of explaining the rationale, procedure, and risks of surgery. The Canadian Medical Protective Agency suggests that one-third of patients in malpractice cases may not have initiated litigation had they received better informed consent. A recent review of 5 years of malpractice lawsuits against ophthalmologists by the Ophthalmic Mutual Insurance Company (OMIC) shows that lack of informed consent was a key allegation in 4% of claims.

Research has shown that residents are often obtaining informed consent for common ophthalmology procedures but that not all residents are confident obtaining consent. This varies by resident post-graduate year (PGY) but also by whether they had prior training in informed consent. The perceived barriers among residents to having a productive informed consent conversation include inadequate time to speak to the patient in a busy clinic, a lack of knowledge about the specifics of the procedure or its risks, as well as patient factors such as poor comprehension.

Therefore, residents must be prepared to obtain informed consent for many ophthalmic procedures. Ensuring proper informed consent processes will enhance the provider-patient relationship and may mitigate the risk of malpractice litigation.

Elements of Informed Consent

In initiating a conversation about a proposed treatment, the resident may find it helpful to think about what he or she would want to know if in the patient's position. Patients are often apprehensive about undergoing a surgical treatment or office procedure, and they may be confused about the terminology being used. For example, patients frequently have misconceptions about the role of lasers in ophthalmology. When considering a laser treatment for glaucoma or a retinal problem, patients often assume this is the same type of the laser that they have heard advertised by refractive surgeons and that it may help to correct their vision. Preemptively pointing this out may reduce the misconceptions and may lead to more active listening during the rest of the informed consent discussion.

Surgical informed consent differs from the consent discussion one might have in the context of a research study as outlined in the Helsinki declaration, which in 1964 set forth the ethical principles for medical research involving human subjects. In obtaining a patient's consent for a surgical procedure, 3 elements are important: preconditions, information, and consent.

Preconditions

Preconditions include patients' competence to make their own healthcare decisions and patient voluntariness for the procedure. Elderly patients with dementia may not be competent to make decisions and often have a family member who makes decisions for them. It is important to involve this caregiver early in the process because they will often be the same family member who will be called upon to provide transport on the day of the procedure and for subsequent follow-up visits. Voluntariness is also an important precondition because patients themselves must be on board with the decision to proceed with surgery. Occasionally, one may encounter family members who are urging a procedure for their relative despite the wishes of the patient.

Information

Information as an element of informed consent includes the specific discussion of the diagnosis and proposed treatment plan. According to guidelines from the Ophthalmic Mutual Insurance Company (OMIC), specific elements of the discussion should include

- discussion of the patient's condition
- rationale for recommending a treatment or procedure
- expected benefits, possible complications, and alternatives to the procedure, including the option of no treatment
- discussion of any comorbid conditions that may increase the risk of a specific complication
- discussion of the anesthesia plan
- discussion of the postoperative care plan including any comanagement by another provider

Consent

The last element, consent, is the process of the patient making a decision to proceed and authorizing the physician to go forward with treatment. It is important to note that the documentation of informed consent is simply one element of the process of consent. Studies have shown that two-thirds of patients do not read the document carefully. Best practices suggest the document should be written at a 12-year-old reading level, which may be difficult to achieve in ophthalmology, given the amount of technology involved in ophthalmic procedures. Viewing the informed consent process in the context of educating patients and having them authorize a treatment should be the overall aim, although documentation is a necessary step.

Putting the Elements Together

One should strive to have the 3 elements—preconditions, information, consent—in every discussion of informed consent, but patients may have different learning styles and levels of health literacy. One way to augment the effectiveness of the informed consent process is to provide patients with supplementary materials such as brochures or videos presented in the office. (See Videos 4-1 and 4-2 for examples of patient clips.) Many patients learn well from visual information, and using this modality has been shown by other authors to enhance patient recall. Another strategy recommended by OMIC is to have the patient repeat back the diagnosis and treatment plan to ensure a basic level of comprehension.

 VIDEO 4-1 Sample, Informed Consent, Panretinal Photocoagulation (01:06)
Courtesy of the American Academy of Ophthalmology, Retina Informed Consent Video Collection

VIDEO 4-2 Sample, Informed Consent, Vitrectomy for Retinal Detachment (00:32)
Courtesy of the American Academy of Ophthalmology, Retina Informed Consent Video Collection

Challenges for Residents Obtaining Informed Consent

Residents face many challenges in the process of obtaining informed consent for ophthalmic procedures, such as taking care of patients with many health problems and limited health literacy. Low health literacy is an increasingly recognized factor that contributes to poor patient outcomes, and nowhere is this more important than a discussion about surgery. The provider needs to recognize that patients may not understand everything written on the informed consent document. This especially applies to visually impaired patients, and particularly if their pupils have been dilated!

The following scenarios illustrate some of the challenging circumstances that residents face in obtaining informed consent.

Scenario 1: The Compromised Patient

The first-year resident is called to the trauma bay of the emergency room in the middle of the night to examine an intoxicated patient who was "minding his own business." The patient is talkative but does not indicate an ability to comprehend the physician well. On examination, his right eye has periorbital ecchymosis, proptosis, and an intraocular pressure of 48 mmHg. His vision is unobtainable but he has an afferent pupillary defect. A computed tomography scan confirms a retrobulbar hemorrhage with an associated fracture of the lateral orbital wall. What do you do?

Discussion

In this scenario, "consenting" the patient is impossible. He is not competent to make his own decisions. It may be worthwhile to ask the trauma team if he has a family member present who can help make decisions for the patient. However, he clearly has a need for urgent intervention, and lateral canthotomy and cantholysis should be performed immediately. This would constitute emergent care and thus pre-procedure informed consent is unnecessary. However, if you are able to obtain informed consent, it is always advisable to do so. If you cannot, document carefully why the patient was unable to provide consent and why the treatment was needed at that particular time.

Scenario 2: The Patient With Dementia

An elderly patient comes to your office at the insistence of her son and daughter, who claim "she is running into walls." The patient has dementia but is pleasant and allows you to examine her eyes. Your exam reveals bilateral dense cataracts with a hazy fundus examination that shows a normal cup-to-disc ratio and normal retina. You explain the findings and tell the patient and family that if she wants to improve her vision, she would need cataract surgery. When she hears the word *surgery,* the patient recoils and begins to get agitated. Despite her agitation, her children insist they want the surgery done and the patient's daughter states that she has power of attorney.

Discussion

This is a difficult scenario. Occasionally, family members want the provider to perform a procedure that the patient may or may not want herself. It can be difficult for the resident to know the right thing to do in this scenario. It is reasonable to start by asking the patient her concerns, which may be relatively trivial such as "Will I be awake the whole time?" In patients with dementia, general anesthesia may be a prudent option for cataract surgery. However, if the patient indicates in some way that she does not want surgery, the provider must respect the patient's autonomy even despite the family's interests. Since the daughter has power of attorney, this is a complex situation. It may be advisable to involve the hospital's Ethics Committee and legal department to determine the best course of action, but it is important as the physician to try to determine the family dynamic while having a complex discussion.

Scenario 3: "How Many of These Have You Done?"

It is July of your third year of residency, and you are seeing patients in the resident-based clinic. A patient comes to your office with a complaint of having a "fog" over her left eye. She is a diabetic, and your examination reveals a dense posterior subcapsular cataract but no diabetic retinopathy. You inform the patient of the findings and offer her the option of cataract surgery if she would like to try to improve her vision. After explaining the rationale of the procedure as well as the expected benefits, potential complications, and alternatives, the patient asks you, "Well, how many of these have you done before?" What do you say?

Discussion

Patients often will ask how much experience you have with a particular procedure. It is an important question that enhances patient autonomy and provides transparency in care. In a training environment, however, it can cause anxiety on the resident's part because cataract surgery has a learning curve. While residents are not expert on the procedure, they need a high case volume in order to become proficient. It is important to be honest with patients in this scenario, but it is also appropriate to inform them that you will be supervised by an experienced physician at all times. The patient has the right to decline your care and to request a more experienced surgeon, but fear of this happening should not bias your informed consent discussion. Falsely claiming a high level of experience with the procedure or having the resident do the surgery despite the patient's request could theoretically result in a charge of battery, according to OMIC.

Scenario 4: "Who's Operating?"

You are seeing patients in an attending's clinic and one of the patients has a moderately dense posterior subcapsular cataract with significant glare symptoms. He has had cataract surgery on his other eye previously, and says, "I want the exact same surgery done on the other side." You explain the surgery to him again and stress that although he experienced no complications on the first eye, this does not imply that the second eye will necessarily have the same result. As your attending physician walks into the room, the patient says "Well, who's going to be doing the surgery, you or the doctor?"

Discussion

Clarifying the role of a trainee can be very unsettling for patients and for the physicians involved. In the setting of a training program, there may be cases in which an attending surgeon allows the resident to perform part or all of the procedure under his or her supervision. Setting expectations with the patient prior to surgery is the best way to avoid potential disappointment after surgery. According to the OMIC guidelines, the provider should clarify who will be performing the surgery and whether there will be involvement of a trainee. In this scenario, one way of handling the patient's question would be to respond that the trainee would be only assisting or, conversely, that the attending physician would be supervising the trainee while he or she performs steps of the surgery. The attending physician and trainee should adhere to the patient's preferences. As mentioned earlier in this chapter, if the surgical team goes against the patient's wishes and has the trainee do the surgery despite a specific request to have the attending physician perform surgery, this could theoretically result in a charge of battery, according to OMIC.

Scenario 5: The Patient Surprised by the Need for Care

A patient comes to your office for an eye examination. He complains, "My vision has been blurry for some time." He has not sought care until now because he just obtained health insurance. He also mentions that he is a diabetic and is "diet-controlled," but he has not had a primary care visit in many years. On examination, you diagnose bilateral dense nuclear sclerotic cataracts, and there is no view to the fundus. Ultrasonography reveals an attached retina and normal optic nerve. After speaking to the attending, you inform the patient that he has cataracts and that you would recommend surgery to improve his vision and the ability to see his fundus to monitor him for diabetic retinopathy. He looks at you concerned because he thought he was just coming in for a routine exam. What do you do?

Discussion

This patient has little insight into his own health problems, but clearly, he is in need of care. Low health literacy is an increasingly recognized factor that contributes to poor patient outcomes. It is important for the provider to recognize that patients may not understand everything you tell them, especially if you use ophthalmic terminology. While you do not want to "talk down" to the patient, you should recognize that his poor self-care is a red flag and may result in unintended consequences after surgery, such as not showing up for follow-up visits or not using post-operative drops. Spending extra time at the front end striving to ensure an adequate understanding of the diagnosis and proposed treatment can potentially mitigate a longer discussion on the back end if a complication or undesired outcome occurs. This may be a patient in which an audiovisual presentation of the diagnosis and treatment of cataracts may be more effective, or a discussion with a close family member or friend if he gives consent to do so. It is important to spend time to build a therapeutic alliance with these patients, as they are more likely to "fall through the cracks."

Summary

Informed consent is a process involving communication between the provider and patients about their diagnosis and proposed treatment. Cultivating the ability to have a productive informed consent discussion with the patient in many different situations is an under-recognized but important aspect of residency training.

Key Points

- Informed consent is a process, not a document, and should be treated as an opportunity to educate the patient.
- Residents are often obtaining consent but may not get specific training; try to understand the procedures and its complications before a discussion with the patient; the OMIC web site is a good starting resource (www.omic.com).
- A proper consent needs a patient with decision-making capacity and a physician who can explain the elements of consent: the rationale for treatment, expected benefits, potential risks, attendant comorbidities, and the anesthesia and postoperative plan. Lastly, one needs to document this in writing.
- In certain situations, the patient may not have decision-making capacity and thus cannot make his or her own healthcare decisions or may have a language barrier. It is important to get a family member or caregiver involved early, as this will likely be the person the physician relies upon to transport the patient for surgery and for postoperative care.
- Striving to educate the patient about his or her condition and the treatment empowers the patient, and learning how to obtain consent prepares residents as they become independent practitioners who are in charge of their patients' care.
- To test your own ability to obtain informed consent, try "consenting" one of your attending physicians for a procedure you are not too familiar with; this may help to illuminate the areas of your knowledge base that need fine-tuning.

American Academy of Ophthalmology in cooperation with Ophthalmic Mutual Insurance Company. "Practice Guidelines for Informed Consent." 2010; revised 2011. Available at http://one.aao.org/patient-safety-statement/informed-consent-guidelines-2. Accessed October 11, 2014.

American Academy of Ophthalmology. "Ethics Course: Informed Consent, Doctor-Patient Relationship and Delegated Services." 2010; revised 2013. Available at http://one.aao.org /ethics-course/ethics-course-informed-consent-doctorpatient-relat. Accessed October 11, 2014.

Chen AJ, Scott IU, Greenberg PB. Disclosure of resident involvement in ophthalmic surgery. *Arch Ophthalmol*. 2012;130(7):932–934.

Eftekhari K, Binenbaum G, Jensen AK, Gorry TN, Sankar PS, Tapino PJ. Confidence of ophthalmology residents in obtaining informed consent. *J Cataract Refract Surg.* 2015;41(1):217–221.

Institute of Medicine. Report Brief. "Health Literacy: A Prescription to End Confusion." Washington, DC: National Academies Press; 2004.

Leclercq WK, Keulers BJ, Scheltinga MR, Spauwen PH, van der Wilt GJ. A review of surgical informed consent: past, present, and future. A quest to help patients make better decisions. *World J Surg.* 2010;34(7):1406–1415.

Lee AG. The new competencies and their impact on resident training in ophthalmology. *Surv Ophthalmol.* 2003;48(6):651–662.

Menke AM. Misunderstanding is common in consent discussions. *OMIC Digest.* 2014:24(4). Available at www.omic.com.

Menke AM. "Informed Consent Obtaining and Verifying: Download Risk Management Recommendations." San Francisco: Ophthalmic Mutual Insurance Group; 2006. Available at www.omic.com/informed-consent-obtaining-and-verifying. Accessed December 17, 2014.

Moseley TH, Wiggins MN, O'Sullivan P. Effects of presentation method on the understanding of informed consent. *Br J Ophthalmol.* 2006;90(8):990–993.

Scanlan D, Siddiqui F, Perry G, Hutnik CML. Informed consent for cataract surgery: what patients do and do not understand. *J Cataract Refract Surg.* 2003;29(10):1904–1912.

Vallance JH, Ahmed M, Dhillon B. Cataract surgery and consent; recall, anxiety, and attitude toward trainee surgeons preoperatively and postoperatively. *J Cataract Refract Surg.* 2004; 30(7):1479–1485.

Self-Assessment

1. Helpful adjunctive elements in the informed consent process include all EXCEPT which one of the following?
   a. viewing video learning materials
   b. reading written brochures
   c. having the patient repeat the information back to you
   d. quoting published data on the rate of posterior capsular tears

2. An elderly patient with moderate dementia has a visually significant cataract and is bothered by her vision. Which of the following is the best practice in obtaining consent?
   a. reading the consent form to the patient
   b. asking the patient if the patient makes his or her own healthcare decisions and then calling the patient's emergency contact to discuss transportation and ask if the contact has any questions
   c. contacting the patient's son to obtain his consent
   d. giving the patient a brochure to take home and signing consent in the office that day

3. A patient has a corneal laceration with uveal prolapse and sustained a concussion at the same time. He nods his head with understanding when spoken

to but does not seem to comprehend the discussion. You smell alcohol on his breath. What is the best course of action?

a. Take the patient to the operating room and repair the laceration.
b. Observe the patient until a family member arrives.
c. Have the patient sign the consent form.
d. Try to get in touch with an emergency contact for the patient to obtain consent and, if unsuccessful, document this in the chart and then perform his surgery.

For preferred responses to these questions, please see Appendix A.

CHAPTER 5

Simulation in Surgical Training

William G. Gensheimer, MD
Yousuf M. Khalifa, MD

Surgical simulation is an important tool available to the beginning ophthalmic surgeon to lessen the stress of transitioning to the operating room and to improve patient safety. The learning curve for ophthalmic surgery is steep, with significantly higher rates of complications during early cases. Simulation provides a safe learning environment for surgeons, where repetition of technical skills can accelerate the learning curve and result in improved comfort and confidence in the operating room. This is particularly important for mastering the difficult steps of surgical procedures and for gaining experience in managing the rare but serious complications encountered during ophthalmic surgery.

Wet Laboratory

Wet laboratories are hands-on surgical training environments. Most wet laboratories contain surgical equipment that is arranged in workstations. Different models are available for intraocular and extraocular simulation in the wet laboratory, including cadaveric human eyes, animal eyes and tissue, and artificial eyes (Table 5-1).

Table 5-1 Models for Simulation in Wet Laboratory

Model	Pros	Cons
Human eyes	Realistic anatomy and tissue consistency	Cost Availability Storage, setup, cleanup, and disposal
Animal eyes	Cost Availability	Low-fidelity anterior segment anatomy and capsule properties Often need to induce cataract Storage, setup, cleanup, and disposal
Model eyes	Increasingly realistic Ease of storage, setup, cleanup, and disposal	Poor simulation of some steps including wound construction

Intraocular Simulation

Human and Animal Eyes

Cadaveric human eyes provide one of the best teaching models for the simulation of ophthalmic surgery. However, the cost and difficulty in obtaining human eyes make animal eyes the preferred model in many wet laboratories. Porcine eyes are the most commonly used animal model but others can be employed, including cow, sheep, and goat eyes (Fig 5-1).

One advantage of animal eyes is the relative ease of availability and low cost from local butcher shops or mail-order scientific supply companies. The disadvantages of animal eyes lie in the anatomical differences between animal eyes and human eyes, the difficulty of obtaining fresh tissue, the risk of infection, and the hassle of storage and disposal.

Fresh animal tissue is excellent for practicing incisions and scleral and corneal suturing. Cataract surgery training using animal eyes falls short when it comes to capsulorrhexis and phacoemulsification. The capsule of the porcine eye is elastic and the lens is quite soft, so the resident practicing on this type of model may fail to develop techniques that are transferrable to the operating room and, even worse, may develop techniques that are counterproductive for a successful transition to human cataract surgery.

In order to use a human or animal eye for simulation, it must be stabilized. Examples of stabilizing devices include a Styrofoam head, Otto device, and the Mandell eye mount.

The Styrofoam head is the most commonly used stabilization device (Fig 5-2). Human or animal eyes are secured in Styrofoam eye sockets using pins. The advantage of the Styrofoam head is the cheap cost. The disadvantages of the Styrofoam head are that it can move during use and that the eye is often not securely fixated by the pins and can also move during surgical simulation. In addition, the eye must be pressurized with fluid or ophthalmic viscosurgical device (OVD); one inserts a 27-gauge needle through the optic nerve or posterior sclera and injects water or OVD.

The Otto device and Mandell eye mount both use vacuum suction to increase stabilization of the globe. The Otto device creates suction in a Styrofoam head mount and the Mandell device has a Plexiglas platform. When animal eyes are used in the wet laboratory, cataracts can be induced using microwave energy or chemicals such as combinations of formalin, ethanol, and 2-propanol.

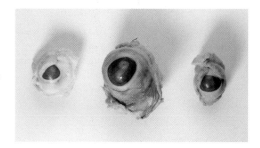

Figure 5-1 Animal eyes. From left to right pig, cow, and sheep eyes. *(Courtesy of Nebraska Scientific.)*

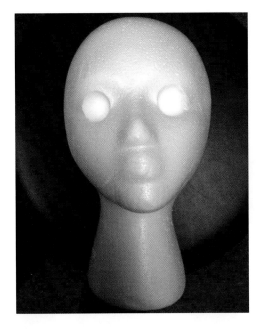

Figure 5-2 Styrofoam head. This type of head can be used to stabilize a human or animal eye for simulation. *(Courtesy of Bob Feathers.)*

Model Eyes

Low-cost models for practicing capsulorrhexis include cherry tomatoes and grape skin. Cherry tomatoes should be boiled and chilled prior to use. Using loupes or a microscope, a cystotome and Utrata forceps can be used to peel the cherry tomato or grape skin in a continuous curvilinear capsulorrhexis.

Model eyes are also commercially available for ophthalmic surgical simulation and have become increasingly more realistic. The advantages of the model eyes include more convenient storage, setup, cleanup, and disposal than human or animal eyes. The disadvantage of model eyes are that they cannot realistically simulate all steps of surgery, such as wound construction.

Other available tools for cataract surgery training are the Kitaro DryLab and WetLab systems (FCI Ophthalmics, Marshfield Hills, MA), Phaco Practice Patient (Gulden Ophthalmics, Elkins Park, PA), and anterior segment and vitreoretinal training models manufactured by Phillips Studio (Bristol, United Kingdom). These tools allow for realistic simulation of the steps of cataract surgery, including realistic simulation of difficult steps such as the capsulorrhexis and nuclear disassembly.

The fidelity of these synthetic systems is changing the role of phacoemulsification training outside the operating theater. The feel of the capsulorrhexis is quite real, and many advanced techniques can be taught, such as saving a capsulorrhexis that is running out or can-opener capsulotomy. Phacoemulsification grooving using the Kitaro WetLab system provides the resident with an opportunity to appreciate depth of field and learn the 3 foot-pedal positions. Nucleus disassembly is a complex bimanual maneuver that can be difficult to master in the operating room. The dissassembly is realistically simulated using the Kitaro training system. Figs 5-3 and 5-4 show examples of the Kitaro systems.

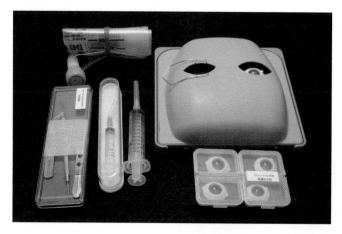

Figure 5-3 Kitaro WetLab Kit. *(Courtesy of FCI Ophthalmics.)*

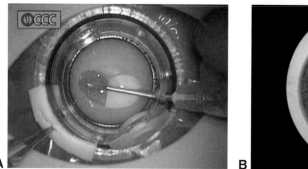 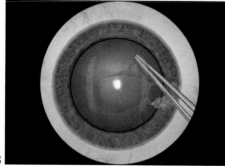

A   B

Figure 5-4 Simulation of continuous curvilinear capsulorrhexis. **A,** Kitaro training system. **B,** Eyesi system. *(Part A courtesy of FCI Ophthalmics and Frontier Medical, Part B courtesy VRmagic.)*

While no comparative studies of the utility of these different models have been published, many programs utilize these simulation devices to ease the resident's transition to the operating room. Surgical practice is most beneficial when a simulation method with reasonable fidelity is incorporated into a well-planned surgical curriculum, and when experienced faculty members are available for teaching, evaluation, and feedback.

Extraocular Simulation

Cadaveric human and animal tissues are also used for extraocular surgical simulation, including strabismus surgery and oculoplastic surgery. Cadaveric human tissue is the most realistic but also the most difficult to obtain. Animal tissue such as pigs' feet and chicken breasts can be used for suturing practice. Other materials such as grapes and bananas can also be used for suturing practice. Suturing models made of synthetic materials are commercially available from several companies (Fig 5-5). There are also commercially available strabismus surgery training models that allow for realistic simulation of horizontal and vertical muscle strabismus surgery.

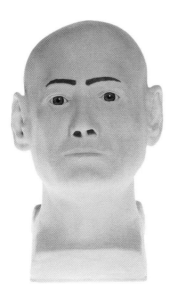

Figure 5-5 Example of a suturing model for practicing advanced flaps and grafts in additional to basic suturing procedures. *(Courtesy of SimSkin.)*

Virtual Reality

Virtual reality (VR) surgical training is a computer-generated 3-dimensional surgical environment that allows interaction between the surgeon and simulated surgical environment through visual and tactile feedback. Virtual reality surgical simulators in ophthalmology have become increasingly more realistic and sophisticated with advances in technology. The major disadvantage of VR simulators is the high cost and lack of comparative data showing that these high cost investments have advantages over other simulation models. The haptic feedback from these systems also still requires further refinement.

The most widely studied and commercially available VR surgical simulator in ophthalmology is the Eyesi surgical simulator (VRmagic, Mannheim, Germany). The simulator includes an Eyesi surgical platform that can be equipped for cataract and vitreoretinal surgical training modules (Fig 5-6). The platform includes an artificial eye, patient head, stereoscopic microscope, adjustable table, and foot pedals. Instruments are inserted into the artificial eye, allowing advanced virtual reality simulation in the steps of ophthalmic surgery. The cataract surgery modules allow simulation of key steps such as capsulorrhexis, hydrodissection, and nuclear disassembly. The vitreoretinal surgery module allows simulation of challenging steps such as posterior hyaloid detachment, internal limiting membrane peeling, epiretinal membrane peeling, and scleral indentation. Complications can be added to training modules to practice the management of complications in a simulation environment.

Other cataract surgery VR simulators include the PhacoVision (Melerit Medical, www.melerit.se) and MicrovisTouch (ImmersiveTouch, www.immersivetouch.com). Both provide a hardware and surgical platform with a microscope, handpieces, and foot pedals. Software modules allow for virtual training in the steps of cataract surgery.

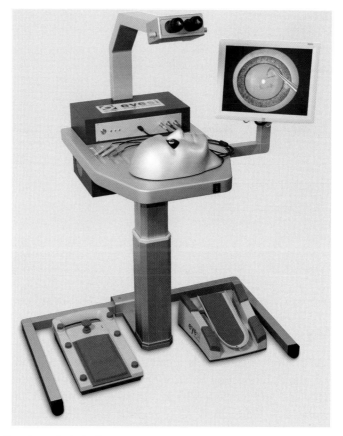

Figure 5-6 Eyesi surgical platform equipped with a cataract interface. *(Courtesy of VRmagic.)*

While resident surgical education in the operating room may be subject to practical limitations, it is encouraging that effective methods of phacoemulsification training are available and should be utilized by the resident during residency training.

Key Points

- Surgical simulation is an important tool available to the beginning ophthalmic surgeon to accelerate the learning curve and improve patient safety.
- Cadaveric human eyes provide one of the best teaching models but are costly and difficult to obtain.
- There are anatomic differences between animal eyes and human eyes such as the more elastic capsule in porcine eyes.
- Model eyes are commercially available for ophthalmic surgical simulation and have become increasingly more realistic, especially for the key steps in cataract surgery such as the capsulorrhexis and nuclear disassembly
- Virtual reality (VR) surgical training provides a simulated surgical environment but the systems are costly to purchase.

Cook DA, Hatala R, Brydges R, et al. Technology-enhanced simulation for health professions education: a systematic review and meta-analysis. *AMA.* 2011;306(9):978–988.

Henderson BA, Grimes KJ, Fintelmann RE, Oetting TA. Stepwise approach to establishing an ophthalmology wet laboratory. *J Cataract Refract Surg.* 2009;35(6):1121–1128.

Khalifa YM, Bogorad D, Gibson V, Peifer J, Nussbaum J. Virtual reality in ophthalmology training. *Surv Ophthalmol.* 2006;51(3):259–273.

Kitzmann A, Oetting TA. The Iowa Ophthalmology Wet Laboratory. EyeRounds.org. Posted December 6, 2012. www.EyeRounds.org/tutorials/Iowa-OWL. Accessed October 13, 2014.

Lee AG, Greenlee E, Oetting TA, Beaver HA, et al. The Iowa ophthalmology wet laboratory curriculum for teaching and assessing cataract surgical competency. *Ophthalmology.* 2007;114(7):e21–26.

Self-Assessment Test

1. Which of the following is true of using porcine eyes for surgical simulation?
   a. can be obtained from mail-order companies
   b. are poor models for practicing incisions and suturing
   c. have a lens capsule that is identical to the human lens capsule
   d. do not require any specialized waste disposal

2. Advantages of model eyes in surgical simulation include which of the following?
   a. ease of storage and setup
   b. realistic simulation of the capsulorrhexis and nuclear disassembly steps of cataract surgery
   c. no specialized waste disposal
   d. all of the above

3. Which of the following is true of using virtual reality training?
   a. has been shown to be superior to other simulation models in randomized controlled trials
   b. does not allow simulation of surgical complications
   c. allows for virtual training in the steps of cataract surgery
   d. are always free for residency programs

4. Which of the following is true of using cadaveric human eyes for surgical simulation?
   a. are always easy to obtain
   b. do not require any specialized waste disposal
   c. have been shown to be superior to other simulation models in randomized controlled trials
   d. are excellent teaching models for ophthalmic surgery

For preferred responses, see Appendix A.

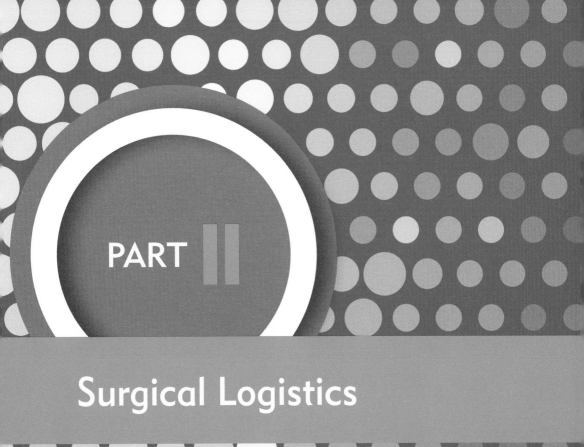

PART **II**

Surgical Logistics

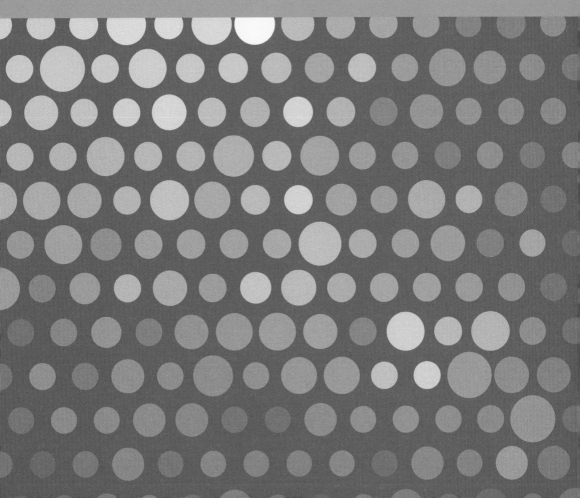

CHAPTER 6

The Importance of Ergonomics for Ophthalmologists

Sandra M. Woolley, PhD, CPE
Anna S. Kitzmann, MD

"Keep your head up and don't let anything get to you. Always keep good posture." This advice, attributed to baseball player Dante Bichette Jr, may resonate with aspiring ophthalmology residents.

The demands on ophthalmologists have changed in recent years. With increasing patient volumes, decreasing reimbursements, transition to electronic medical records, and changing procedures, ophthalmologists are exposed to musculoskeletal disorders (MSDs) earlier in their careers. Surveys sent to ophthalmologists and optometrists have indicated that younger providers, with fewer years in practice and females are more likely to experience MSDs. Another factor to take seriously is the contributing role of the design of the physical environment in both the clinic and procedural setting and its relationship to the development of MSDs. Furthermore, ergonomic recommendations focusing on the elimination and reduction of ergonomic risk factors should be initiated during ophthalmology training to maintain the longevity of individual's career.

A seasoned ophthalmologist will probably not take long to name an ophthalmology colleague who has been affected by work-related musculoskeletal pain.

There is often little time spent toward caring for oneself, given the demands of residency. However, in embarking on a career in ophthalmology, it is important to learn about steps to take to prevent musculoskeletal problems. These steps may seem small, but they are worth following to prevent the large future costs of time away from work to have surgery or physical therapy due to musculoskeletal pain and its impact on quality of life outside of work.

Ergonomics and Ergonomic Risk Factors

According to the Board of Certified Professional Ergonomists, ergonomics is the scientific study of people at work. It is the discipline that applies scientific data and principles about people to the design of equipment, products, tasks, devices, facilities, environments, and systems to meet the needs for human productivity, comfort, safety, and health. The goal is to design work tasks so that they fall within the worker's capabilities.

Work-Related Musculoskeletal Disorders

Work-related MSDs are defined as disorders of the muscles, nerves, tendons, ligaments, joints, cartilage, or spinal discs. These disorders are also known as cumulative trauma disorders, repetitive strain disorders, repetitive motion disorders, or overuse syndromes. They occur as a result of cumulative exposure to ergonomic risk factors over a prolonged period of time. The common risk factors that predispose an individual to work-related MSDs are exertions or force, awkward postures or static or sustained postures, repetitive behaviors, contact stress, vibration, or extreme temperatures, particularly cold environments. Job tasks that involve multiple risk factors have a higher probability of causing work-related MSDs.

The signs of work-related MSDs include loss of function, decreased grip strength, decreased range of movement, and deformity. The symptoms include stiffness, cramping, pain, tingling, and numbness. Examples of these disorders include carpal tunnel syndrome, herniated spinal discs, low back pain, tarsal tunnel syndrome, epicondylitis, sciatica, ganglion cysts, tendinitis, rotator cuff tears, stenosing tenosynovitis (trigger finger), and DeQuervain tendinitis.

Over the last 20 years, research has found that ophthalmologists are exposed to a number of common ergonomic risk factors in the office, the clinic and the operating environments. These risk factors include high levels of static loads, extreme or awkward postures, lack of head and arm support, repetition of the same task, bending and twisting of the back, prolonged visual focus, and high cognitive load and mental stress.

The prevalence of ophthalmologists and optometrists who have expressed work-related complaints of pain or discomfort range between 35.9%–82%. The most common sites reported were lower back (21.4%–81%), neck (8.2%–69%), both back and neck (55.4%–62.4%), shoulder (31%–50.2%), upper extremity including elbow/arm (17%–33%), hand/wrist (17%), and leg pain (14.5%). Between 32%–62.5% of the practitioners sought no medical treatment. Those who sought treatment primarily took non-steroidal anti-inflammatory medications (56%). Others required physical therapy (23%–32.1%), sought alternative treatment from a chiropractor or osteopath (8%), or required surgery (2.7%–7.6%). A number of ophthalmologists who have experienced work-related musculoskeletal disorders have had to modify their practices to accommodate the pain, and it is estimated that 9.2% have discontinued operating. Table 6-1 summarizes some of the areas in which injuries can emerge over time.

Adopting Ergonomically Friendly Practices

In the Operating Room

It is estimated that 72% of ophthalmologists experience pain associated with operating. Use of loupe magnification and use of headlamps account for 61% and 43% of the pain, respectively. Activities associated with ergonomic risks in the operating room include laser surgeries, use of operating microscope, limited freedom to reposition instruments, and focus on the video monitor while using a foot pedal. Chapter 7 covers many recommendations about the proper positioning in the operating room, in particular the crucial aspects of surgeon positioning at the operating microscope. Table 6-2 provides a brief

Table 6-1 Selected Injury Pathways Toward Musculoskeletal Disorders of the Trunk and Extremities[a]

Area of Anatomy	Injury Pathway
Back	Maintaining an unbalanced posture for long periods of time produces static loading of the soft tissues and ischemic accumulation of metabolites in them. This can accelerate disk degeneration and lead to disk herniation.
Neck	Repeated flexion or extension of the neck while at the slit lamp, operating microscope, or computer terminal can cause chronic pain and severe spasms.
Arms, shoulders	Extended periods of holding the bent arms too high, too low, or unsupported while with a patient, or while entering data into a computer, can produce shoulder pain, swelling of tendons and ligaments in the carpal tunnel, and tingling and numbness of the fingers and hands from tendinitis and tenosynovitis.
Arms	Repeatedly resting the elbows or forearms on a hard surface during procedures, or on malpositioned armrests, can lead to ulnar neuropathy.

[a] Frequently, pathways interact to create a complex collection of symptoms that can worsen and/or become chronic over time. Symptoms can vary from day to day, depending on the work activity. Musculoskeletal disorders also are multifactorial, potentiated by everything from lifestyle and psychological stress to small changes in the way the office or surgical suite is arranged. Often, people say they were fine until their normal routines changed because of a new job, new equipment, or expanded duties. Some studies have linked musculoskeletal disorders to personal factors such as gender, height, and genetic predisposition, but others have not.

Reproduced with permission, *EyeNet* 2009;13(8):49–50.

Table 6-2 Surgical Activities, Ergonomic Risk Factors, and Potential Solutions

Surgical Activity	Ergonomic Risk Factors	Potential Solutions
Patient preparation	Forceful exertions and awkward postures associated with laying down and sitting up the patient	Select a bed/cart with a pneumatic backrest.
	Forceful exertions associated with raising the bed/cart to a working height	Select a bed/cart with a pneumatic height adjustment.
	Forceful exertions and awkward postures while boosting the patient on the bed/cart	Select a bed/cart in which the head is appropriately placed prior to laying the patient down. Have lifting equipment available.
	Awkward and sustained postures associated with injections and patient draping	Raise the height of the bed to reduce forward bending.
During the procedure	Awkward and sustained postures with the back erect and the neck extended while looking into the microscope	Adjust the microscope eyepieces (oculars) so that the eyepieces rest just below the eyes and the neck should be bent no more than 10° to 15° below horizontal.
	Awkward and sustained postures in the shoulder while stabilizing the hand/wrist position	Relax the shoulders and keep the upper arms close to the body with the elbows flexed at 90°. Use a stool that has forearm support rests, which will support both the shoulders and forearms.

(Continued)

Table 6-2 *(continued)*

Surgical Activity	Ergonomic Risk Factors	Potential Solutions
	Awkward posture of the lumbar spine resulting in lumbar kyphosis	Select a stool that has a height-adjustable backrest to support lumbar lordosis and a seat pan that has a slight forward tilt to maintain lumbar lordosis. Ensure that the seat pan is long enough to support the thighs.
	Awkward posture with the spine tilted due to the different height profiles of the foot pedals for the microscope and the foot pedals for other machines, such as the phacoemulsification machine	Raise the height of the microscope foot pedal to be at the same height as the other machine foot pedals.
	Forceful, sustained, and repetitive precision pinch grip on the instruments	Relax the grip as much as possible. Use a wrist rest.
After the procedure	Awkward postures associated with documentation	Place the monitors and keyboard on a height-adjustable arm. The eyes should look to the top of the monitor or slightly below, and the hands should be at or slightly lower than the elbows.

summary of the ergonomic issues associated with various surgical procedures and outlines potential solutions to eliminate or reduce exposures to these risk factors.

In general, the goal is for the ophthalmologist to maintain the normal spinal curvature whatever the task, with lordosis (concavity) of the cervical and lumbar spine and kyphosis (convexity) of the thoracic and sacral spine, as seen from the side (Fig 6-1).

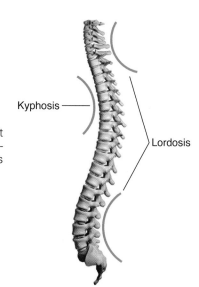

Kyphosis ——

Lordosis

Figure 6-1 Good posture is shown, with a normal slight kyphosis of the thoracic spine and lordosis of the cervical and lumbar spine. Try to keep these natural curvatures throughout the day. *(Courtesy of Sandra M. Woolley, PhD, CPE.)*

Various surgical activities have ergonomic risk factors associated with them. These areas include

- preparing the patient (Figs 6-2–6-6)
- performing the procedure (Figs 6-7–6-11)
- documenting the procedure (Fig 6-12)

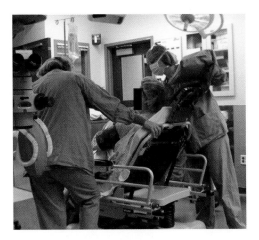

Figure 6-2 Lifting/lowering the bed/cart height. Both health care providers are exhibiting awkward postures with their trunks bent. The provider on the left is exerting force to pump up the bed. Using a cart with a pneumatic height adjustment would reduce these ergonomic risk factors. *(Courtesy of Sandra M. Woolley, PhD, CPE.)*

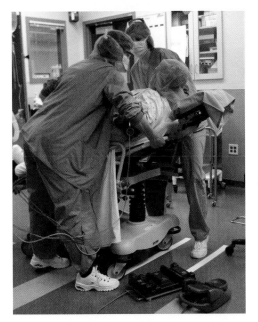

Figure 6-3 Manually lifting/lowering the patient. Look at the stance of the health care provider on the left. The back is twisted to the side and she is bent forward. Both are exerting considerable force attempting to raise the patient from a supine position. A pneumatic bed would eliminate these issues. *(Courtesy of Sandra M. Woolley, PhD, CPE.)*

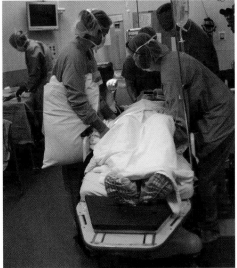

Figure 6-4 Boosting the patient on the bed/cart. Awkward postures and forceful exertions are being used to boost the patient on the cart. Raising the cart would reduce the amount of back flexion. *(Courtesy of Sandra M. Woolley, PhD, CPE.)*

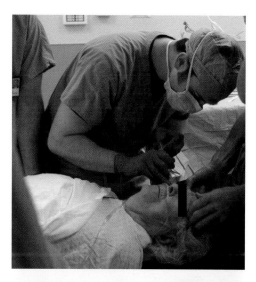

Figure 6-5 Injecting the patient. The physician's back is bent forward and being held in this position for some period of time. Raising the bed would help in reducing this awkward posture. *(Courtesy of Sandra M. Woolley, PhD, CPE.)*

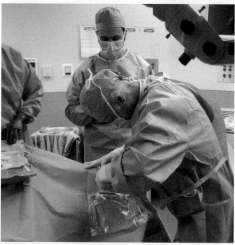

Figure 6-6 Draping and preparing the patient. The physician has his back bent forward and his arms abducted. Raising the height of the cart would reduce this posture. *(Courtesy of Sandra M. Woolley, PhD, CPE.)*

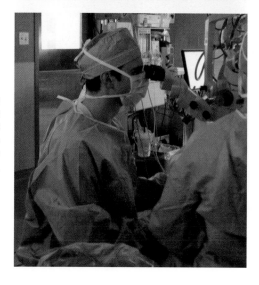

Figure 6-7 Back and neck position while using the microscope. The physician's neck is in extension. Having microscope eyepieces that have a vertical height adjustment and adjusting them so that they are slightly below sitting eye height would be an improvement. *(Courtesy of Sandra M. Woolley, PhD, CPE.)*

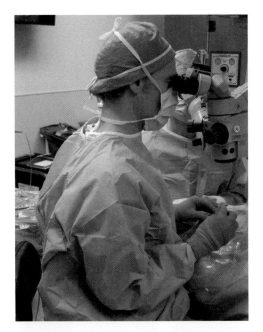

Figure 6-8 Sustained shoulder retraction. Holding the shoulders in this position provides stability to the hands, but puts stress on the trapezius muscles and may lead to shoulder and neck pain. Armrests on the stool would provide support for the forearms, alleviating the need for shoulder stabilization. *(Courtesy of Sandra M. Woolley, PhD, CPE.)*

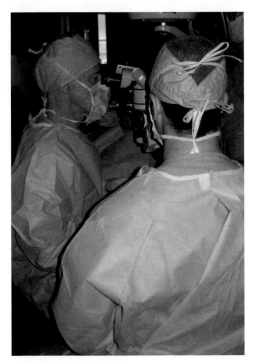

Figure 6-9 Lumbar kyphosis while sitting. Without a backrest on the stool, the back is placed in lumbar kyphosis. A backrest and a seat that tilts slightly forward would eliminate this posture. *(Courtesy of Sandra M. Woolley, PhD, CPE.)*

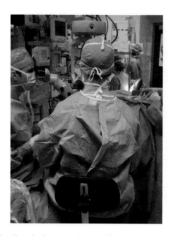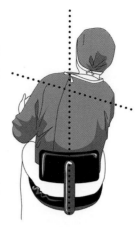

Figure 6-10 Back tilted due to the different height profiles of the foot pedals. Raising the microscope foot pedal slightly would place the feet at a similar height and reduce tilting of the trunk. *(Courtesy of Sandra M. Woolley, PhD, CPE.)*

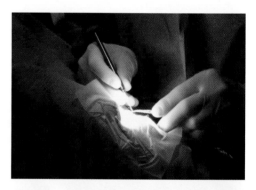

Figure 6-11 Prolonged precision gripping of the instruments. Attempt to be as relaxed as possible while using the instruments. *(Courtesy of Sandra M. Woolley, PhD, CPE.)*

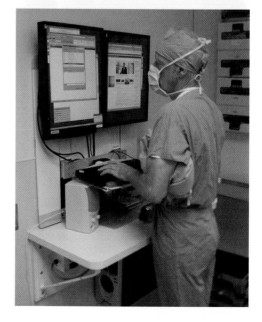

Figure 6-12 Hands are above the elbows while documenting and the eyes are lower than the top of the monitor. Placing the monitors and keyboards on a height-adjustable sliding arm is important. *(Courtesy of Sandra M. Woolley, PhD, CPE.)*

In the Office

Many people spend a significant amount of time on the computer, and steps also need to be taken to assure proper position when using the computer. Office ergonomics come down to 3 critical features: eyes, hands, and feet. The eyes should be level with the top of the monitor or slightly lower, particularly if one is wearing bifocals. The hands should at the level of the elbow or slightly below. The feet should be supported flat on the floor or on a footrest (Fig 6-13).

Monitors

Monitor(s) should be located at or slightly below sitting/standing eye height. Monitor(s) should be no closer to the eyes than the length of the arm extended forward. The monitors should be positioned directly in front of the eyes, in line with the keyboard and mouse.

Keyboard and mouse

The keyboard and mouse should be located at or slightly below seated elbow height. The hands should be in a neutral position, in line with the forearms, while resting on the keyboard. The keyboard and mouse should be located on the same horizontal surface.

Chair

Select a height-adjustable chair with height-adjustable armrests to support the forearms. The chair should have a height-adjustable backrest with lumbar support. There should be approximately 3 fingers of width between the back of the knees and the front of the chair. Most chairs have a seat pan that allows the depth of the seat to be adjusted to achieve the 3 fingers of distance. The chair should have comfortable padding and be rounded in the front with a waterfall (slopes down slightly) front. Sit back in the chair using the backrest, with the thighs parallel to the floor and the lower legs perpendicular to the floor with knee flexion of approximately 90°. If the chair seems too high, use a footrest to support

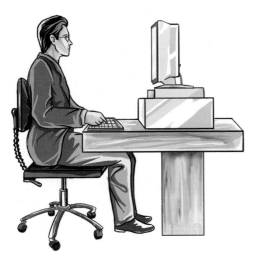

Figure 6-13 Ideal seated posture. This includes feet supported on the floor, the knees flexed to 90°, the thighs parallel with the floor, the upper arms positioned close to the trunk, the elbows flexed at 90° or less, and the head looking forward without any flexion or extension.

the feet. Avoid putting the feet behind the knees. Also avoid sitting with the trunk twisted (Fig 6-14), or sitting at an angle to the keyboard and monitor (Fig 6-15).

In the Clinic

Research has shown that there is a positive relationship between the number of eye exams performed per day and the reported incidence of pain and discomfort. It has been suggested that more than 11 eye exams per day are associated with a 50% increase in the risk of neck, shoulder, upper/lower back pain, and elbow/arm discomfort. Tasks such as slit-lamp biomicroscopy, indirect ophthalmoscopy, and direct ophthalmoscopy exhibit ergonomic risk factors such as non-neutral postures, and prolonged static muscle contractions in the neck, shoulders, trunk, and upper extremities. Table 6-3 provides a brief summary

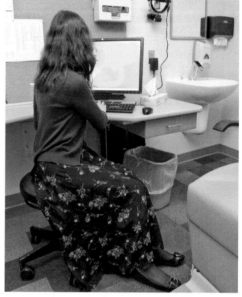

Figure 6-14 Avoid sitting with the trunk twisted. *(Courtesy of Lucas T. Digman.)*

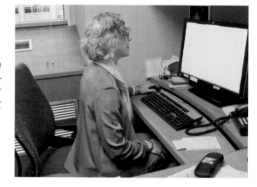

Figure 6-15 Sit back in your chair to take advantage of the backrest. Lower the monitor so that the top of the monitor is level or slightly below eye height. *(Courtesy of Lucas T. Digman.)*

Table 6-3 Clinical Activities, Ergonomic Risk Factors, and Potential Solutions

Clinical Activity	Ergonomic Risk Factors	Potential Solutions
Slit lamp	Forward trunk flexion, shoulder protraction, forward head, neck extension, lumbar kyphosis	Raise the stool so that the eyes are positioned just above the eyepieces. Maintain a neutral posture of the trunk, with the cervical and lumbar spine in lordosis and the thoracic spine in kyphosis. It may be helpful to visualize the ischial tuberosity (the "sit bones" of the pelvic girdle), the bony parts you feel under you when sitting up straight on a firm surface. Relax your shoulders and sit up straight. Your feet should be positioned flat on the floor.
	Arm controlling the slit lamp: upper arm is close to the body, the elbow is leaning on the sharp edge of the slit-lamp table, the wrist is flexed and the hand exhibits a lateral grip.	Provide a padded surface to reduce the contact stress at the elbow. Increase the size of the dial control to reduce hand pinching.
	Arm with the lens: unsupported shoulder flexion and abduction, elbow flexion with contact stress at the elbow or the elbow being unsupported above the slit-lamp table surface, wrist extension, ulnar deviation, and pinch grip on the hand with the lens	Move closer to the slit-lamp table surface to reduce the amount of unsupported arm flexion. Provide a padded support surface for the elbow.
Indirect ophthalmoscopy	Forward trunk flexion and excessive neck flexion. The weight of the ophthalmoscope tends to pull the head and neck into flexion.	Raise the height of the chair to reduce neck flexion.
Direct ophthalmoscopy	Trunk flexion, one shoulder is higher than the other, and neck flexion. The trunk is also twisted.	Raise the patient's chair to reduce the amount of trunk flexion.

of the ergonomic risk factors associated with various clinical activities and lists potential solutions to eliminate or reduce exposures to these risk factors.

The following figures depict various clinical activities and the associated ergonomic risk factors. These areas include

- the slit lamp (Figs 6-16–6-19)
- indirect ophthalmoscopy (Figs 6-20, 6-21)
- direct ophthalmoscopy (Figs 6-22, 6-23)

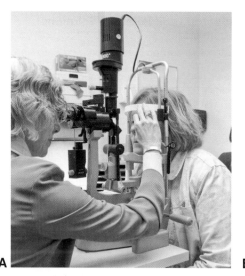 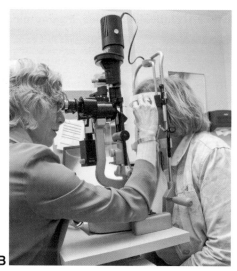

A   **B**

Figure 6-16 **A,** Notice the flexion and abduction of the arms, the neck extension, and forward head position. **B,** With the elbow supported, less stress is being placed on the shoulder and neck muscles. *(Parts A and B courtesy of Lucas T. Digman.)*

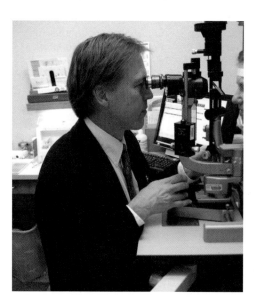 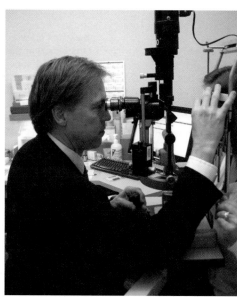

Figure 6-17 Notice that the hands are above the elbows and unsupported on the slit-lamp surface. *(Courtesy of Sandra M. Woolley, PhD, CPE.)*

Figure 6-18 The arm with the lens is abducted, flexed, and unsupported. Providing padded supports would reduce the strain on the shoulder muscles. *(Courtesy of Sandra M. Woolley, PhD, CPE.)*

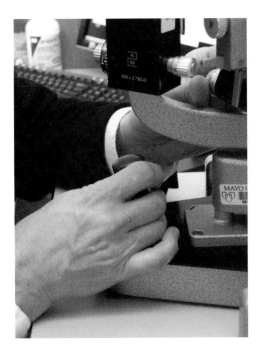

Figure 6-19 Notice the contact stresses on the right wrist and the left forearm, where the tissues are compressed between the bones and the sharp edge of the slit-lamp table. Consider padding or rounding of the edges. *(Courtesy of Sandra M. Woolley, PhD, CPE.)*

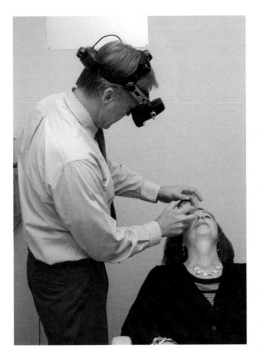

Figure 6-20 Use of the indirect ophthalmoscope results in neck and trunk flexion. Raise the chair. *(Courtesy of Lucas T. Digman.)*

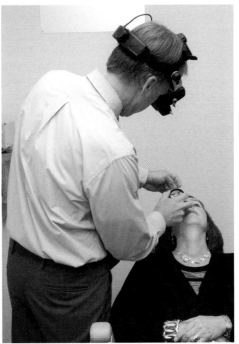

Figure 6-21 The trunk is twisted. *(Courtesy of Lucas T. Digman.)*

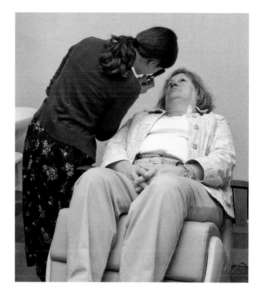

Figure 6-22 Note that the back is bent forward and twisted. Raising the chair will reduce the amount of forward back flexion. *(Courtesy of Lucas T. Digman.)*

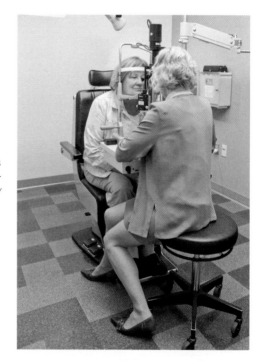

Figure 6-23 Wearing a skirt or dress results in the physician assuming a side-saddle position with the back and neck twisted. *(Courtesy of Lucas T. Digman.)*

Reducing the Risk of Developing Musculoskeletal Disorders

The research literature suggests taking a comprehensive approach to preventing the development of work-related MSDs. A first step is to recognize the ergonomic risk factors in the work area and redesign the work layout, equipment, and work practices to reduce exposure to these risk factors. Consideration should also be given to one's personal lifestyle choices. Incorporating stress management techniques can be very helpful, as demonstrated by the following suggestions:

- Exercise programs with a strengthening component can increase muscular strength gains and significantly reduce pain scores, the number of days absent from work, and the prevalence of work-related MSDs.
- It has been suggested that ophthalmologists who exercise 5 hours per week are significantly less likely to experience pain associated with performing surgery and are less likely to need to modify their surgical practice.
- Yoga may be helpful in reducing physical and mental stresses, thereby reducing the severity and potential incidence of MSDs.
- Although the outcomes from exercise-stretching programs have had mixed reviews on preventing work-related MSDs, there appear to be some positive effects of routine stretching.
- Another factor to consider is the recognized association between high perceived work-related and non–work-related stress and the development of work-related MSDs. There is also evidence of a link between high job demands and work-related MSDs.

Key Points

- Pay attention to maintaining your normal body curves.
- Rest elbows and wrists on cushioned surfaces.
- Avoid maintaining positions with extremities suspended in the air and unsupported.
- Perform stretching exercises throughout the day.
- Maintain a healthy lifestyle with regular exercise and include stress management techniques.
- If you are experiencing signs and symptoms of WRMSDs, seek medical advice early on.

American Academy of Ophthalmology, Ergonomics Task Force. "Ergonomics Best Practices." Course. Available at http://one.aao.org/course/ergonomics-best-practices. Accessed October 28, 2014.

Ang BO, Monnier A, Harms-Ringdahl K. Neck/shoulder exercise for neck pain in air force helicopter pilots. *Spine.* 2009;34(16):E544–E551.

Ayanniyi AA, Olatunji FO, Majengbasan T, Ayanniyi RO, and Danfulani M. Ophthalmic practice health hazards among ophthalmologists in a resource-limited setting. *Asian Pac J Trop Dis.* 2011;1(1):17–20.

Board of Certified Professional Ergonomists. Bylaws. Available at www.bcpe.org/about-bcpe /bylaws/. Accessed October 28, 2014.

Bongers PM, Kremer AM, ter Laak J. Are psychosocial factors, risk factors for symptoms and signs of the shoulder, elbow or hand/wrist? a review of the epidemiological literature. *Am J Ind Med.* 2002;41(5):315–342.

Centers for Disease Control and Prevention. Ergonomics and musculoskeletal disorders. Available at http://www.cdc.gov/niosh/topics/ergonomics. Accessed October 28, 2014.

Chams H, Mohammadi SF, Moayyeri A. Frequency and assortment of self-reported occupational complaints among Iranian ophthalmologists: a preliminary survey. *MedGenMed.* 2004;6(4):1.

Chatterjee A, Ryan WG, Rosen ES. Back pain in ophthalmologists. *Eye.* 1994;8(Pt 4): 473–474.

Chengalur SN, Rodgers SH, Bernard TE. *Kodak's Ergonomic Design for People at Work.* 2nd ed. Hoboken, NJ: John Wiley & Sons; 2003.

Chiang A, Baker PS, Miller, EA, Garg SJ. Fellows' focus: ergonomics for the retina specialist. *Retina Today.* 2010;July/August:25–26.

Da Costa BR, Vieira ER. Stretching to reduce work-related musculoskeletal disorders: a systematic review. *J Rehabil Med.* 2008;40(5):321–328.

Dhimitri KC, McGwin G Jr, McNeal SF, et al. Symptoms of musculoskeletal disorders in ophthalmologists. *Am J Ophthalmol.* 2005;139(1):179–181.

Gundewall B, Liljeqvist M, Hansson T. Primary prevention of back symptoms and absence from work. A prospective randomized study among hospital employees. *Spine.* 1993;18(5): 587–594.

Kitzmann AS, Fethke NB, Baratz KH, Zimmerman B, Hackbath DJ, Gehr KM. A survey study of musculoskeletal disorders among eye care physicians compared with family medicine physicians. *Am Acad Ophthomol.* 2012;119(2):213–220.

Long J, Naduvilath TJ, Hao LE, et al. Risk factors for physical discomfort in Australian optometrists. *Optom Vis Sci.* 2011;88(2):317–326.

Marx JL, Wertz FD, Dhimitri KC. Work-related musculoskeletal disorders in ophthalmologists. *Tech Ophthalmol.* 2005;3(1):54–61.

Marx JL. Ergonomics: back to the future. *Ophthalmology.* 2012;119 (2):212–213.

National Institute for Occupational Safety and Health. *Elements of Ergonomics Programs. A Primer Based on Workplace Evaluations of Musculoskeletal Disorders.* U.S. Department of Health and Human Services . CDC DHHS (NIOSH) Publication No. 97-117. 1997.

Occupational Safety & Health Administration. Ergonomics. Available at www.osha.gov /SLTC/ergonomics. Accessed October 28, 2014.

Roach L. Ergonomics, part one: is the job you love a pain in the neck? *EyeNet.* www.aao.org /publications/eyenet/200907/practice_perf.cfm. Accessed October 28, 2014.

Roach L. Seven risk factors for injury, and seven solutions: ergonomics, part two. *EyeNet.* www.aao.org/aao/publications/eyenet/200909/practice_perf.cfm%20. Accessed October 28, 2014.

Silverstein B, Clark R. Interventions to reduce work-related musculoskeletal disorders. *J Electromyogr Kinesiol.* 2004;14(1):135–152.

Sivak-Callcott JA, Diaz SR, Ducatman AM, Rosen CL, Nimbarte AD, Sedgeman, JA. A survey study of occupational pain and injury in ophthalmic plastic surgeons. *Ophthal Plast Reconstr Surg.* 2011;27(1):28–32.

U.S. Department of Labor, OSHA. eTools: Computer workstations. www.osha.gov/SLTC /etools/computerworkstations/index.html%20. Accessed October 28, 2014.

U.S. Department of Labor. OSHA proposed rule 64:65768-66078 29 CFR 1910.900. Ergonomics Program. http://goo.gl/DBs9AP. Accessed October 28, 2014.

U.S. Department of Labor. OSHA Final rule 29 CFR Part 1910. Ergonomics Program. http://goo.gl/nvW97u. Accessed October 28, 2014.

Self-Assessment Test

1. During surgery or a procedure, which of the following is an important consideration?
   a. Adjust the eyepieces so that they are just above the eyes.
   b. Maintain the arms away from the body to strengthen the deltoids.
   c. Use a stool without a backrest.
   d. Use a wrist rest.

2. While working on the computer, which of the following is incorrect?
   a. If you are using the computer only for a short time, it is acceptable to twist your trunk so that your arms and legs are not aligned above one another.
   b. The chair height should be adjustable and you should sit back in the chair and use the backrest.
   c. The monitor should be positioned directly in front of your eyes, at or slightly below the eye height, with the monitor extended an arm's length away.
   d. Place your feet flat on the floor and avoid putting your feet behind your knees.

3. As a resident, what is the relevancy of understanding ergonomic issues?
   a. Survey studies have reported that about 50% of ophthalmologists experience or suffer from work-related musculoskeletal disorders.
   b. The costs of lost work time due to musculoskeletal disorders can be significant for the doctor, patients, and the employer.
   c. There are some steps one can take to help prevent work-related musculoskeletal disorders.
   d. All of the above.

For preferred responses to these questions, see Appendix A.

CHAPTER 7

The Operating Microscope and Surgical Loupes

Norman A. Zabriskie, MD
Daniel I. Bettis, MD

The development of the surgical microscope revolutionized ophthalmic surgery. Historically, cataract surgery was performed without magnification. The modern surgical microscope makes possible the current standard of small-incision phacoemulsification with capsulorrhexis, complete nuclear and cortical removal, preservation of the posterior capsule, and in-the-bag placement of a foldable intraocular lens. Most vitreoretinal surgical procedures are wholly dependent on the high magnification, lighting, and depth perception that the microscope affords. Surgical loupes provide magnification as well, with unique advantages and disadvantages when compared to the microscope. This chapter describes the practical use of both instruments in the operating room.

Just as a smooth cataract operation depends on the successful completion of a series of maneuvers in their proper order, maximal benefit from the operating microscope is obtained by repeating certain steps carefully and effectively every time. These include proper positioning of the patient and surgeon, hand positioning that reduces tremor and fatigue, and efficient operation of the microscope controls. Refer to Chapter 6 for additional information about the importance of ergonomics for the ophthalmologist.

Advantages and Disadvantages of Magnification

The many advantages of the modern-day surgical microscope may seem intuitive. Its lighting is excellent and uniform throughout the surgical field, and a good red reflex is usually readily obtained. Newer illumination systems can even enhance the red reflex in difficult cases, such as those with small pupils. The light intensity is adjustable, and filters protect the patient and surgeon from phototoxic effects. The optical system provides the surgeon with an excellent binocular wide-field stereoscopic view. Most microscopes can provide a stereoscopic view through an assistant arm as well, usually by way of a beamsplitter that splits the light between the surgeon and the assistant, historically in a 70/30 ratio. However, the newest generation microscopes provide 100% stereovision and 100% illumination to both the surgeon and the assistant via independent light sources.

Such an advancement is particularly useful for teaching institutions where residents perform surgery while faculty supervise through the assistant arm of the microscope.

Magnification itself is obviously a significant advantage in ophthalmic surgery, but the control and variability of this magnification are the key benefits. Most microscopes offer a range of magnification from approximately 10×–30× and foot pedal controls. Thus, the surgeon can focus on the posterior capsule and then into the anterior chamber, or from the mid-vitreous to the retinal surface, with a simple touch of the foot pedal. Motors on the microscope also provide motion control of the optical system in the x-y axes. This allows adjustment of the microscope to compensate for minor patient movements that change the operating axis.

The benefits of the microscope far outweigh the disadvantages, but several disadvantages deserve mention. Because of the high magnification, even the slightest vibration can disturb the view through the microscope. For this reason, operating rooms that house surgical microscopes must be constructed to very high vibration-dampening standards. Even maintenance or construction in adjacent rooms or floors can cause excessive vibration. In such cases it is not uncommon to have to search out the source of the vibration (usually a construction or maintenance worker) and have them stop their work until completion of a surgical case. High magnification also places greater demands on the surgeon. Any hand tremor or surgical misstep is magnified along with the ocular tissues. Controlling tremor and nerves can be more difficult in such a setting. This is particularly true for the beginning surgeon.

Another disadvantage of the operating microscope is that procedures requiring the surgeon to view the surgical field from multiple angles (ie, oculoplastic, strabismus, or scleral buckle surgeries) are not easily performed. Fortunately, surgical loupes provide a good alternative because of the flexibility of their viewing angle and magnification that is well suited to these tasks. The main disadvantage of loupes is their fixed focal length, which results in a fixed working distance for the surgeon.

Patient Positioning

Good patient positioning is essential for proper use of the surgical microscope. The goals of patient positioning, as related to the microscope, are to (1) maximize the view of the surgical field, especially the red reflex, (2) minimize the need for microscope adjustment during surgery, (3) facilitate good patient fixation on the microscope light for procedures under topical anesthesia, and (4) avoid excess light exposure to the patient.

Careful positioning of the surgical eye relative to the microscope is the first step in a successful surgery. Position the patient so that the corneal surface of the operative eye is parallel to the floor (Fig 7-1). This recommendation holds whether the surgical approach is temporal or superior, and whether using retrobulbar or topical anesthesia. Positioning the eye surface parallel to the floor is most easily accomplished if the surgical bed has a separate headrest with its own adjustment system (Fig 7-2). Usually one can adjust both the tilt and the vertical position of the headrest without affecting the patient's overall position. With this flexibility, the surgeon can be very precise in adjusting the head of the

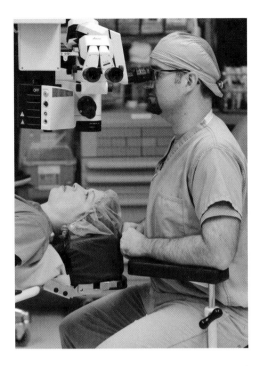

Figure 7-1 Good patient positioning with the "eye parallel to the floor." This maximizes the view for the surgeon and allows the patient to better fixate on the microscope light. *(Courtesy of Daniel I. Bettis, MD.)*

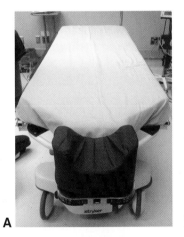

A

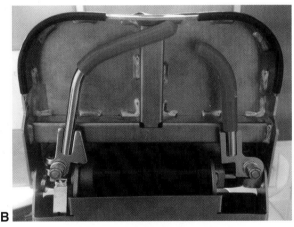

B

Figure 7-2 Surgical bed. **A,** Outpatient surgical bed with separate headrest and independent headrest controls. **B,** Levers on underside of headrest allow for independent adjustment of elevation (vertical position) and tilt of the headrest. *(Courtesy of Daniel I. Bettis, MD.)*

patient even when anatomic challenges, such as kyphosis, might make proper positioning very difficult on a traditional operating room bed.

Having the surgical eye parallel to the floor is very important for proper use of the microscope, especially for topical anesthetic procedures. Such positioning allows the visual axis to be centered between the upper and lower eyelids when the patient fixates on the microscope light. This maximizes the quality of the surgical view as well as the red reflex, and it helps the patient to maintain proper fixation on the microscope light. If the patient is positioned so that her chin is up (Fig 7-3) and the superior limbus of the eye tilts toward the floor, fixation on the microscope light by the patient drives the eye toward the lower lid, This can hinder the surgical view, surgical access, and the red reflex. Conversely, if the patient is in the chin-down position, with the inferior limbus tilting toward the floor, fixation on the microscope light drives the eye toward the upper lid, causing similar problems (Fig 7-4). This latter problem is particularly true for a right-handed surgeon performing cataract surgery on a left eye from a temporal approach; the chin-down patient position must be avoided in this case. Failure to position the patient far enough onto the headrest is a common cause of the chin-down position. Before starting, ensure that the patient's head is fully seated within the headrest. This will not only result in better patient positioning for surgery, but also greater comfort for the patient, because the head and neck are much better supported.

Pearls and Pitfalls of Patient Positioning

If the patient is positioned properly at the start of the case, then any subsequent movement of the eye out of the surgical field is unwanted, and the cause should be ascertained and corrected. In most cases, excessive movement of the operated eye is due to improper hand position by the surgeon, a point to be discussed later; however, sometimes the patient simply moves. If the case is being performed under topical anesthesia, the patient simply may have lost fixation on the microscope light. A gentle reminder from the surgeon to "look at the light" or "find the light" will correct this problem. However, if after refixation on the microscope light, the upper lid still partly obscures the surgical eye, the patient has probably dropped her chin, and if the surgical eye is covered by the lower lid, the patient has lifted her chin. The surgeon need simply ask the patient to "lift your chin" or "drop your chin," and the problem is corrected.

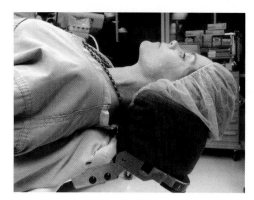

Figure 7-3 The "chin-up" patient position. This posture drives the eye to the lower lid when the patient fixates on the microscope light. *(Courtesy of Daniel I. Bettis, MD.)*

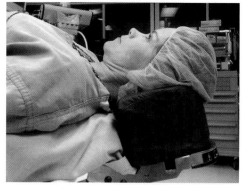

Figure 7-4 The "chin-down" patient position. This position drives the eye to the upper eyelid. This is a particularly troublesome position for a right-handed surgeon operating on a left eye from the temporal approach. *(Courtesy of Daniel I. Bettis, MD.)*

The surgical eye moving away from the surgeon is another very common position-ing problem during surgery from the temporal approach. For example, if the surgeon operates on a left eye temporally from the 3 o'clock position, the eye may move toward the 9 o'clock position, requiring the surgeon to repeatedly use the x-y control on the foot pedal to move the microscope in that direction and center the image. Although this is usually due to the surgeon displacing the eye nasally with improper hand position (lift-ing on the surgical wound and/or paracentesis), there is also a common tendency for the patient to rotate his head away from the temporal incision site. To correct this head rota-tion, either ask the patient to rotate his head back toward you or take your nondominant hand and gently rotate the head back toward you in a very slow and controlled fashion. The latter approach is safer and more effective. Some patients have such a strong tendency to roll away from the incision site that the surgical assistant or scrub nurse must hold the patient's head in place.

Some patients are not able to tolerate lying flat. This may be due to difficulty breath-ing in the supine position, dizziness, or the patient's body habitus, including obesity and spinal kyphosis. One strategy for such patients is to elevate the head of the bed to about 30°. Raise the entire bed, and then use the Trendelenburg pedal to lower the head into position (Fig 7-5). This method maintains the 30° angle of the patient, while putting the head flat and into position for the microscope. This "V-position" reduces the patient's sensation of being in a completely flat position and therefore results in better tolerance and cooperation with the surgery. This method also works well for patients who are sig-nificantly kyphotic, in whom the head seems to dangle in midair above the headrest when the patient is placed in the supine position. This maneuver brings the head into contact with the headrest and allows for good "eye parallel to the floor" positioning.

Infants and small children can also pose unique positioning problems. Due to anes-thesia requirements, these cases are often performed in main hospital operating rooms, on traditional surgical beds without separate headrests and independent controls. The main problem stems from the fact that the infant head is bigger in proportion to the body than in adults, resulting in an exaggerated chin-down position. A shoulder roll (usually a rolled towel of appropriate size) placed under the child's shoulders extends the neck and places the head in the "eye parallel to the floor" position. The microscope can then be positioned

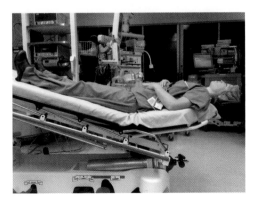

Figure 7-5 The patient unable to lie flat can be successfully positioned using this strat-egy. The head of the bed is elevated, the bed is raised, and then a Trendelenburg position places the eye properly for the microscope. *(Courtesy of Daniel I. Bettis, MD.)*

as usual. This method can also be used in adults when a surgical bed with independent headrest controls is not available.

Surgeon Positioning

Proper positioning of the surgeon in relationship to the microscope allows easy control of the microscope foot pedal without disturbing the surgical field and maintains the surgeon's comfort throughout the case. Most forms of intraocular surgery that use an operating microscope are performed with the surgeon sitting at the head of the patient. Therefore, the patient's bed must be raised enough to allow the surgeon's legs to slide under the patient's head. This can be thought of as placing the head of the patient in the lap of the surgeon. This assures that when the microscope is brought into position directly over the patient, the surgeon does not have to lean too far forward or back to view through the microscope oculars. This positioning promotes surgeon comfort during the case and places the surgeon's hands in the most ergonomically favorable position.

The microscope pedal is positioned to allow manipulation by the foot without altering the position of the surgical field. With the surgeon at the 12 o'clock position, the microscope pedal can be placed slightly to the side of the patient and the table. A second control pedal, for example one controlling a vitrectomy unit, can be placed at the other side. The surgeon's legs are then not directly under the bed itself and therefore it is easy to use the pedals without inadvertently bumping the surgical table and changing the position of the surgical field (Fig 7-6).

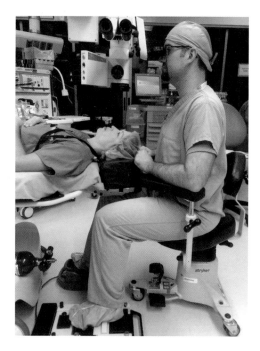

Figure 7-6 Surgeon positioning at the 12 o'clock position. The pedals are positioned just to the sides of the patient and table. At the 12 o'clock position, it is relatively easy for the surgeon to avoid inadvertent contact with the overlying table. *(Courtesy of Daniel I. Bettis, MD.)*

The Temporal Approach

Proper surgeon positioning for the temporal approach is more difficult. As with other approaches, the surgeon's legs need to be far enough under the head of the patient. This again ensures that the surgeon has good ergonomic posture, without leaning too far forward or back. (See Chapter 6.) The challenge comes in placing the control pedals for the microscope and phacoemulsification unit. At the temporal position, one leg of the surgeon will be directly under the surgical bed. For example, when operating on the right eye of a patient from the temporal approach, the right leg of the surgeon is completely under the bed (Fig 7-7); temporal surgery on a left eye places the left leg in a similar position, with difficulty keeping the leg clear of the table (Fig 7-8). This is especially difficult for the taller surgeon. In the temporal approach, as compared with the 12 o'clock position, the bed must be raised to accommodate the surgeon's legs. Because the bed must be higher, the microscope must also be raised to allow proper focus. However, the surgeon's chair cannot be raised the same amount or again the surgeon will bump the bottom of the table. Thus, the surgeon must assume a quite erect torso posture to reach the oculars of the microscope. This can be particularly true for a surgeon with a short torso relative to leg length. However, as discussed later in this chapter, this erect torso posture is an important step in stabilizing the hands.

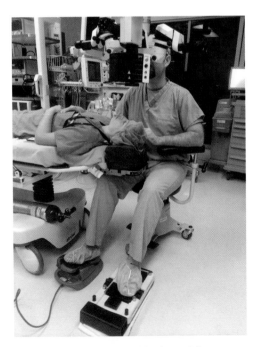

Figure 7-7 Surgeon positioning while operating on a right eye at the temporal position. Note that the right leg is completely under the surgical bed. *(Courtesy of Daniel I. Bettis, MD.)*

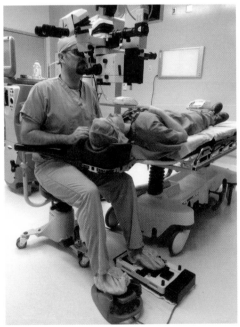

Figure 7-8 Surgeon positioning for a temporal approach to the left eye. Here, the left leg must be completely beneath the surgical bed. *(Courtesy of Daniel I. Bettis, MD.)*

Pearls and Pitfalls of Surgeon Positioning

In summary, good positioning starts by making sure that the surgeon's body is sufficiently under the head of the patient. This is true at either the 12 o'clock or temporal position. If the surgeon is not close enough to the patient, and the head of the patient does not overlie at least the knees and perhaps the thighs of the surgeon, the surgeon must lean too far forward to reach the microscope oculars. This is uncomfortable for the surgeon and extends the arms away from the body, which makes it more difficult to stabilize the hands. In the proper surgeon position relative to the patient, the surgeon will have an erect torso posture with a slight forward lean at the waist to reach the microscope oculars.

Positioning the Bed

The most common positioning error the beginning surgeon makes when operating from the temporal position is failing to raise the bed high enough. This is typically not a problem at the head of the patient, since at the 12 o'clock position the surgeon's legs are positioned on either side of the patient's head when controlling the foot pedals. However, as mentioned before, in the temporal position one leg has to be under the table. This creates a problem when the bed is not high enough and during pedal maneuvers the surgeon bumps the underside of the table with his or her leg (Fig 7-9). This action elevates the bed slightly, which causes the surgical field to go in and out of focus under high microscopic magnification.

The bumping action can be a major problem for the beginning surgeon. It is far more common while controlling the microscope pedal than the phacoemulsification unit pedal,

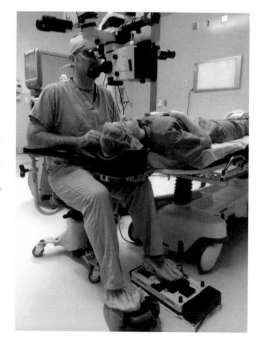

Figure 7-9 In this case, the left leg of the surgeon is in contact with the overlying bed. This creates a problem as the surgeon's leg elevates the bed during foot pedal maneuvers and defocuses the surgical field. *(Courtesy of Daniel I. Bettis, MD.)*

as the latter requires a downward motion on the foot pedal, lowering the knee and avoiding contact with the surgical bed. The microscope pedal, on the other hand, requires a rocking motion with the foot as the focus tab is controlled with the toe and the zoom tab is controlled with the heel. When the foot is flat on the pedal, both the toe-down position controlling the focus tab and the heel-down position required for the zoom tab elevate the knee, and it is during these maneuvers that the bed is most likely to be bumped.

Three steps prior to starting the surgical case can help you avoid this problem:

1. Initially determine the proper bed height so that your legs may slide comfortably under the patient's head.
2. Make sure that the clearance is still adequate when your feet are on the pedals. Commonly, beginning surgeons set the bed height with their feet flat on the floor. Then when the feet are placed on the pedals, the bed is obviously too low.
3. If the microscope pedal is the one directly under the patient, rock your foot back and forth, controlling the focus and the zoom while assuring proper clearance. It is also common for the beginning surgeon to have the leg extended all the way to the joystick of the pedal when setting the bed height. Once the case starts, and the surgeon has to bring the foot back to use either the focus or zoom tabs, the knee elevates dramatically and the bed is disturbed.

For surgeons with a relatively short torso or long legs, it can sometimes be a challenge to achieve the necessary clearance of the bed over the legs. One option involves flaring the knee out slightly, operating the microscope pedal with the outside of the foot (Fig 7-10). This lowers the leg significantly and allows the foot to work the pedal with very little elevation of the knee and therefore little disturbance of the surgical bed. Another option for

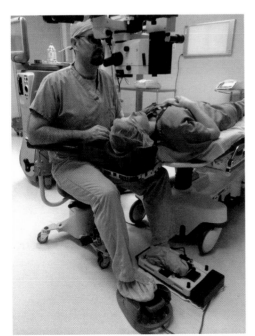

Figure 7-10 Flaring the left leg out and operating the foot pedal with the outside of the left foot drops the leg significantly and improves clearance under the bed. See Chapter 7 for additional information on positioning. *(Courtesy of Daniel I. Bettis, MD.)*

certain body types is to use newer microscope oculars that extend down from the microscope head. Because this allows the microscope to be higher relative to the surgeon's eye level, the bed can also be raised more. For some, this results in better clearance of the legs under the operating table. Simple experimentation is often best to determine which setup is best for a given surgeon.

Stabilizing the Hands

The greatest advantage of the operating microscope also creates the biggest surgical challenge. The high magnification provides excellent visualization of fine tissues and delicate maneuvers, but it exaggerates any aberrant hand movement. Learning to properly stabilize the hands and thereby decrease hand tremor is one of the greatest challenges facing the novice surgeon. (See also Chapter 3.) It can be a vicious cycle. Understandable nervousness from the surgeon causes a minor tremor, which when viewed under the microscope appears much greater than it actually is. This in turn fosters more nervousness, with even greater tremor, and so on. Keeping the hands well stabilized dramatically increases your comfort level.

Stabilizing the hands involves 4 steps:

1. The large arm and shoulder muscles must be stable enough to be quiet and nearly motionless throughout the case; they should not really participate.
2. The hands should be stabilized, usually at the wrist.
3. The small hand muscles must be kept loose and relaxed while working.
4. Any tremor may be dampened with counter touch from the nondominant hand.

Stabilizing the Large Arm and Shoulder Muscles

Stabilizing the hands begins by removing the large muscles from the surgical equation. Two important signs indicate that the large muscles are being used: elevation of the shoulders and elevation of the elbows. Lifting the shoulders, as in a "shrug," tightens the muscles all the way down the arms and increases tremor. An erect torso posture drives the shoulders down into a relaxed position (Fig 7-11). If, on the other hand, the surgeon has the chair too high, he or she must crouch to position at the microscope oculars (Fig 7-12). This position is much more conducive to shrugging the shoulders, causing arm and hand tightness. If you begin to feel tense during surgery, try consciously "dropping the shoulders." This creates a relaxed position with a profound effect on hand stability.

Raised elbows are another sign that the large muscles are too active. This position also elevates the wrists off their support, which greatly destabilizes the hands. There are 2 ways to ensure that the elbows are staying low and in a relaxed position: The first involves use of a surgical chair that has armrests (Fig 7-13). This allows excellent support for the entire forearm, from the elbow to the wrist, with the elbow in constant contact with the armrest. If the surgeon becomes aware that the elbow is not in contact with the armrest, he or she knows that the elbows are raised and should be dropped into a better position.

A second method is use of a wrist rest. Again, elevation of the elbows lifts the wrists off the rest and, on recognizing this, the surgeon should drop the elbows and shoulders if necessary and reposition the wrists back onto the rest.

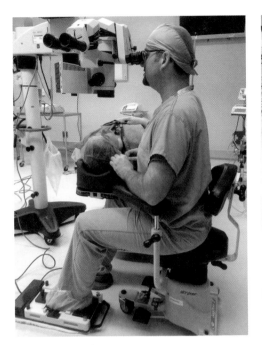

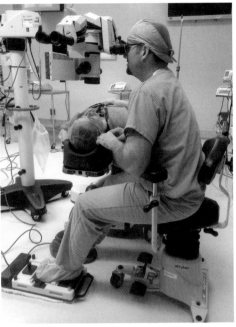

Figure 7-11 Sitting with an erect torso posture lowers the shoulders into a comfortable position. This helps to relax the large shoulder and arm muscles. See Chapter 6 for additional information on positioning. *(Courtesy of Daniel I. Bettis, MD.)*

Figure 7-12 If the surgeon's chair is too high, he or she must crouch to reach the oculars. This causes the shoulders to shrug, which tends to tighten the shoulder and arm muscles. *(Courtesy of Daniel I. Bettis, MD.)*

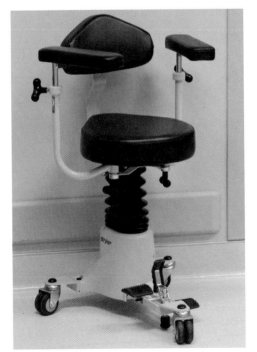

Figure 7-13 Surgical chair with adjustable armrests. *(Courtesy of Daniel I. Bettis, MD.)*

Stabilizing the Hands at the Wrists

It is critical that the hands be stable at the wrists. A chair with armrests provides excellent stabilization of the forearm and wrist. Often the armrests are sufficient and no separate wrist rest is needed, but a wrist rest can also be used separately. This will also help to quiet the arms and shoulders. It is important to understand that the wrist rest (and/or armrests) must be set at different heights depending on the surgeon's position. When working at the 12 o'clock position, the surgeon's hands have to come over the brow and then "down" to the eye. The wrist support must therefore be set high enough to accomplish this (Fig 7-14). Conversely, when operating temporally, the wrist support can be set lower. The surgeon should have the mental image of the wrists set low and the hands coming "up" to the eye (Fig 7-15).

Relaxing the Small Hand Muscles

The next step in reducing tremor is to relax the small hand muscles and keep them tension-free. This is extremely difficult without first quieting the large muscles and supporting the wrists. The enemy of such relaxation is a tight grip on the instruments. The beginning cataract surgeon sometimes grips the phacoemulsification handpiece like a vise. It is impossible to reduce tremor with such a grip. Hold the instrument like a pencil and with a light grip (Fig 7-16). This allows the hand to relax. A good practice maneuver is to take a large diameter pen, grip it normally with the thumb and first 2 fingers of the dominant hand, and practice rotating the pen back and forth as gently as possible. Keep

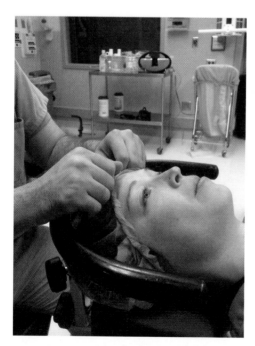

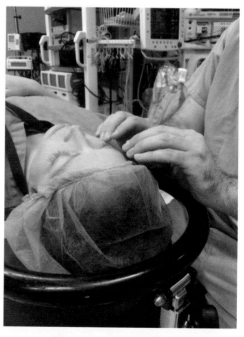

Figure 7-14 At the 12 o'clock position, the wrist rest is set a little higher to allow the hands to come over the brow and "down" to the eye. *(Courtesy of Daniel I. Bettis, MD.)*

Figure 7-15 At the temporal position, the wrist rest is set lower and the hands come "up" to the eye. *(Courtesy of Daniel I. Bettis, MD.)*

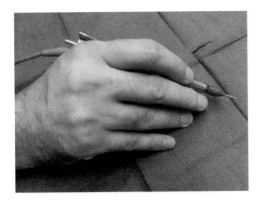

Figure 7-16 The instrument should be held like a pencil with a light grip. This helps to relax the muscles in the hand and reduce tremor. *(Courtesy of Daniel I. Bettis, MD.)*

the rest of the hand still, and only move the thumb and 2 fingers in a gentle rotating motion. This mimics the required maneuvers of cataract surgery, in particular the irrigation and aspiration step during cortical removal, and teaches the surgeon to keep the hands relaxed.

Dampening Tremor With Counter Touch

One of the most effective means of reducing hand tremor is to touch the instrument with the nondominant hand. For example, if the surgeon is holding an instrument in his or her dominant right hand, using the left index finger to lightly touch the instrument greatly reduces tremor. This obviously is not possible when both hands are being used, but during one-handed maneuvers the technique is very important and effective. The classic example is during the capsulorrhexis step of cataract surgery, which is a one-handed maneuver usually involving forceps. Grasp the forceps lightly, like a pencil, with the thumb and first 2 fingers of the dominant hand. Next, take the index finger of the nondominant hand and touch the forceps just below the fingers of the dominant hand (Fig 7-17). This is a very stable hand position and can dramatically reduce hand tremor.

Pearls and Pitfalls of Hand Stabilization

Incorrect hand position causes several common microscope problems. The first is the tendency for the operative eye to move away from the surgeon during the case, making it difficult to keep the eye centered in the surgical field through the microscope. As discussed previously, this problem can occur if the patient is having trouble fixating on the microscope light or if the patient has rolled her head away from the surgeon. However, the most common cause by far is poor hand position, specifically lifting the hands.

Incorrect hand position, particularly hand lifting, causes several problems, especially during cataract surgery. First, lifting the hands causes the phacoemulsification handpiece to angle downward in the eye. This creates a downward vector during lens sculpting, which is not desirable for zonule preservation. Second, the downward angle of the instrument opens the incision. This allows fluid to escape the eye too quickly, allowing the anterior chamber to shallow, thus increasing the risk of breaking the posterior capsule. Third and most important in the context of the microscope, hand lifting persistently pushes the operative eye away from the surgeon, either down toward the

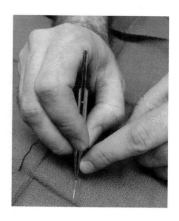

Figure 7-17 Counter touch with the nondominant hand significantly dampens tremor. It can be used during one-handed maneuvers such as capsulorrhexis. *(Courtesy of Daniel I. Bettis, MD.)*

lower lid if the surgeon is at the 12 o'clock position or toward the nose if the surgeon is operating temporally. This requires more and more adjustment of the microscope position. Beginning surgeons can learn to recognize this problem if they are repeatedly using the foot pedal joystick to move the microscope away from them. The remedy is to drop the hands, bringing the wrists and hands back into contact with the wrist rest or armrest.

Another common microscope problem caused by poor hand position is excessive side-to-side eye movement. This can happen at either the 12 o'clock or temporal position. The most common cause is failure to keep the surgical instrument centered in the incision. This is one of the most difficult concepts for the new surgeon. The natural tendency is to move the instrument laterally in the incision. Eventually, the end of the incision is reached and at that point the whole eye moves in that direction. The proper technique is to keep the instrument centered in the incision and pivot around that point, like a fulcrum. A good visual concept is to picture the instrument like the oar of a boat. At the wound entrance into the eye, the instrument is locked into place, like the oarlock on the side of the boat. At this point the instrument (or oar) cannot move laterally, it can only pivot. Learning this technique for intraocular surgery, especially cataract surgery, is essential if the eye is to remain centered in the microscope field. This technique also reduces corneal striae, which improves visualization and safety—especially when creating the capsulorrhexis.

Microscope Function

Once the patient is well positioned, the surgeon is comfortable, and the hands are stabilized, attention is directed to the microscope itself. Four key points in the proper operation of the microscope include

1. gross maneuvering of the microscope and centering of its axes
2. positioning and setting the oculars
3. adjusting the microscope during the case
4. controlling the lighting

Gross Maneuvering of the Microscope

Modern microscopes can be either ceiling- or floor-mounted. Ceiling-mounted micro-scopes are useful when there is a dedicated operating room for microsurgery. They pose less of a physical obstacle within the operating room and do not have to be repositioned with each new patient. Nevertheless, floor-mounted microscopes are equally effective. When the surgeon is positioned at the 12 o'clock position, the floor-mounted microscope is usually placed on the side of the surgeon's nondominant hand. This allows the surgical instruments to be at the ready for the surgeon's dominant hand. Alternatively, the micro-scope may always be placed on one side or the other regardless of the operated eye, and it functions very well in this manner. For the temporal approach, the microscope is typically positioned opposite the surgical eye. For example, when operating on a right eye from the temporal approach, the microscope is brought in from the patient's left. Floor-mounted microscopes provide a great advantage in that they can be moved from room to room. Ceiling- and floor-mounted microscopes share most other technical features.

The microscope head is positioned on an elaborate swinging positioning arm (Fig 7-18). The various pivot points in the arm can be changed to allow great flexibility in positioning the head of the microscope. Each break point typically has a tightening mech-anism so that the arm can be fixed at that position if desired. The optimal adjustment of the positioning arm is unique for every surgical room and patient orientation. Another important control on the microscope arm, the counterweight setting, determines the ver-tical excursion of the microscope head when it is positioned and released. This control should be set so that the microscope head remains in place when released.

The centering button, located on the microscope head (Fig 7-19), centers it in the x-y axes and should be depressed at the beginning of each surgery, thus giving the microscope full excursion in all directions at the start of the case. The head of the microscope is also equipped with large positioning handles. There are 2 or 3 handles, usually one on each

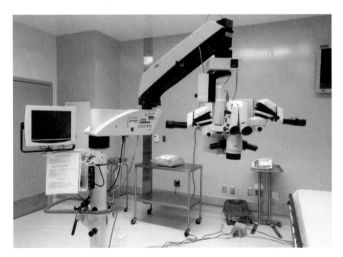

Figure 7-18 Typical operating microscope positioning arm with pivot point controls and coun-terweight control. *(Courtesy of Daniel I. Bettis, MD.)*

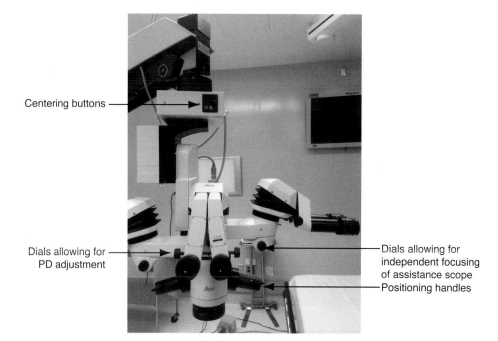

Centering buttons

Dials allowing for PD adjustment

Dials allowing for independent focusing of assistance scope

Positioning handles

Figure 7-19 Microscope head with centering buttons to center both the x-y axes and level of magnification, positioning handles, dials allowing for pupillary distance adjustment, dials allowing for independent focusing of assistant microscope head. *(Courtesy of Daniel I. Bettis, MD.)*

side of the oculars and sometimes a third on the positioning arm. Typically, the handles are fitted with slide-on covers that can be sterilized. A final important initial adjustment is the centering of the microscope focus in the up and down axis. Older microscope models may have a scale on the side of the microscope head showing the midpoint of the focus. At the beginning of the case, the microscope focus should be adjusted via the foot pedal to lie in the middle of the focus axis to slightly above center. Because most of the focusing during surgery is downward, sufficient excursion in this direction must be available to start. Newer microscope models have a second button, alongside the x-y centering button, to center the focusing mechanism. This too should be depressed at the beginning of each case to allow full excursion.

Positioning and Setting the Oculars

The important parameters to be set for the microscope oculars are the pupillary distance (PD), the diopter setting, and the tilt. The PD is set either with a small knob on the side of the oculars or simply by manually spreading the oculars to the proper distance. If more than one surgeon will use the microscope during a case or during the course of a day, it may be necessary to adjust the PD intraoperatively under sterile conditions. This is accomplished either with a sterilizable cap over the adjusting knob, or with sterile covers over the oculars themselves.

The oculars can be set to a specific diopter setting to match the refractive error of the surgeon. Most oculars have a range of +/– 5.00 diopters, and each can be set independently to accommodate anisometropia. Alternatively, the surgeon may set the oculars at zero and wear spectacles; this is a good option at teaching institutions where 2 surgeons may need to view through the primary microscope oculars during the same case.

The oculars also may be tilted vertically. The main use of the vertical tilt is to allow the surgeon to assume the upright torso posture discussed earlier.

Reviewing the Sequence of Setup Steps

To review, the sequence of important steps at the start of the typical case is as follows:

1. Both the patient and surgeon are properly and comfortably positioned.
2. The surgeon checks that his or her feet are on the pedals, the hands are stabilized, and posture is correct.
3. The circulating nurse swings the microscope into position, having first pushed the x-y and zoom centering buttons.
4. The oculars are set.
5. The surgeon then grasps the sterile handles of the microscope, positions the microscope over the surgical eye with low light intensity, and achieves gross focus by manually adjusting the microscope up or down. The microscope focus scale (if present) is checked to ensure that the focus is at the midpoint or slightly above.
6. The surgeon then uses the foot pedal to achieve fine focus in the up and down axis. The foot pedal is then used to set the desired magnification level, and again to adjust the fine focus.

With some experience, the entire sequence can be completed in a very short time, and the surgeon is ready to start the case.

Maneuvering the Microscope

Proper use of the foot pedal is the key to efficient and smooth use of the microscope. Most surgeons find that they cannot feel the microscope pedal well enough with shoes. Many elect to wear shoes that can be easily kicked off, placing surgical shoe covers over their socks and operating the pedals with their stocking feet. Removing the shoes also lets the knee ride a little lower, which helps in clearing the underside of the surgical table.

Most pedals consist of the same basic elements: a joystick to maneuver the scope in the x-y axes, a rocker switch to control the fine focus, and a rocker switch to control the magnification or zoom (Fig 7-20). Some pedals also offer a switch to turn the illumination on and off. Newer generation foot pedals allow for high levels of surgeon customization, including variable control of the illumination.

An efficient surgery, if properly set up and executed, requires little maneuvering of the microscope with the joystick, because the eye remains well-centered within the microscope's field of view. In fact, technique may be measured to some degree by how little the microscope needs to be adjusted during a case. However, there will inevitably be some

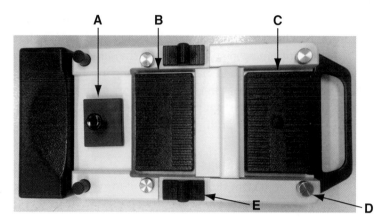

Figure 7-20 Typical microscope foot pedal with **(A)** x-y joystick, **(B)** the fine focus tab, **(C)** the magnification (zoom) tab, **(D)** the illumination on/off switch, and **(E)** independent illumination level control tabs. *(Courtesy of Daniel I. Bettis, MD.)*

maneuvering required, and always some focus and magnification changes during the case. Thus, it is essential that the beginning surgeon learn to smoothly operate the microscope foot pedal.

As mentioned earlier, the foot pedal is usually positioned so that the joystick is away from the surgeon, placing the controls for the focus and zoom under his or her foot. A recommended position involves the surgeon's heel on the magnification tab and the ball of the foot on the focus tab. In this position, each can be controlled with little foot movement, with a toe-down position controlling the focus and a heel-down position controlling the zoom. Slightly extending the leg and manipulating the joystick either with the side of the toes or the ball of the foot controls the joystick. Experience will allow all of these movements with little or no movement of the surgical field or change in hand position. It is recommended that the surgeon always use the same foot, either right or left, to control the microscope pedal, irrespective of the eye undergoing surgery.

Pearls and Pitfalls of Maneuvering the Microscope

The resident surgeon tends to accommodate through the microscope. This can be fatiguing for the new surgeon, and it hinders the senior mentor's ability to maintain focus while looking through the assistant scope (which typically has little independent focusing ability). In the initial setup, it is helpful to focus up with the fine adjustment tab on the foot pedal until the field is just out of focus, and then focus down until the image just comes into focus. This fogging and refocusing limits accommodation through the scope. Because the effect of accommodation is more apparent at high magnification, this maneuver should be performed at high magnification.

Staying in proper focus is also very important. It is common for the beginning surgeon to alter the focus inadequately. This hesitancy usually relates to a lack of comfort with foot pedal manipulation. For example, the surgeon may maintain good focus on the surface of the lens during the initial sculpting step of cataract surgery but fail to focus down into the lens substance when sculpting more deeply. The focus should concentrate on the point of action. Specifically, the phaco tip must be kept in focus. When coming up into the anterior chamber to remove an air bubble, focus must be adjusted upward, and on moving the instrument down to crack the nucleus, focus is readjusted downward.

Maintaining the proper focus during a typical intraocular case requires multiple adjustments with the focusing tab. If the foot is kept on the microscope foot pedal throughout the entire case, it is easier to make the many small focusing adjustments required.

The level of magnification depends on surgeon preference. Lower magnification allows a wider field of view and greater depth of focus, but it may not offer maximum visualization. High magnification, on the other hand, provides excellent tissue visualization but reduces the field of view. Maintaining precise focus is also more demanding at higher magnification. The modern microscope offers such easily adjustable magnification that different levels may be used during the same case. For example, dissection of the scleral flap during a trabeculectomy might best be performed under high magnification because tissue visualization is paramount. Suturing the conjunctival peritomy in the same case might be done with low magnification because a wider field of view might be advantageous during this step. Excessive magnification changes, however, are usually not necessary and can be fatiguing for the surgeon and particularly for the assistant viewing through the side arm.

Finally, control of the microscope light intensity not only helps reduce the risk of retinal phototoxicity, but also helps to ensure patient cooperation throughout the case. It is not necessary to increase the microscope light to the maximal level to perform good surgery. Indeed, excessive illumination can result in corneal reflections that may obscure the surgical view and hinder the ability to perform good surgery.

For topical cataract surgery, the intensity can be set very low to start. One approach involves turning the microscope light completely off and then nudging the dial up until the light just comes back on, using this intensity as the initial lighting level. All steps up to hydrodissection, including capsulorrhexis, can be performed at this low lighting level. Once hydrodissection is complete, the patient will be less photophobic, and the intensity can be turned up, but not much more is needed. For other anterior segment procedures, such as trabeculectomy, the light intensity can be kept low throughout the entire case.

Surgical Loupes

Surgical loupes provide one great advantage over the surgical microscope. With loupes, the surgeon has the flexibility to view the surgical field rapidly from several angles and positions. For example, many oculoplastic and strabismus surgeries require the surgeon to operate from multiple positions during the same case. These procedures are particularly amenable to surgical loupes, and in the oculoplastics and pediatric ophthalmic disciplines, loupes are commonly used. Proper use of surgical loupes requires understanding of the principles of magnification, working distance, and field of view.

Magnification

Surgical loupes provide magnification typically ranging from 2× to 6×. Unlike the surgical microscope, this magnification is fixed. The surgeon must decide on what power of loupes to use based on the intricacy of the surgery to be performed. For most ophthalmic procedures, magnification of at least 2.5× is required; some surgeons recommend at least 3.5×. Higher magnification, however, reduces the field of view, and equally important, the depth of field. For example, a 2× loupe may have a depth of field of 4 inches whereas a 6× loupe may have a depth of field less than 1.5 inches. Higher magnification loupes require the surgeon to keep the head very still in order to maintain focus, because even slight head movement can translate into a blurred image.

Working Distance

The working distance is also set and not adjustable once the loupes are made. It is important therefore to make sure that this variable is correct. Many factors determine the proper working distance for surgeons, including height and simply where they like to work with their hands. At lower magnification levels (2.5× and less) manufacturers typically offer a few different working distances, ranging from about 10 to 20 inches. At higher magnification levels (3.5× and higher) the demands of the optics do not allow such flexibility, and often the manufacturer offers only one working distance.

Field of View

The field of view varies with the magnification level. The field of view can also be changed optically at the same magnification level. For example, manufacturers can provide different fields of view at the 2× magnification level, ranging from around 4 inches to 10 inches. Again, however, at the higher magnification levels, the field of view is usually set. The working distance also affects the field of view. A shorter working distance tends to have a smaller field of view.

Pearls and Pitfalls of Surgical Loupes

The most important lesson to learn while working with surgical loupes is to maintain a constant working distance. It is certainly possible to look away from the surgical field over the loupes, but while performing a particular surgical maneuver, it is important to keep the head still to maintain proper focus. When asking for a surgical instrument, the surgeon should keep his or her eyes focused on the tissues and let the scrub nurse hand over the instrument. Although this is not possible in every instance, it should be common practice.

As with surgery through the microscope, good lighting is essential for surgery performed with loupes. Overhead surgical lights provide good illumination and can be easily adjusted by operating room personnel. Many surgeons who use loupes prefer to wear a headlight, which provides bright and even illumination and is always centered on the desired area. It can be particularly helpful when operating within the orbit or nasal cavity.

Key Points

- Proper patient positioning includes stabilizing the head neither chin-up nor chin-down in the headrest, ensuring that the eye is parallel to the floor and centered in the microscopic field, while supporting the back and legs in a comfortable position.
- Proper surgeon positioning includes ensuring freedom of movement of the legs under the operating table, comfortable access to the microscope foot pedal, and a posture allowing for stabilization of the shoulders and hands.
- The surgeon must be familiar with gross maneuvering of the microscope and centering of its axes; positioning and setting the oculars; adjusting the microscope during the case; and controlling the lighting.
- With surgical loupes, the surgeon has the flexibility to view the surgical field rapidly from several angles and positions. Knowledge of magnification, field of view, and working distance are critical.

Byrnes GA, Antoszyk AN, Mazur DO, Kao TC, Miller SA. Photic maculopathy after extracapsular cataract surgery. A prospective study. *Ophthalmology.* 1992;99(5): 731–737; discussion 737–738.

Gorn RA. Ophthalmic microsurgery: instrumentation, microscopes, technique. *Arch Ophthalmol.* 1987;105(6):759.

Lim AS. Ophthalmic microsurgery: adjustment problems. *Aust N Z J Surg.* 1980;50(4): 335–338.

Macsai MS, Jensen AA, Yang JW. Principles and Basic Techniques for Ocular Microsurgery. In: Duane TD, Tasman W and Jaeger EA eds. *Duane's Ophthalmology on CD-ROM.* Philadelphia: Lippincott Williams & Wilkins, 2006.

[No authors listed.] Operating microscopes in ophthalmic surgery. *Health Devices.* 1988; 17(5):168–169.

Technical manual for the surgeon's specific microscope.

Self-Assessment Test

1. Which of the following steps are included in optimal patient positioning relative to the operating microscope?
   a. ensuring that the corneal surface is parallel to the floor
   b. avoiding the chin-up and chin-down positions
   c. ensuring that the patient's head is fully onto the headrest
   d. all of the above

2. Which of the following are common pitfalls in surgeon positioning? (Choose all that apply.)
   a. surgeon too far away from patient (legs not sufficiently under the table)
   b. table too high
   c. shoulders and elbows too low
   d. pedals poorly positioned

3. Which of the following are included in proper setup of the operating microscope? (Choose all that apply.)
   a. oculars set
   b. the x-y control decentered toward head
   c. microscope manually positioned and grossly focused
   d. fine focus set in down-focused position
   e. foot pedal used for fine focus
   f. foot pedal used to set magnification
4. Which of the following can be said of surgical loupes? (Choose all that apply.)
   a. They provide increased mobility for the surgeon requiring magnification.
   b. Higher magnification loupes also provide increased depth of focus and working distance.
   c. Head movement during surgery increases depth perception with loupes.
   d. A headlight may be worn with loupes to improve focal lighting of the surgical field.

For preferred responses to these questions, see Appendix A.

CHAPTER **8**

Surgical Instruments and Blades

Jay M. Lustbader, MD
Robert B. Dinn, MD

One of the most important aspects of becoming a proficient ophthalmic surgeon is gaining an understanding of the use of the many instruments and blades ophthalmologists employ. Although the number of surgical instruments can initially be quite daunting, being able to identify and use surgical instruments and blades properly is an essential skill. This chapter introduces you to the major categories of instruments and blades.

The choice of instruments is quite individualized, and in time each surgeon develops a favorite tool for performing a given task. Many ways exist for performing the same procedure, and the best way is the one that allows a particular surgeon to accomplish the task with minimal trauma to the tissues. Having a detailed and thorough knowledge of the surgical instruments needed and required in your operating room will help instill confidence in yourself, the operating room personnel, and the patient. Additionally, being well prepared with the names and purposes of the different instruments will aid in efficiency and communication, particularly during stressful times (eg, complications) in the operating room. Although detailed discussion of surgical instrumentation and machinery is beyond the scope of this book, equipment company representatives and other experienced surgeons are valuable sources of information in this area.

Surgical Instruments

Retractors

Retractors are used to help open the eyelids, both in the office and in the operating room. The wide variety of retractors introduced in medical school for general surgery are not discussed here, but a wide variety of modifications exist that are commonly employed in oculoplastic surgery.

Figure 8-1 Desmarres lid retractor. Often used when the lids cannot otherwise be opened (eg, lid edema) or in double everting of the lid to look for foreign bodies. This is a very useful instrument to have available in evaluating trauma and is a vital component of many "on-call bags." Like many of the instruments shown in this chapter, the Desmarres lid retractor comes in different sizes.

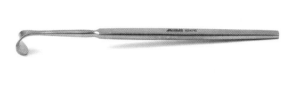

Figure 8-2 Jaffe wire retractor. Pair shown. Used in ruptured globe surgery to avoid applying undue pressure to the globe. Also can be used in many oculoplastic surgeries to retract tissues. Attached to the surgical drapes with a rubber band and a hemostat.

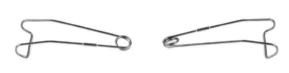

Figure 8-3 Jaeger lid plate. Often used to retract tissues away from the globe in orbital procedures, protect the eye during eyelid procedures, and used to help evert the eyelid. Come in a wide variety of sizes and styles. Available in plastic and stainless steel (malleable). Shown is the Berke-Jaeger lid plate, with stainless steel matte finish. Some lid plates have a special coating to prevent reflection of the CO_2 laser. When coated properly, the Jaeger lid plate can be inserted under the eyelid to protect the globe while making laser incisions into the eyelid.

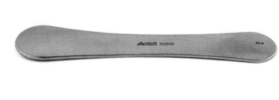

Speculums

Speculums are used to hold the eyelids apart, in order to have better access to the eyeball during a surgical procedure. The main types of eyelid speculums are *rigid* (often with screws for setting a fixed palpebral width) or *wire*. In addition to numerous other indications, wire speculums are most commonly used during phacoemulsification and intravitreal injections. Rigid speculums are useful when wide exposure is necessary (eg, enucleation or strabismus surgery); however, opening the palpebral fissure too far can place extra pressure on the globe, increasing intraocular pressure. Further, care should be taken to avoid undue tension to prevent damage to the eyelids in the form of postoperative ptosis or lid laxity. Many speculums come with an "open loop" that inserts around the lid margin. Similar designs have "guards" that insert around the lid margin to retract the eyelashes as well. The guards have become less useful because of the increased utilization of plastic drapes over the eyelashes during surgery. Eyelid speculums come in pediatric and adult sizes.

Figure 8-4 Barraquer wire. Commonly used in many anterior segment procedures. The traditional Barraquer speculum is designed to be placed with the hinge temporal. The hinge is bent so that it angles away from the eye while in position. This allows greater access to the temporal aspects of the eye. A modification is available where the hinge angles in the opposite direction (ie, anterior), and the speculum is placed with the hinge pointed toward the nose, allowing much greater access to the temporal aspects of the eye. This modification works well for most patients' anatomy but some patients' noses may interfere with the placement of a speculum orientated in this direction.

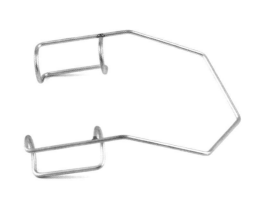

Figure 8-5 Kratz-Barraquer speculum with open blades to allow easy insertion and removal of the phacoemulsification handpiece.

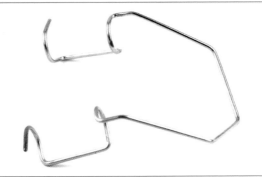

Figure 8-6 Varieties of rigid/screw-type speculums, which can be adjusted to the dimensions of the lid fissure as needed. **A,** Cook. **B,** Lancaster. **C,** Williams. The Cook speculum is useful in patients with a strong blink reflex. Many surgeons like to use this speculum during muscle surgery as the sutures used during strabismus surgery can easily be tangled by other designs of speculums. The example of the Cook speculum in this picture has a guard style (as opposed to the wire loop style pictured for the Barraquer speculum) area for retracting the eyelid, which helps secure the eyelashes out of the sterile field. Both the Lancaster and Williams speculums are useful for patients with strong blink reflexes and can be particularly helpful in cataract surgery in patients when the Barraquer speculum is not adequate or desired.

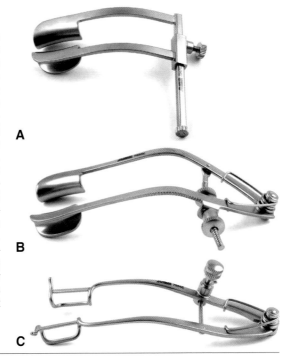

A

B

C

Figure 8-7 McNeill-Goldman scleral fixation ring and blepharostat. Example of a speculum used in corneal transplant surgery. In addition to opening the eyelids, the ring is sutured to the episclera to provide support to the globe after the patient's cornea is removed.

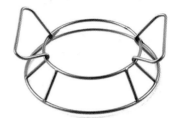

Chalazion Instruments

Clamp and curette are the primary tools used in excising chalazions. The individual shape and size chosen will vary with the size and location of the chalazion. A chalazion clamp is extremely useful as it provides for hemostasis, easy inversion of the eyelid, and stabilization of the eyelid. The clamp can be slowly loosened toward the end of the procedure to make sure adequate hemostasis is achieved. The chalazion clamps are traditionally placed with the open end on the posterior aspect of the eyelid, allowing easy access to the posterior lamella when the eyelid is everted. The chalazion clamp can also be placed with the plate on the posterior eyelid and the open side on the skin; this prevents inadvertent trauma to the globe when incising the skin. Many medical specialties use curettes and these instruments are available in most surgery centers.

Figure 8-8 Chalazion eyelid clamp. The clamp is used to hold the lid and provide some hemostasis around the chalazion. Such clamps include variations in cross action, dimensions, and sizes and shapes of the upper and lower "plates." **A,** Desmarres chalazion forceps with 31 mm solid lower plate, 12 × 20 mm open upper plate. **B,** Lambert chalazion forceps with large, round, solid lower plate, 15-mm open upper plate. **C,** Desmarres chalazion forceps with 20-mm solid lower plate, 12 × 14 mm open upper plate.

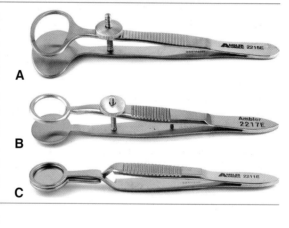

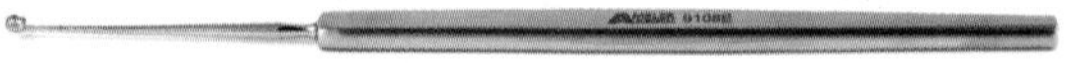

Figure 8-9 Curette used to scoop out the contents of the chalazion; available in sizes of 0 (1.5 mm) to 4 (3.5 mm).

Lacrimal Instruments

This group of instruments is used to locate and clear obstructions of the tear duct. Lacrimal sets may group a dilator to enlarge the punctum, a syringe and a blunt cannula to introduce solution into the duct, and a lacrimal probe to clear the duct. Some surgeons include a sterile safety pin in their lacrimal set to be prepared for any cases of punctal agenesis that may be encountered during a planned nasolacrimal duct intubation in infants; however, a safety pin or needle should be used with extreme caution to open the punctum, as a false passageway can easily be created.

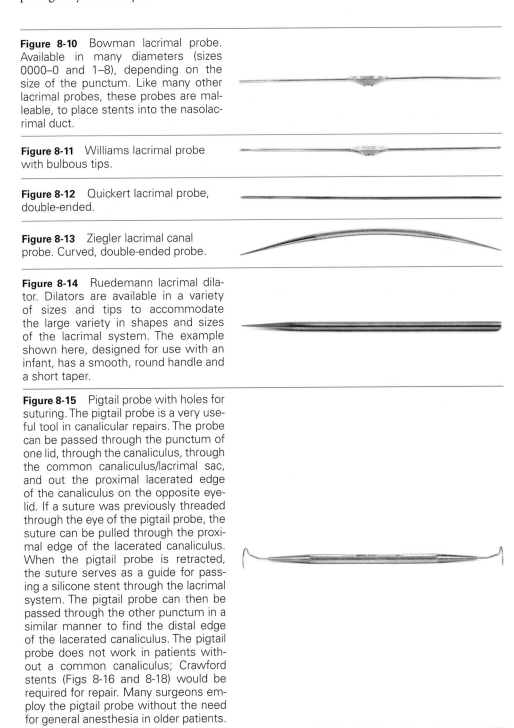

Figure 8-10 Bowman lacrimal probe. Available in many diameters (sizes 0000–0 and 1–8), depending on the size of the punctum. Like many other lacrimal probes, these probes are malleable, to place stents into the nasolacrimal duct.

Figure 8-11 Williams lacrimal probe with bulbous tips.

Figure 8-12 Quickert lacrimal probe, double-ended.

Figure 8-13 Ziegler lacrimal canal probe. Curved, double-ended probe.

Figure 8-14 Ruedemann lacrimal dilator. Dilators are available in a variety of sizes and tips to accommodate the large variety in shapes and sizes of the lacrimal system. The example shown here, designed for use with an infant, has a smooth, round handle and a short taper.

Figure 8-15 Pigtail probe with holes for suturing. The pigtail probe is a very useful tool in canalicular repairs. The probe can be passed through the punctum of one lid, through the canaliculus, through the common canaliculus/lacrimal sac, and out the proximal lacerated edge of the canaliculus on the opposite eyelid. If a suture was previously threaded through the eye of the pigtail probe, the suture can be pulled through the proximal edge of the lacerated canaliculus. When the pigtail probe is retracted, the suture serves as a guide for passing a silicone stent through the lacrimal system. The pigtail probe can then be passed through the other punctum in a similar manner to find the distal edge of the lacerated canaliculus. The pigtail probe does not work in patients without a common canaliculus; Crawford stents (Figs 8-16 and 8-18) would be required for repair. Many surgeons employ the pigtail probe without the need for general anesthesia in older patients.

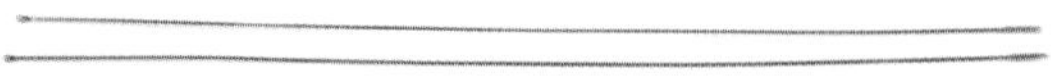

Figure 8-16 Crawford stent (shown without silicone tubing). This instrument is used in cases of nasolacrimal duct or canalicular stenosis/obstruction, trauma repair, reconstruction, and dacryocystorhinostomy (DCR). The Crawford stents have an olive-shaped tip at the end of a metal probe connected by silicone tubing. The olive-shaped tip is passed through the canalicular system of each eyelid down the nasolacrimal duct. The tip of each stent is retrieved from the nasal cavity and the silicone portion of the stent is tied to the other end of the stent, leaving the lacrimal system intubated.

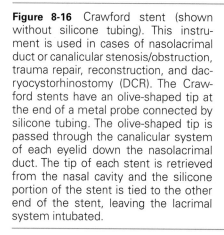

Figure 8-17 Crawford hook. This hook is designed for retrieving the Crawford stent from the nasal cavity.

Figure 8-18 Mono-Crawford stent. This stent is similar to the Crawford stent but does not require intubation of the opposite eyelid. It is used in canalicular laceration repairs and in congenital nasolacrimal duct obstruction. The punctual plug on the end is designed to help in anchoring the stent.

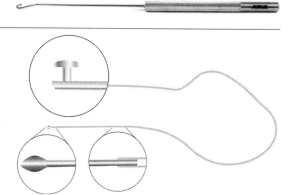

Scissors

A variety of scissors are available for use in ocular surgery. Depending on the surgical purpose, scissors may be blunt or sharp, curved or straight, and may feature either spring or direct action. Straight scissors are often used for cutting sutures and straight lines. Curved scissors are often used for tissue dissection. Notice that the typical scissors used under the microscope are shorter than the scissors used in medical school. This helps in making the instrument steadier in the surgeon's hand and avoids bumping the microscope. Although such scissors may seem awkward at first, ophthalmologists quickly appreciate the steadiness that they feel with Westcott scissors in their hands. Plastic surgery sets often have longer scissors that fit the normal hand better and allow for easier dissection into deeper tissues.

Figure 8-19 Stevens tenotomy scissors. Come in blunt, sharp, curved, and straight. Often used by the surgical assistant to cut sutures.

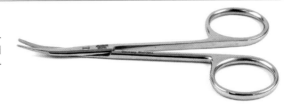

Figure 8-20 Westcott tenotomy scissors with blunt or sharp tips are all-purpose ophthalmic surgery scissors. They are typically curved to facilitate tissue dissection, which is the primary function of these scissors. Note the serrations on the handle that aid in holding the scissors. You will inevitably find a spring-action instrument that has been damaged because the handles were bent too far, making the instrument much less facile to use.

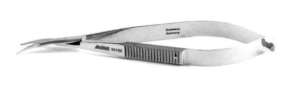

Figure 8-21 Westcott conjunctival scissors. Smaller than tenotomy scissors, also with blunt or sharp tips.

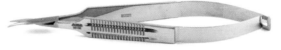

A

B

Figure 8-22 Suture scissors are available in many styles. **A,** Fine, straight stitch scissors. **B,** Jaffe type with flat 3-hole handle. A blunt "stopper" on the inside of spring-action "finger" instruments, visible in this image, prevents the instrument from being closed too tightly and bending the handles. **C,** Needle point with ribbon-style ring handle. **D,** Westcott type with flat handle. **E,** Westcott type with wide, serrated handle.

C

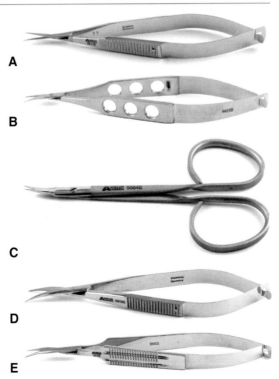

D

E

Figure 8-23 Vannas scissors with sharp pointed tips, available curved or straight. Commonly used scissors for cutting sutures, iris, or fine tissues. Versions with longer tips are helpful for cutting within the eye, but smaller corneal incisions have led many surgeons to use microsurgical scissors and sets (see below) for use in the eye.

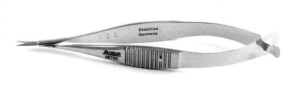

Figure 8-24 Katzin corneal transplant scissors, lower blade of 11 mm, upper blade with left, strong curve. Corneal scissors are more curved than corneoscleral scissors. Corneal scissors are used to cut the corneal button in corneal transplant surgery. Designed to curve to the left or to the right.

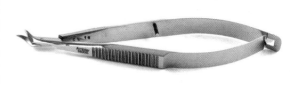

Figure 8-25 Enucleation scissors. Specially designed to reach to the posterior globe to cut the optic nerve during enucleation. This example shows a medium curve; strong and light curves are also available.

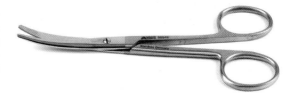

Forceps

Forceps are used for grasping tissues or sutures. Teeth or serrations in forceps help the surgeon grasp ocular tissues to allow suturing, fixation, or dissection. Forceps with serrations in the edges are typically referred to as *smooth forceps* despite the fact that the edges are not really smooth. They are also often referred to as *dressing forceps* because they are still used to apply dressings on wounds. Smooth forceps generally cause more trauma than forceps with teeth because smooth forceps tend to crush tissue. An exception is in handling the conjunctiva during glaucoma surgeries, where forceps with teeth would have a high tendency to leave holes in the conjunctiva. Forceps with teeth are often referred to as *tissue forceps*. These forceps often have 2 teeth on the distal end of one arm and a single tooth on the other arm. You will often find that you are able to use one of the teeth of the forceps to retract tissue delicately in a similar fashion to a skin hook. Tying forceps typically have flat arms and nontoothed tips that aid the surgeon in tying sutures. Some instruments may contain a locking device in the handle.

Figure 8-26 Cilia forceps for removal of aberrant cilia. Available in different angles and types of jaws. The examples shown here have a wide, blunted tip to aid in grouping the cilia. **A,** Barraquer. **B,** Beer. **C,** Douglas. **D,** Ziegler.

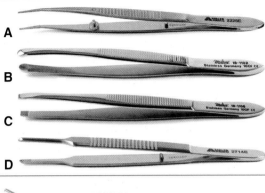

Figure 8-27 Superior rectus forceps are used to grasp the rectus muscles for placement of traction sutures.

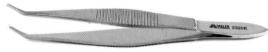

Figure 8-28 Castroviejo suturing forceps, toothed. Available with a tying platform for suture tying. The 0.12-mm (".12") forceps are widely used in a variety of ophthalmic surgeries. They are excellent for grasping and holding fine tissues. The 0.3-mm and 0.5-mm forceps are used when a larger grasp of tissues is needed than is possible with a 0.12-mm forceps.

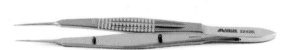

Figure 8-29 Colibri corneal forceps. A 0.12-mm forceps with a curved shaft and tying platform.

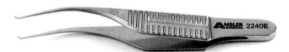

Figure 8-30 Bishop-Harmon forceps. The example shown has serrated tips. Many surgeons prefer serrated tips for handling the delicate conjunctiva, because forceps with teeth can leave holes in the conjunctiva. The Bishop-Harmon style of forceps comes with a variety of tips. Bishop-Harmon forceps with larger teeth (eg, 0.7 mm) are often used in oculoplastic procedures and are generically referred to as "Bishop-Harmons." Manufacturers list Bishop-Harmon forceps based on the style of the handle, not the teeth.

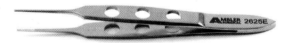

Figure 8-31 Graefe iris forceps. Without teeth, with serrated tips. Smaller version of the standard 0.12-mm forceps, also good for grasping tissue.

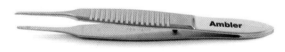

Figure 8-32 Jeweler forceps. Sharp, fine-tipped forceps available in a variety of designs and sizes, beyond the examples shown here. Many comprehensive ophthalmologists find the sharp-pointed jeweler forceps to be the most useful forceps in clinic. They can be used on both the eye and eyelid for removing foreign bodies and sutures. The fine tips allow for corneal debridement of loose epithelium and dendrites. Additionally, the fine, sharp tips can be used to remove a rust ring in lieu of a drill. Office personnel must be careful with the sharp tips to avoid poking themselves and also avoid damaging the tips. Ophthalmologists should take due diligence in informing their staff of the dangers with sharp tips and take appropriate actions to avoid inadvertent trauma to their staff from contaminated instruments left in exposed areas. In addition to their other properties, jeweler forceps tend to be relatively inexpensive. **A,** Straight, strong points. **B,** A variation in width and thickness. **C,** Curved with fine points. **D,** Simple, short, stubby with medium points.

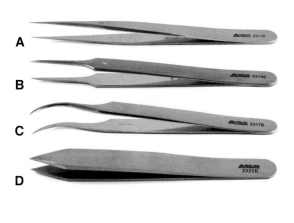

Figure 8-33 McPherson tying forceps. Many styles of tying forceps are available, including straight and angled designs. Some surgeons prefer to tie sutures with a straight tying forceps in one hand and a curved tying forceps in the other hand.

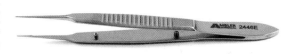

Figure 8-34 Tennant tying forceps. Another example of tying forceps. Round handle with guide pins and platform, for 9-0 to 11-0 sutures.

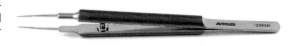

Figure 8-35 Kelman-McPherson angled tying forceps. Angled tying forceps are most commonly used for intraocular manipulations (for example, placing the superior haptic with intraocular lens insertion). They are also useful for grasping intraocular tissues.

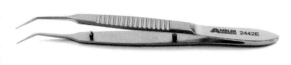

Figure 8-36 Capsulorrhexis forceps. Used to grasp the anterior capsule flap to create the circular curvilinear capsulorrhexis in cataract surgery. The tips can be sharp, cupped, or blunt. Sharp tips can be used to both initiate and complete the capsulorrhexis without the need for a cystotome. This Kraff-Utrata example shows a 3-hole handle and delicate tips. There has been a rapid expansion of styles of capsulorrhexis forceps. Many of the older-style capsulorrhexis forceps are designed for larger wounds and are difficult to fit through some of the smaller cataract wounds used today. If the capsulorrhexis forceps are too large, it is difficult to create an appropriate-sized capsulorrhexis. Several of the newer capsulorrhexis forceps have markings on them to guide the surgeon in making an appropriate-sized capsulorrhexis.

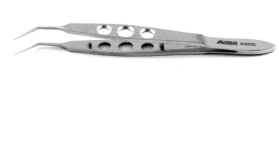

Figure 8-37 Fechtner conjunctival forceps. The tips of these forceps have specially modified tips to prevent damage to conjunctiva while handling the conjunctiva.

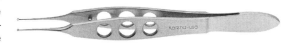

Figure 8-38 Watzke sleeve spreading forceps. These forceps are used during scleral buckling procedures.

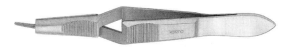

Iris Retractors

Iris retractors are designed to retract the iris during anterior segment or vitreoretinal surgery in cases of trauma, small pupils, or intraoperative floppy iris syndrome. Some are designed to be inserted though corneal wounds to retract the iris during intraocular surgery. Some iris retractors can be used to retract the capsule in cases of zonular weakness; however, modifications are available for retracting the capsule (next section). Iris retractors come in disposable and reusable designs. They are often placed in the Oetting diamond configuration to retract the iris. When using this configuration, it is important to place a single hook just subincisional.

Figure 8-39 Example of iris retractor. Typically, an iris retractor can fit through a tract created with a 27-gauge needle, although a 27-gauge needle usually becomes dull after the second tract is created. Marking the planned locations of the needle tracts prior to creating the tracts is helpful, as the tract created by a 27-gauge needle can be difficult to visualize and find when first learning to do surgery.

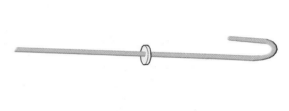

Figure 8-40 Malyugin Ring. Disposable instrument used for retracting the iris during surgery. Comes in a 6.25-mm or 7.0-mm size. Comes with its own inserter.

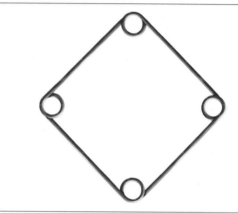

Figure 8-41 Osher/Malyugin Ring manipulator (close-up image plus full view). Reusable instrument designed for manipulation of the Malyugin ring inside the eye. The end of the instrument is similar to other instruments used in cataract surgery with a "mushroom-shaped button."

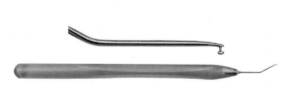

Capsule Support/Retractors

Capsular tension rings are designed to stabilize the capsular bag both during and after surgery. They are made by several companies and come in different sizes. There are modifications available that allow the capsule tension ring to be sutured into position (eg, Cionni capsular ring and Ahmed capsular tension segment). Capsule retractors are designed to support the capsular bag during cataract surgery. There are a few modifications available.

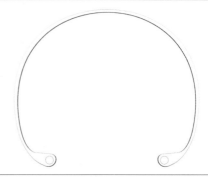

Figure 8-42 Morcher capsular tension ring. The traditional design for a capsule tension ring. Can be injected through an injector, using the Little fishtail technique or the fishtail on a line technique. (See Fig 8-44.)

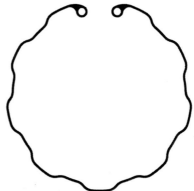

Figure 8-43 Henderson Capsule Tension Ring. Modification of the traditional capsule tension ring. Designed in case the capsule tension ring needs to be inserted prior to cortical cleanup. The indentations allow for easier cortical removal.

Figure 8-44 Geuder Capsule Tension Ring Inserter. Used to insert a capsular tension ring. The injector has a small hook used to capture the eyelet of the capsule tension ring. When tension is brought off the plunger, the ring is loaded into the injector. The injector can be used with one hand to inject the capsule tension ring into the capsular bag, or a second instrument (eg, Sinskey hook) can be used to guide the capsule tension ring in order to minimize trauma to the zonules. Preloaded injectors are also available. An alternative to using a capsule tension ring injector is to use the Little fishtail technique, where forceps are used to gently bend the capsule tension ring into the configuration of a fishtail before inserting the capsule tension ring into the capsular bag. Another alternative is the fishtail on a line technique where a 10-0 nylon suture is threaded through the leading eyelet prior to loading the capsule tension ring in the injector. This technique allows the surgeon to retract the leading eyelet as it is injected into the capsule to prevent undue tension on the capsule.

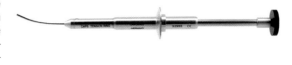

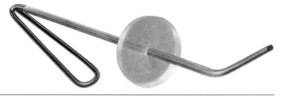

Figure 8-45 MST Capsule Retractor. A temporary capsule retractor designed to provide a broad range of support at its tip.

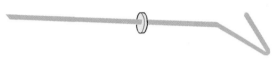

Figure 8-46 Mackool Capsular Retractor. Inserted through the cornea/limbus during cataract surgery for capsular support in cases of weak zonules.

Hooks

Hooks are curved tools used for holding, lifting, or pulling on tissue and intraocular lenses.

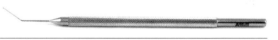

Figure 8-47 Sinskey hook. A small hook used in a variety of applications, including IOL positioning, tissue displacement, corneal marking, and many others. The Sinskey hook can be straight or angled. Modifications of the Sinskey hook are used in creating the flap for endothelial keratoplasties.

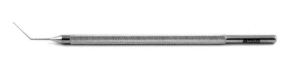

Figure 8-48 Lester IOL manipulator.

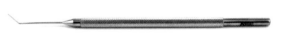

Figure 8-49 Kuglen iris hook (to manipulate the iris) and lens manipulator.

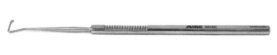

Figure 8-50 Bechert nucleus rotator for phacoemulsification. The y-shaped rotator tip, not obvious in this image, allows the rotator to embed in the nucleus for rotation.

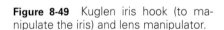

Figure 8-51 Jamison muscle hook used in strabismus surgery. The bulb on the end helps prevent the muscle from slipping off the hook. It also allows the surgeon to inspect the end muscle ensuring the entire muscle is hooked and not "split."

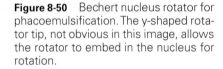

Figure 8-52 Stevens hook used in strabismus surgery. No bulb on the end.

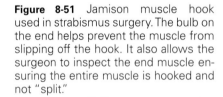

Figure 8-53 Gass retinal detachment hook. Muscle hook with a hole in the end for passing suture around a muscle.

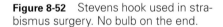

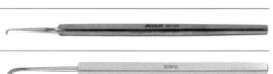

Spatulas

Spatulas are useful in a variety of applications in ophthalmic surgery. They allow gentle, controlled manipulation of tissue.

Figure 8-54 Cyclodialysis spatulas are used primarily to sweep across the anterior chamber, particularly through the anterior chamber angle. Also useful when checking for residual vitreous in the anterior chamber or manipulating the lens nucleus in cataract surgery. The spatula can be flat, as shown in this example (Castroviejo cyclodialysis spatula).

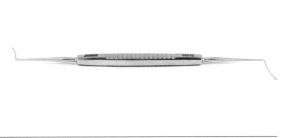

Figure 8-55 Example of a round cyclodialysis spatula, also referred to as an *iris spatula* (Barraquer iris spatula in this example).

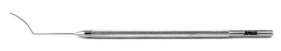

Figure 8-56 Koch phaco spatula. Very useful in rotating and manipulating the lens nucleus in cataract surgery.

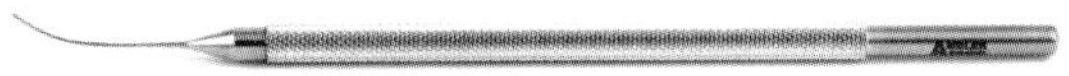

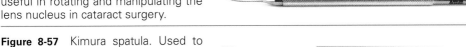

Figure 8-57 Kimura spatula. Used to scrape the cornea when culturing corneal ulcers.

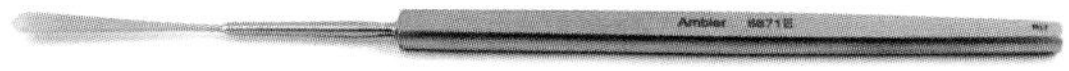

Needle Holders

Needle holders are used to hold the suture needle, which provides the surgeon with more control of the suturing process. In use, the needle holder is often cradled like a pencil. Ophthalmologists tend to prefer spring-action needle holders. Locking needle holders are helpful when handing suture back and forth between the surgeon and the assistant. The surgeon should be very cognizant of the style of needle holder being used prior to placing a suture or handing the suture back. In particular, surgeons typically unlock the needle holder just prior to placing the needle through eye tissues to avoid any inadvertent movement and trauma caused by unlocking the needle holder after the suture is in the tissue. Additionally, the surgeon should be cognizant of the size of the tip of the needle holder, because larger tips bend smaller needles and smaller tips provide for less control over larger needles. Curved tips are often easier to use in delicate ophthalmology procedures.

Figure 8-58 Needle holders for suturing can be straight or curved. Additionally, they can be supplied with or without a lock, to hold the needle in place in the jaws. The example shown here is a curved Barraquer needle holder.

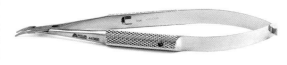

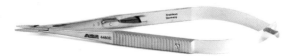

Figure 8-59 Example of a straight needle holder with straight, standard jaws and lock (Castroviejo).

Cannulas

Cannulas are small, tube-like instruments frequently used in ophthalmic surgery to inject or extract fluid or air. Cannulas are used for a variety of purposes, from irrigating the lacrimal system, to hydrodissection, to keeping the cornea wet. The wide variety of available instruments reflects the wide variety of applications. Disposable, single-use cannulas are now widely available and are preferred by many surgeons since reusable cannulas have been implicated in toxic anterior segment syndrome (TASS). The gauge of the cannula affects the force of fluid that is expelled from the tip based on the pressure the surgeon places on the syringe. The smaller tip of a 30-gauge cannula provides a strong force with a small amount of fluid, which is why many surgeons prefer to use a 27- or 25-gauge cannula for hydrodissection. On the other hand, the 25-gauge tip is too large to hydrate the corneal wounds in cataract surgery, making the 30-gauge tip more preferable for this application.

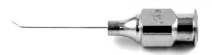

Figure 8-60 Anterior chamber irrigating cannula. Example of Knolle irrigating cannula with 45° angled tip, available in different gauges.

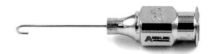

Figure 8-61 J-shaped hydrodissection cannula. Hydrodissection cannulae are available with a variety of tip designs, allowing improved access under the subincisional anterior capsular edge. Subincisional hydrodissection can improve subincisional cortex removal and can also allow the nucleus to prolapse anteriorly during hydrodissection. Additionally, the J-shaped hydrodissection cannula allows for easier removal of subincisional cortex.

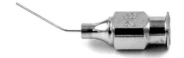

Figure 8-62 Example of a flat-shaped hydrodissection cannula (Seeley).

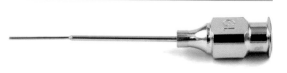

Figure 8-63 Lacrimal cannula. Used to irrigate through the lacrimal system. Available in various gauges and styles of opening. This example is 23-gauge cannula with a front opening.

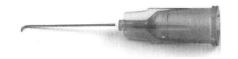

Figure 8-64 Chang Hydrodissection Cannula. This is a dual-purpose instrument that can hydrodissect, including in the subincisional space, and then used to rotate the nucleus.

Nucleus Choppers and Splitters

Nucleus choppers are designed to fragment the lens during nucleus disassembly. Although there is broad overlap, there are 2 main styles of choppers: horizontal and vertical. Horizontal choppers are placed under the capsule between the nucleus and an epinuclear cushion. Utilizing the phacoemulsification tip for stabilization, the horizontal chopper is then brought "horizontally" toward the phaco tip for fragmentation. In contrast, the vertical chopper is placed under the capsular bag after the nucleus is engaged and vacuum is applied with the phaco tip to secure the nucleus. The vertical chopper is then directed posteriorly to crack the nucleus, similar to chopping wood. The "quick" chop (also known as *diagonal chop*) combines elements of horizontal and vertical chopping. Many choppers are double-sided with a horizontal chopper on one side and a vertical chopper on the other. Choppers can be made to suit right-handed or left-handed surgeons. Nucleus splitters are designed to crack the lens. When learning the "divide and conquer" technique, surgeons often find that using a nucleus splitter facilitates cracking after a central groove is created.

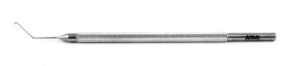

Figure 8-65 Standard phaco chopper. Nucleus choppers are available in several angles (45°, 60°, 90°) and designs. Used in phaco-chop cataract surgery to break the lens nucleus into small pieces.

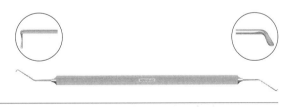

Figure 8-66 Chang-Seibel chopper. Double-armed chopper with the Chang MicroFinger on one end and the Seibel vertical safety chopper on the other end. Styles are available for use in the right or the left hand.

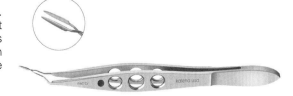

Figure 8-67 Akahoshi prechopper. Designed to split the nucleus without sculpting. When the forceps handles are closed, the tips of the forceps open to split the lens after it is placed inside the nucleus.

Capsule Polishers

Capsule polishers are designed to remove residual debris, plaques, and cells from the capsule. Disposable, single-use capsule polishers are preferred by many surgeons, particularly if the instrument has a tube-like ending (eg, cannula) that can be difficult to clean.

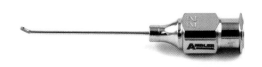

Figure 8-68 Posterior capsule polishers and scrapers come in many designs. Used to remove residual material from the posterior capsule prior to intraocular lens insertion in cataract surgery.

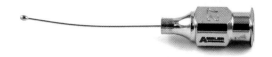

Figure 8-69 Jensen posterior capsule polisher.

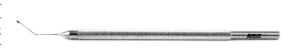

Figure 8-70 Drysdale nucleus manipulator and polisher. Blunt instrument designed to manipulate the lens and crack the nucleus. Can also be used to polish the posterior capsule.

Microsurgical Forceps and Handles

With the advent of smaller-incision intraocular surgery and more complex anterior segment surgery, a wide variety of forceps and scissors have been designed for insertion through small corneal wounds. The basic principles of the instruments previously described apply to these smaller instruments. Several of the forceps that have been developed by various companies allow for different heads to be placed on handles, leading to greater flexibility.

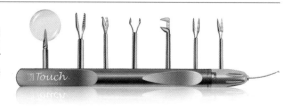

Figure 8-71 MST System. Designed to be inserted through small corneal incisions for intraocular use. The MST system has changeable heads for the handles.

Corneal Markers

Corneal markers have many purposes. Several were originally developed for penetrating keratoplasty to aid in suture placement. Some are now used to leave a circular mark on the cornea to aid in capsulorrhexis creation, centration and sizing, although capsulorrhexis forceps are available with markings to allow for appropriate sizing as well. Others are used in refractive corneal surgery (eg, LASIK) to make sure the corneal flap is repositioned in the exact right place. With the advent of toric intraocular lenses, there has been substantial increase in designs of corneal axis markers.

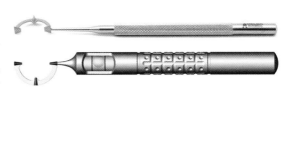

Figure 8-72 Toric reference marker. Used to mark the axis of 0°, 270°, and 360° prior to surgery. The patient is brought to a seated position and the eye is marked with this instrument (usually after the edges have been marked with sterile ink). The instrument has markings on each side so that the same instrument can be used for both eyes. This instrument is designed to avoid off axis placement of a toric intraocular lens since the eye is known to rotate once a patient lies supine. Similar models have "level" markers with air bubbles to make sure the instrument is placed parallel to the ground. Although imaging software is available to serve as reference marks, many surgeons still prefer this method. Care should be taken that the eye is not covered with a viscous substance, gel, or ointment just prior to marking the cornea.

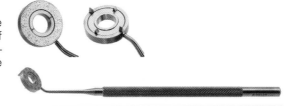

Figure 8-73 Intraoperatve reference marker. Used to mark the axis of planned toric intraocular lens placement after the patient is supine and the eye has been prepped and draped.

Corneal Trephines and Punches

Trephines and punches are instruments used during corneal transplant surgery.

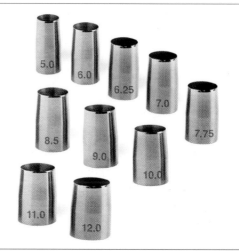

Figure 8-74 Corneal trephines. Blades are used to excise the donor cornea and diseased patient cornea during corneal transplantation.

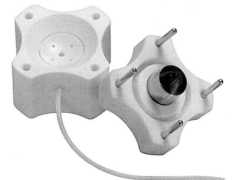

Figure 8-75 Barron vacuum punch. A variant of the standard donor punch in which vacuum is applied to the donor cornea prior to the cutting of the tissue. This provides improved stability and centration.

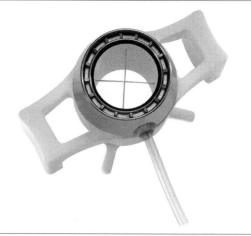

Figure 8-76 Barron radial vacuum trephine. An alternative to the standard handheld corneal trephine. Suction is applied to the patient's cornea, and a rotary blade is gradually applied to the cornea. This device can provide improved centration and control while excising the recipient cornea.

Other Specialized Surgical Instruments

This section includes selected examples of other specialized instruments used in ophthalmic surgery. Discussion of corneal shields, strips, and sponges is beyond the scope of this book. Discussion of some instruments, such as lamellar dissection instruments, is beyond the scope of this chapter.

Figure 8-77 Kelly Descemet membrane punch with serrated squeeze action handle. Used to excise portions of trabecular meshwork during trabeculectomy.

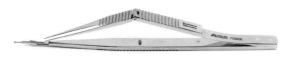

Figure 8-78 Castroviejo caliper. Used in a variety of surgical procedures to measure distances on the eye. This example measures 0–20 mm in 1-mm increments. Fixed "calipers" (more technically called rulers or standards) are available. Some are used in retina surgery to mark for planned sclerotomies. A curved ruler is used in strabismus surgery to more accurately measure distances along the globe (eg, distance from a muscle insertion).

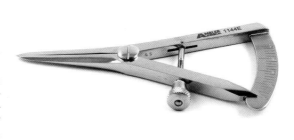

Figure 8-79 Standard lens loop. Lens loops are used to help in removal of the nucleus in extracapsular cataract extraction.

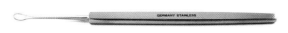

Figure 8-80 Sheets irrigating vectus (another example of a lens loop). Allows irrigation of fluid into the anterior chamber during nucleus extraction.

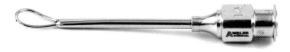

Figure 8-81 Fine-Thornton fixation ring. Used to fixate the globe while making incisions. Fixation rings come in a variety of styles and sizes.

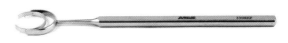

Figure 8-82 Flieringa scleral fixation ring. Sutured to the episclera prior to corneal transplantation in some patients. The ring provides support to the globe before removing the patient's cornea. Most commonly used in aphakic and pseudophakic patients. The ring comes in a variety of sizes.

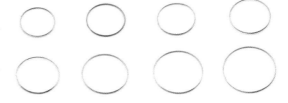

Figure 8-83 Halsted mosquito clamp. Multipurpose clamp. Can be used for securing drapes, for blunt dissection (eg, during a temporal artery biopsy), for passing suture, and so on.

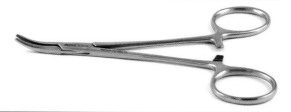

Figure 8-84 Schocket scleral depressor. Used for scleral depression to allow for adequate examination of the peripheral retina. Some scleral depressors can be autoclaved.

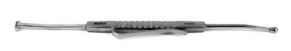

Figure 8-85 Schepens scleral depressor. Thimble-style scleral depressor. Available in different sizes.

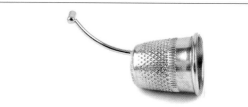

Figure 8-86 Freer periosteal elevator. Used in orbital procedures for elevating the periosteum off bone and for fracturing thin bone. One end is sharp and the other end is blunt.

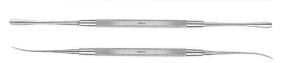

Figure 8-87 Serrefine. Used for clamping sutures. Also known as a "bulldog."

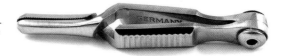

Figure 8-88 Schepens orbital retractor. Commonly used during vitreoretinal surgeries.

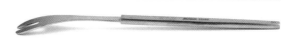

Figure 8-89 Cystotome. Used for creating a capsulorrhexis. Can be made by manually bending a 27- or 25-gauge needle or can be purchased prebent. Available in a variety of shapes and sizes. A cystotome can be inserted onto a syringe filled with balanced salt solution or a viscoelastic material allowing fluid to be inserted into the anterior chamber without removing the cystotome from the eye.

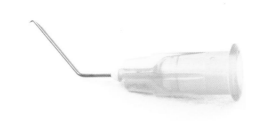

Surgical Blades

Surgical blades are supplied presterilized and are disposable. They either can be supplied preloaded on a handle or inserted into a standard surgical scalpel handle. Blades for standard surgical scalpels are available in various sizes and shapes (Nos. 10–5, Nos. 20–23). Numbers 10 and 15 tend to be the most commonly used in ophthalmology. Blades typically are made of rib-back carbon steel or stainless steel.

Stab Knife Blades

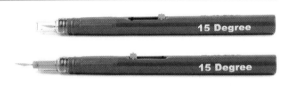

Figure 8-90 A stab knife is used for controlled entry to the anterior chamber for paracentesis and other purposes. A variety of blades and angles are available, including 15° ("supersharp"), 22.5°, 30°, and 45°.

Corneal and Scleral Blades

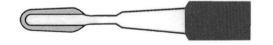

Figure 8-91 Crescent blade. Used for tunneling through the sclera into clear cornea. Straight or angled design.

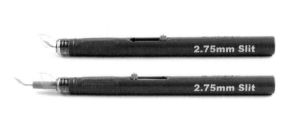

Figure 8-92 Keratome (phaco slit knife). A variety of blade diameters are available depending on the desired incision size for the phacoemulsification procedure. Sharp-tip keratomes (shown) penetrate the cornea easily and provide an optimal fit for the phaco tip. Blunt-tip keratomes are used to enlarge the phaco incision for intraocular lens insertion. This keratome follows the slit blade incision and the cutting edge creates a precise opening for lens insertion.

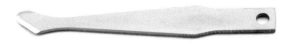

Figure 8-93 Blade No. 57. Also called a *hockey-stick blade* due to its unique shape. Often used for creating scleral flaps.

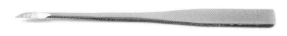

Figure 8-94 Blade No. 59. Also called a *Ziegler knife*. Used to make a precise entry into the anterior chamber through the limbus.

Figure 8-95 Blade No. 64. This blade has both a straight edge and a rounded edge. In addition to creating scleral incisions, also used for scraping the corneal epithelium.

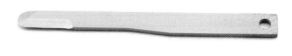

Figure 8-96 Blade No. 66. Available angled or straight. Used to create lamellar dissections of sclera or cornea.

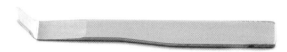

Figure 8-97 Blade No. 69. The blade is curved all the way around. Useful for creating extracapsular cataract incisions, as well as corneal scraping.

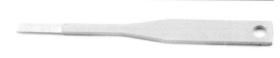

Figure 8-98 Microvitreoretinal (MVR) blade. Also called a *needle knife*. A sharp, diamond-shaped, pointed blade, usually 19 or 20 gauge. Used in vitreous surgery to create the sclerotomies.

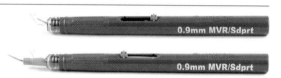

Adjustable Depth Blades

Figure 8-99 Many widths and angles are available. Can be made of steel or diamond. Frequently with depth markings to ease the creation of clear cornea incisions, limbal relaxing incisions, and scleral pockets and tunnels.

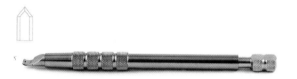

Key Points

- Scissors for microscopic use have specific design characteristics for the type and direction of incision and tissue involved for dissection. Depending on the surgical purpose, scissors may be blunt or sharp, or curved or straight, and may feature either spring or direct action.
- Forceps are used for tissue stabilization and suture tying; they vary in size and tip characteristics depending upon desired function. Teeth or serrations in forceps help grasp ocular tissues. A broad, flat, nontoothed tip aids the surgeon in tying sutures. Some instruments may contain a locking device in the handle.
- Surgical blades vary in size and shape according to tissue dissection and type of incision. They include designs for stab incision, curvilinear incision, and dissection of deep tissue layers.

About the diamond configuration to retract the iris: Oetting TA, Omphroy LC. Modified technique using flexible iris retractors in clear corneal cataract surgery. *J Cataract Refract Surg.* 2002;28(4):596–598.

About the pigtail probe: Graff JM, Allen R. "Canalicular Laceration—Dog Bite." Available at: http://webeye.ophth.uiowa.edu/eyeforum/cases/case26.htm. Accessed November 17, 2014.

About the capsular tension ring: Angunawela RI, Little B. Fish-tail technique for capsular tension ring insertion. *J Cataract Refract Surg.* 2007;33(5):767–769.

About the fishtail on a line technique: Rixen JJ, Oetting TA. Fishtail on a line technique for capsular tension ring insertion. *J Cataract Refract Surg.* 2014;40(7):1068–1070.

Self-Assessment Test

1. Which statement is inaccurate?
   a. It is the surgeon's responsibility to know about the surgical instruments before surgery begins.
   b. Many ophthalmic instruments come in different sizes.
   c. Variations in ophthalmic surgical instruments are often subtle but nonetheless important.
   d. The eyelid speculum that can create the most force in opening the eyelids is often the most appropriate in intraocular surgery for greater exposure.

2. Which forceps is most appropriate for handling the conjunctiva during glaucoma filtering surgery?
   a. 0.12 toothed forceps
   b. smooth forceps
   c. Fechtner forceps
   d. jeweler forceps

3. Which of the following is the LEAST appropriate instrument to sweep vitreous away from an incision?
   a. cyclodialysis spatula
   b. Barraquer spatula
   c. Kimura spatula
   d. Castroviejo spatula

4. Which ring is appropriate to use for fixation when making a clear corneal temporal incision for cataract surgery?
   a. Fine Thornton Ring
   b. Malyugin Ring
   c. Flieringa Ring
   d. McNeill-Goldman Ring

5. Which of the following is not typically a single-use instrument?
   a. keratome
   b. capsule tension ring
   c. cystotome
   d. mosquito clamp

For preferred responses to these questions, see Appendix A.

The Academy appreciates the contributions of the following companies that supplied photographs for this edition. Their websites contain wide-ranging collections of product images for further study, including close-ups of tips and edges. For complete figure credits, please refer to the acknowledgments after the Preface.

Ambler Surgical: www.amblersurgical.com
Asico: www.asico.com
FCI Ophthalmics: www.fci-ophthalmics.com
Katena Eye Instruments: www.katena.com
MST: www.microsurgical.com
Wilson Ophthalmic: www.wilsonopthalmic.com

CHAPTER **9**

Suture Materials and Needles

Jennifer Lee, MD
Keith D. Carter, MD

Surgical techniques for reapproximation of skin edges and support of wounds vary widely; the broad array of suture material allows ophthalmic surgeons individual preferences in ocular surgery. This chapter introduces the characteristics of suture and needle construction that the beginning surgeon must understand in order to minimize tissue damage and maximize wound support. (Chapter 15 reviews the mechanics of proper knot tying and suturing.)

Characteristics of Sutures

An ideal suture should have ease of handling, correct tensile strength, minimal tissue reactivity, and minimal promotion of bacterial infection. The surgeon must select a suture material with the characteristics that are most appropriate for the cutaneous or ocular wound.

The following definitions are helpful in understanding characteristics of sutures.

- *Suture-size nomenclature.* A number followed by a dash and a zero describes suture size. In ophthalmology, you will probably use sutures between 2-0 and 10-0. A smaller number indicates a larger suture. The size of the suture affects the tensile strength.
- *Handling.* The ease of manipulating and tying a suture.
- *Coefficient of friction.* The force required to move 2 sliding surfaces over each other, divided by the force holding them together. It is reduced once the motion has started.
- *Tensile strength.* The amount of force required to break a suture divided by its cross-sectional area. It is a specific feature of the suture composition itself. Strength of the suture also depends on its size; for example, a 6-0 suture is typically more resistant to breakage than a 10-0 suture.
- *Tissue reactivity.* The amount of inflammatory response evoked by the presence of suture material.

Classification of Sutures

Sutures are classified by the kind of material from which they are made (natural, synthetic, metallic), their internal structure (monofilament versus multifilament), whether or not they are absorbable, and their diameter.

Material

Suture is composed of natural fibers (silk or gut), synthetic material (nylon, polyglycolic acid, polypropylene), or stainless steel. Selection of suture material involves consideration of absorbability, tensile strength, and handling needs for the situation. No suture is ideal from all standpoints; therefore, the choice of suture material remains the surgeon's preference.

Internal Structure

Monofilament sutures are made of a single strand of material, while multifilament sutures involve braided strands of single filaments. Monofilament suture causes less scarring and tissue reaction. It is easier to remove and has less tissue drag. With monofilament sutures, a 3-1-1 tying sequence is used for throws (a *throw* is the tying down of one or more loops. (See Chapter 15 for techniques of wound closure.) The number of throws used also depends on the memory of the material. Polypropylene (Prolene) is very resilient to being deformed and sometimes requires a 3-1-1-1 sequence as opposed to nylon that may be tied with a 2-1-1 sequence. Braided suture is easier to manipulate, has higher tensile strength, and maintains tension on a wound after the first throw. With braided sutures, a 2-1-1 or 1-1-1 sequence can be used. Silk sutures are braided and are considered the easiest to handle and tie because the suture deforms exceptionally well.

Absorbability

Absorbable sutures degrade by an enzymatic process or hydrolysis by tissue fluid, occurring from 5 days to 3 months. Common absorbable sutures include gut, chromic gut (treated with a chromic salt to increase its resistance to absorption), synthetic polyester (Biosyn), polyglactin (Vicryl), and polyglycolic acid (Dexon). Absorbable sutures cannot be used where extended approximation of tissue is required. These sutures absorb more quickly in areas of infection and inflammation. They should be used with caution in patients suffering from conditions that may cause delayed wound healing. All absorbable sutures cause a slight foreign body response that causes the gradual loss of tensile strength and suture mass as the enzymatic process dissolves the suture until it is completely gone. This process can cause increased scarring.

Nonabsorbable sutures allow for extended approximation of tissues. Common nonabsorbable sutures are nylon (Surgilon, Monosof, Dermalon), polyester (TiCron, Mersilene), polypropylene (Prolene), silk (Sofsilk), and stainless steel. Nonabsorbable sutures elicit a minimal acute inflammatory reaction that is followed by a gradual encapsulation of the suture by fibrous connective tissue. Some nonabsorbable sutures, such as polypropylene, can remain indefinitely in a deep closure. However, they must be removed if used on the skin.

Absorbable suture material

There are 4 types of absorbable suture material: gut/chromic, polyglactin and polyglycolic acid (Vicryl/Dexon), glycolide/lactide polyester (Polysorb), and polydioxanone and polydioxanone/glycolide/trimethylene carbonate (PDS II/Biosyn). Table 9-1 summarizes each category.

Table 9-1 Examples of Absorbable Sutures

Type	Primary Material	Filament Type	Tensile Strength	Wound Support	Complete Absorption	Comments
Natural						
Gut; gut chromic	Collagen	Monofilament	Poor at 7–23 days	4–8 days	Variable	Absorbs more rapidly in inflamed or infected tissue
Synthetic						
Vicryl, Dexon	Polyglactin; polyglycolic acid	Multifilament	75% at 14 days, 5% at 30 days	7–10 days	60–90 days	Less tissue reaction than gut
Polysorb	Glycolide/lactide polyester	Multifilament	70% at 14 days, 55% at 21 days	15–20 days	56–70 days	—
PDS II; Biosyn	Polydioxanone; polydioxanone/glycolide/ trimethylene carbonate	Monofilament	70% at 14 days, 25% at 42 days	15–20 days	90–110 days	May need additional throws

Gut suture is composed of strands of collagenous material prepared from the submucosal layer of the small intestine of healthy sheep or from the seromucosal layer of the small intestine of healthy cattle. It is packaged in a solution of isopropanol, water, and triethanolamine. The suture dries out quickly and becomes stiffer and more difficult to handle; therefore, gut should be opened immediately before usage. Chromic gut is treated with chromic salt solution, which allows maintenance of its tensile strength for a longer time. Care should be taken to avoid crushing or crimping this relatively fragile suture material. Gut is useful in situations where tissues need to be approximated for 4–8 days. It is not useful in the closure of sites subject to expansion, stretching, or distention unless other sutures are used deeper in the tissue for structural support. This suture should be avoided in patients with sensitivity to collagen or chromium.

There are many synthetic absorbable polyester and polyglycolic acid ophthalmic sutures, the most common of which are outlined in Table 9-1 in order of fastest absorption to slowest absorption. Vicryl (polyglactin 910) and Dexon (glycolic acid) are braided sutures with similar absorption properties. They elicit lower tissue reaction than gut suture. These sutures offer wound support for 7–10 days. Absorption is complete in 60–90 days. Skin sutures may cause localized irritation after 7 days. Polysorb (glycolide/lactide polyester) is a braided suture and offers wound support for 15–20 days. Absorption is complete in 56–70 days. PDS II (polydioxanone) and Biosyn (glycolide, dioxanone, trimethylene carbonate) are monofilament sutures and are similar in absorption properties. They offer wound support for 15–20 days and are completely absorbed by 90–110 days. Additional throws may be necessary for these monofilament sutures.

Nonabsorbable sutures

There are 5 types of nonabsorbable sutures: silk, Prolene/Surgipro, nylon, TiCron/Mersilene, and stainless steel. Table 9-2 summarizes each category.

Silk suture (Sofsilk, Perma-Hand) is considered the gold standard for handling and is made from natural proteinaceous silk fibers called *fibroin*. The material is derived from the domesticated silkworm species *Bombyx mori*. Silk suture is braided and coated with a wax

Table 9-2 Examples of Nonabsorbable Sutures

Type	Primary Material	Filament Type	Tensile Strength	Degradation	Comments
Natural					
Sofsilk, Perma-Hand	Fibroin	Multi	None in 365 days	Some	Gold standard for handling
Stainless steel	Stainless steel	Mono or multi	Permanent	None	Telecanthus repair
Synthetic					
Prolene, Surgipro	Polypropylene	Mono	Permanent	None	Resists involvement in infection
Nylon (many brands)	Nylon	Mono or multi	20% per year	Some	
TiCron, Mersilene	Polyethylene terephthalate	Multi	Permanent	None	

mixture to reduce capillarity and increase the ease of passage through tissue. Silk sutures are not absorbed, but progressive degradation of the proteinaceous fiber may cause a very gradual loss of the suture's tensile strength over time. This suture enhances bacterial infectivity.

Polypropylene (Surgipro, Prolene) is a monofilament suture with no change in tensile strength over time. This suture resists involvement in infection and has been successfully employed in contaminated and infected wounds to eliminate or minimize later fistula formation and suture extrusion. The lack of adherence to tissue has facilitated the use of polypropylene suture as a pull-out suture. This material does not deform easily and may require extra throws to avoid knot slippage.

Nylon sutures are available in both monofilament (Monosof, Dermalon, Ethilon) and braided (Surgilon, Nurolon) forms. The braided suture is coated with silicone to increase the ease of passage through tissue and to reduce capillarity. This suture is not absorbed, but progressive hydrolysis of the suture may result in gradual loss of tensile strength over time. Nylon has easier handling than polypropylene, but may still require an extra throw with the monofilament version.

Polyester suture composed of polyethylene terephthalate (TiCron, Mersilene) is a braided suture that is not absorbed and does not degrade over time. It has a higher coefficient of friction and maintains tension on a wound after the first throw.

Stainless steel suture is composed of 316L stainless steel, a type of molybdenum-bearing steel that is more resistant to corrosion than the conventional chromium-nickel stainless. Stainless steel suture is available in both monofilament and multifilament forms. This type of suture offers extremely high tensile strength and is used for telecanthus repair.

Suture Size

The diameter of sutures may range from thread-like to microscopically thin: the larger the suture, the smaller the number that is assigned to it. Tables 9-3 and 9-4 list the sizes of sutures commonly used for extraocular and intraocular surgery.

Needles

Suture needles are classified by 2 primary characteristics: curvature and shape (Figs 9-1 and 9-2). Shapes include 1/8 circle (45°), 1/4 circle (90°), 3/8 circle (135°), 1/2 circle (180°), 5/8 circle (225°), bi-curve, compound curve, and straight. Different diameters are available, usually selected to match the diameter of the suture material being used. The 3/8 needle is used most commonly. The 1/2 needle is useful in tight spaces. Straight needles are used in the anterior chamber to suture without disturbing the lens.

Points are classified as either taper or cutting. Cutting needles can be conventional cutting, reverse cutting, or spatula. The needle point determines how easily sutures are passed through tissue. Taper points push through tissue. In ophthalmology, these needles are usually labeled "BV" for blood vessel repair and are used primarily for delicate tissue (eg, the conjunctiva in a trabeculectomy procedure, in which the seal around each suture pass is essential to prevent leaking). Cutting needles are more commonly used; their cutting action facilitates the needle penetration of tissue. Reverse cutting needles are the most versatile and cut on the outside curve of the needle. Conventional cutting needles cut on

Table 9-3 **Examples of Sutures for Extraocular Surgery**

Suture Size	Type and Use
2-0	2-0 polyglactin (Vicryl): strong stitch to use as deep anchoring sutures on cheek flaps
3-0	3-0 expanded polytetrafluoroethylene (Gore-Tex CV-3): for indirect browplasty
	3-0 silk: to loop the rectus muscles in scleral buckle surgery
	3-0 polyglactin: strong stitch to use as deep anchoring sutures on cheek flaps or for subcutaneous closure of forehead and scalp
4-0	4-0 silk: reverse cutting needle for traction sutures
	4-0 silk: taper needle for bridle sutures under extraocular muscles
	4-0 polyglactin: short half-circle reverse cutting needle, especially useful for lateral tarsal strip
	4-0 polyglactin: long reverse cutting needle for thicker subcutaneous closure or as an anchoring suture
	4-0 polyglactin: used on a P-2 needle for tight areas like lateral canthus during eyelid tightening
	4-0 chromic: for Quickert suture and suturing oral mucosa
	4-0 chromic: short half-circle needle useful for suturing the flaps for external dacryocystorhinostomy
	4-0 polyester fiber (Mersilene): S-2 1/2-circle needle for eyelid tightening
5-0	5-0 nylon: for brow skin closure
	5-0 polypropylene (Prolene): blue color especially useful for repair of lacerations in the brow hairs
	5-0 polyglactin: for subcutaneous and orbicularis muscle closure
	5-0 chromic: for medial spindle operation used double armed, Quickert sutures (entropion)
	5-0 fast-absorbing gut: for skin closure
	5-0 polyester (Dacron): for scleral buckle attachment to the sclera, superior oblique tuck, or posterior
	5-0 fast-absorbing gut: for skin closure
	5-0 polyester: for scleral buckle attachment to the sclera, superior oblique tuck, or posterior fixation sutures in strabismus
6-0	6-0 polyglactin: double armed for tarsal fracture operation and Jones tube anchoring suture
	6-0 nylon: for skin closure of eyelid and periocular skin and to intubate and tie stent used with pigtail probe for repair of canalicular lacerations
	6-0 fast-absorbing plain gut: for conjunctival closure and for skin closure (blepharoplasty)
	6-0 polypropylene: used with P-1 needle for skin closure
7-0	7-0 polyglactin: for closure of conjunctiva and skin

Table 9-4 **Examples of Sutures for Intraocular Surgery**

Suture Size	Type and Use
4-0	4-0 silk: traction suture that can be passed under muscles and through the lids
5-0	5-0 polyglactin: suture on a spatula needle for strabismus surgery used double armed to pass a locking stitch through the muscles and one-half thickness through the sclera
7-0	7-0 polyglactin: suture for traction through the cornea
8-0	8-0 polyglactin: on a taper-point BV needle (Ethicon) for the conjunctival wound in a trabeculectomy
	8-0 silk: used for scleral closure in open globes
9-0	9-0 polypropylene (Prolene): iridodialysis repair with a straight or large curved needle
	9-0 nylon: used for scleral closure near the limbus
	9-0 polyglactin: suture on a BV needle for bleb revision or conjunctival defects
10-0	10-0 nylon: closure of cornea and flap of trabeculectomy. Must be a dark color in order to identify the suture for postoperative laser suture lysis
	10-0 polypropylene: iris or scleral fixation suture of intraocular lens

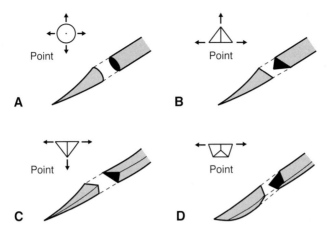

Figure 9-1 Four basic shapes of needle points used in ocular surgery. **A,** Taper point. A cone-shaped single point on a round shaft; used for delicate tissues. **B,** Cutting. A triangular point with 2-sided cutting edges and an upper cutting edge; largely replaced by the reverse-cutting needle. **C,** Reverse cutting. A triangular point with 2-sided cutting edges and a lower cutting edge; used for resistant tissue. **D,** Spatula. A rhomboid-shaped point with 2-sided cutting edges; used in the cornea and the sclera where the plane of penetration must be precise. *(Reprinted, with permission, from Newmark E,* Ophthalmic Medical Assisting: An Independent Study Course, *5th ed. San Francisco: American Academy of Ophthalmology; 2012.)*

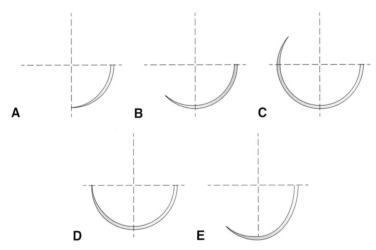

Figure 9-2 Basic shapes of curvature of needles used in ocular surgery. **A,** 1/4 circle. **B,** 3/8 circle. **C,** 5/8 circle. **D,** 1/2 circle. **E,** Compound curve. *(Illustration by Mark M. Miller.)*

the inside curve and can create a bigger hole as the needle tends to move superiorly out of the wound. Spatula needles facilitate lamellar passes. They are commonly used in scleral buckle surgery or strabismus surgery; the flat bottom surface facilitates partial thickness passes through the thin sclera without penetrating the interior scleral wall.

When suturing, always grasp the needle one-third of the way from the suture end in order to avoid damaging the functional integrity of the needle or dulling the cutting surfaces. When handling 7-0 size suture or smaller, always grasp the suture to pull it through the tissue rather than the needle, as you can easily snap the needle off the end of the suture.

Key Points

- Suture material is classified by composition, internal structure, absorbability, and size.
- Common nonabsorbable sutures include silk, nylon, and polypropylene.
- Common absorbable sutures include gut/chromic, polyglactin (Vicryl)/glycolic acid (Dexon), and glycolide/lactide (Polysorb).
- Surgical needles are classified by shape, size, and point.

Covidien. "Wound Closure Materials and Accessories." http://surgical.covidien.com/products /wound-closure. Accessed October 10, 2014.

Ethicon. "Sutures: By Needle Type." Features a printable true-to-scale needle template and includes needle numbers such as P-2. www.ecatalog.ethicon.com/sutures-by-needle-type. Accessed October 10, 2014.

Ethicon. "Wound Closure Overview." www.ethicon.com/healthcare-professionals/products /wound-closure. Accessed October 10, 2014.

Lutchman CR, Leung LH, Moineddin R, Chew HF. Comparison of tensile strength of slip knots with that of 3-1-1 knots using 10-0 nylon sutures. *Cornea*. 2014;33(4):414–418.

Self-Assessment Test

1. What are the advantages of monofilament suture?
   a. less tissue reaction and scarring
   b. slower passage through tissue
   c. requires fewer throws for stability in knots
   d. rapidly absorbed
2. Which of the following is an absorbable suture?
   a. silk
   b. nylon
   c. polyethylene (Prolene)
   d. polyglactin (Vicryl)
3. Which best describes one of the properties of polyglactin (Vicryl) and glycolic acid (Dexon)?
   a. This suture material maintains tissue support for 7–10 days.
   b. This suture material incites a greater tissue reaction than gut suture.
   c. This suture material is absorbed in 30–60 days.
   d. This is a monofilament suture.
4. Which statement best describes spatula needles?
   a. They are flat needles.
   b. They are useful for vascular repair.
   c. They facilitate lamellar passes in tissue.
   d. They are commonly used in multilayered skin repair.

For preferred responses to these questions, see Appendix A.

CHAPTER 10

Lasers

Jonathan D. Walker, MD

This chapter discusses the fundamental principles of laser surgery, with an emphasis on the approach to retinal photocoagulation. For guidelines regarding specific treatments, such as panretinal photocoagulation or posterior capsulotomy, please see the companion volume, *Basic Techniques of Ophthalmic Surgery.*

Laser Physics

Laser stands for **L**ight **A**mplification by **S**timulated **E**mission of **R**adiation—an acronym that is remarkably self-explanatory. Recall that electrons orbiting the atomic nucleus prefer to be at the lowest energy level possible. When they drop to a lower orbital, they give off photons. The energy of the photon is precisely determined by the difference in energy between the higher orbital and the lower orbital, and the orbitals are in turn determined by the atom in which the electron resides. Electrons can also be bumped up to a higher orbital if they absorb a photon having the energy that matches the difference between the lower and upper orbitals. If a bunch of electrons are bumped up to a given orbital—a process referred to as *pumping*—and then are encouraged to drop back down to a specific lower level under special circumstances, the result is laser light.

Making this happen involves the Stimulated Emission part of the acronym. If a photon happens to have the same energy as the difference between the higher orbit and the next-lowest orbit, and if the photon happens to pass by one of these pumped-up electrons—without hitting it—the photon will stimulate the electron to drop into the lower orbit and produce a second photon that is coherent (meaning the peaks and troughs of the waves of both photons occur at the same time). This rather amazing property allows for the production of laser light from a host of stimulated electrons. Furthermore, a given photon can stimulate any number of electrons as it passes, and each photon released will in turn stimulate even more photons (the Light Amplification part of laser).

In ion gas lasers of the past, a gas such as argon or krypton was used as the laser medium to provide the high-energy electrons population. Excimer (excited dimer) lasers use a combination of argon and fluorine gas, and electrical energy is used to stimulate the argon to form high-energy dimers with fluorine. With the exception of excimer lasers (and CO_2 laser used on skin), typical modern ophthalmic solid state and semiconductor lasers generate coherent light from a light-emitting diode; such lasers tend to be much smaller and more efficient than gas lasers. Stimulated emission occurs at the junction of the diode, and the diode itself is sandwiched between mirrors, with a fully reflective mirror at one end and a partially reflective mirror at the other. The photons bounce back and forth, which ensures that as many electrons as possible are stimulated to drop to a lower orbit and release a photon. The photons escaping through the partially reflective mirror produce the laser output beam.

Lasers used to treat retinal diseases are known as "continuous wave" or CW lasers because their output beam is generated in a continuous fashion. The user sets the duration of the beam exposure, and the power output is titrated for a gradual, controlled response in the target tissue. This is in contrast to the "pulsed" lasers that are also used in ophthalmology—such as the excimer laser and the neodymium:yttrium-aluminum-garnet laser (Nd:YAG). These types of lasers concentrate all of their energy output into a very brief period. Because the energy is the power per unit of time, a laser pulse released in a very short time can have a very high peak power, which can reach an extremely high power density (irradiance) in the target tissue and can essentially cause bubble formation and be explosive, as described later in this chapter.

The frequency and correlated wavelength (λ) of the light generated by a laser depend on the substance being used as the lasing medium. If the frequency produced is not ideal for the chosen application, it can be changed by using either harmonic generation or organic dyes. An organic dye laser can produce a spectrum of tunable wavelengths, but such lasers are rather inefficient—a lot of energy is required from the primary "pumping" laser to excite and lase the organic dye fluorescence spectrum in the dye laser cavity and produce a modest tunable wavelength output power.

Harmonic generation is a far more common technique for changing a laser's fundamental frequency. In this case, the laser light is passed through a special crystal that will vibrate at the laser's frequency and generate harmonics that are multiples of the laser's frequency. Such crystals are commonly used to double the frequency of the output of an Nd:YAG laser in order to halve its fundamental infrared wavelength into a visible green beam (ie, from 1064–532 nm). A typical diode-laser-pumped, frequency-doubled Nd:YAG green laser generates light in this fashion.

Laser/Tissue Interactions

There are 3 main types of tissue interactions, depending on the nature of the laser: *photodisruption, photocoagulation,* and *photoablation.* These categories are a bit arbitrary because they are really part of a spectrum of tissues' photothermal responses to laser energy. It is convenient, though, to use these terms to distinguish the tissue effects of the different types of ophthalmic lasers.

Photodisruption

Photodisruption occurs when performing peripheral iridectomy or capsulotomy with Q-switched Nd:YAG lasers. This is more of a mechanical effect that results from tightly focused, high-power laser light, which produces an explosively expanding vapor bubble of ionized plasma. This bubble then quickly collapses, producing acoustic shockwaves that ablate the tissue being treated. A variation of this is the femtosecond Nd:YAG laser, which uses a much shorter time interval to deliver the laser energy compared to typical anterior segment Nd:YAG lasers. This allows for very controlled photodisruption of tissue, which is useful for creating corneal stromal flaps in LASIK surgery. The femtosecond laser is also being used more and more in cataract surgery. When coupled with image guidance systems using high-resolution anterior segment OCT, the laser can create very precise corneal incisions and capsulotomies. It can even be used to create cuts in the crystalline lens to make phacoemulsification easier (Fig 10-1).

Photocoagulation

Photocoagulation is widely used for traditional retinal laser treatments. In this case the laser literally cooks the tissue at a microscopic level. Specifically, chromophores such as melanin in the retinal pigment epithelium (RPE) cells absorb the laser energy and convert it into heat. As the heat spreads to equilibrate with surrounding cooler tissue, it raises the temperature in the outer and inner retina, producing coagulation of proteins that results in loss of the natural transparency of the retina. This starts backscattering the slit-lamp light, showing the intended grayish-white burn endpoint, a change typically associated with thermal elevations of 20°–30°C above baseline body temperature. The burn then induces scar formation that in turn creates the desired clinical effect. The degree of scarring required depends on the disease being treated, ranging from very mild applications to treat macular edema to hotter burns designed to control proliferative retinopathy or to increase retinal adhesion around a retinal tear. Because traditional retinal photocoagulation results in some degree of damage, it is incumbent on the treating physician to optimize the laser settings to minimize potential short- and long-term complications from excessive treatment. Fig 10-2 shows an example of how heat spreads up into the retina from the pigmented regions of the RPE and choroid. Fig 10-3 is a series showing retinal photocoagulation burns of different intensities.

Photoablation

Photoablation is the third form of laser tissue interaction. Photoablation refers to the use of laser energy to ablate or break chemical bonds. The excimer laser used for corneal refractive surgery generates a wavelength of 193 nm (in the ultraviolet range) to break chemical bonds, which allows very precise removal of corneal tissue with only minimal damage to the surrounding structures.

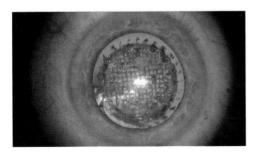

Figure 10-1 An example of treatment with femtosecond laser prior to cataract surgery. A matrix fragmentation pattern is present within the crystalline lens (along with cavitation bubbles). *(Courtesy of Alcon.)*

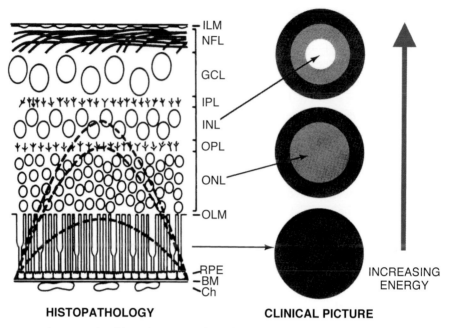

HISTOPATHOLOGY   CLINICAL PICTURE

Figure 10-2 An example of how heat spreads up into the retina from the pigmented regions of the RPE and choroid. As the energy is increased, the damage extends higher and higher into the retina. When more of the retina is damaged the clinical appearance of the laser spot becomes whiter as the involved tissue loses its transparency and scatters more light. Ch, choroid; BM, Bruch's membrane; RPE, retinal pigment epithelium; OLM, outer limiting membrane; ONL, outer nuclear layer; OPL, outer plexiform layer; INL, inner nuclear layer; IPL, inner plexiform layer; GCL, ganglion cell layer; NFL, nerve fiber layer; ILM, inner limiting membrane. *(Modified from Weingest, T, et al, Laser Surgery in Ophthalmology: Practical Applications, Copyright © 1992;17, with permission of the McGraw-Hill Companies.)*

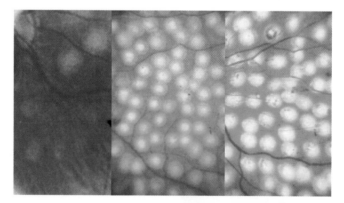

Figure 10-3 A series showing retinal photocoagulation burns of different intensities. The left image shows very mild burns with only light graying of the retina—the lower burns are very light and the ones at the top of the image are more powerful. This is the type of treatment often used for macular edema. The middle image shows burns that are typical for that used for panretinal photocoagulation. There is more whitening in the center and choroidal details are not seen beneath the opacified retina. Note that even with a standard power and spot size there is variable uptake as indicated by the different amount of whitening at the center of each burn. The image on the right shows much heavier burns that are almost entirely white. These burns are too hot for most treatment indications. *(Courtesy of Ingolf H.L. Wallow, MD.)*

For completeness, there is a fourth tissue interaction—photochemical—wherein a very low-power laser is used to activate a specific chemical to obtain the desired effect in the tissue. In this case the laser has no direct effect on the tissue itself; the clinical response depends on the chemical being activated. The use of a red laser to activate verteporfin (Visudyne) in order to treat neovascular age-related macular degeneration is the best example of this in ophthalmology.

Wavelength

The wavelength of the laser is a very important factor for safe and effective treatment. Fig 10-4 shows how certain ocular chromophores absorb various wavelengths. For example, there is a marked drop-off in hemoglobin uptake and a gradual drop-off in melanin uptake as the wavelength increases, moving into the red and infrared end of the spectrum. This explains in part why red and infrared burns require more power and tend to penetrate deeper through the RPE into the more pigmented choroid. When using an infrared laser for retinal treatment, it is important to become familiar with the difference in absorbance in order to avoid complications—do not assume techniques that work for a green laser can be directly applied to an infrared laser.

A more subtle difference in treatment effect is felt to exist between yellow and green wavelengths. Note that yellow coincides with an absorption peak of oxyhemoglobin, and

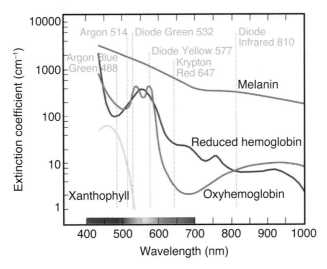

Figure 10-4 The absorption of different laser wavelengths by xanthophyll, melanin, deoxyhemoglobin, and oxyhemoglobin. Note that, in general, there is less absorption as one moves to the redder end of the spectrum. This explains the need for more power and a resultant deeper burn with longer wavelengths. Note that diode yellow hits a peak of oxyhemoglobin absorption relative to diode green. This results in a slightly different effect between the 2 colors when treating microaneurysms. It is not clear if the difference is clinically significant. Finally, the graph shows why it is dangerous to use blue wavelengths to treat the retina, given the profound uptake of that color by xanthophyll pigment in the macula. *(Based on data from Mainster MA. Wavelength selection in macular photocoagulation. Tissue optics, thermal effects, and laser systems.* Ophthalmology. *1986;93:952–958.)*

some investigators feel that this creates a clinically significant difference in how diabetic microaneurysms respond to each wavelength. However, no one has definitely proven that there is a huge difference in the ultimate treatment effect, regardless of the wavelength used. Most of the studies involving retinal laser photocoagulation were performed using some sort of green wavelength—usually argon green (514 nm) or diode green (532 nm)—and that is the wavelength that is generally available to most clinicians.

The one thing to remember with any wavelength is that darker tissue will absorb much more of the laser energy than lighter tissue. In other words, if treatment needs to be carried into a pigmented area such as a nevus or a previous laser scar it is crucial to turn down the power to avoid a dangerously hot burn. Alternatively, a very pale area will require increased power, but the power will need to be reduced when the treatment returns to areas of normal pigmentation.

Controlling the Energy

It is important for the ophthalmic surgeon to understand how to modify the settings on the laser to control the energy that is being delivered to the target tissue. For an Nd:YAG capsulotomy, the device has a fixed pulse duration and spot size so one can only modify the one setting, which is typically the energy in millijoules. For retinal photocoagulation using a continuous wave laser, the surgeon must select a spot size, an exposure time, and a power setting. In order to understand the amount of energy delivered with these settings, the surgeon must know the following irradiance and fluence equations (also called *power density* and *energy density*):

irradiance (W/cm^2) = power (watts)/spot area (cm^2)
fluence (J/cm^2) = energy (joules)/spot area (cm^2)

Because the energy (joules) equals the power (watts) times the exposure duration in seconds, the form for the fluence equation that is most useful clinically is

fluence (J/cm^2) = power (watts) × exposure time (seconds)/spot area (cm^2)

Lasers used for photocoagulation allow the surgeon to control multiple variables, and for these lasers the fluence or the energy density is very important to manipulate and understand. Note that changes in power (watts) or exposure duration (time) create a linear increase or decrease in the energy delivered. As an example, if a given laser setting is providing an adequate burn and the duration is doubled, then one has to decrease the power to avoid a dangerously hot burn. The clinical effect from altering these variables tends to be intuitive—a mild increase in the power or duration will result in a mild increase in the burn, and vice versa.

Heat Transfer

Because the treatment is being applied to a biological system and not a photometer, it turns out that the relationship between the energy delivered and the type of burn is more complex. The exact same energy can result in different burns because the burn depends on how the laser is absorbed and how the heat is transmitted by the tissue. In other words, changing the laser power and duration *generally* results in a commonsense change in the degree of uptake—a little more time or power results in a little more burn and a lot more time or power results in a lot more burn. But this relationship is not always consistent.

For example, although the equation for fluence suggests a linear relationship between power and duration and the degree of uptake, the actual laser effect is determined not only by the fluence but also by the rate of heat transfer out of the burn area. Heat transfer is governed by complex factors that include the nature and thickness of the tissue, the rate of absorption of laser energy, and the degree of vascularity. The rate of heat transfer explains why it is easy to get a burn in the retina but hard to get a burn on a large retinal blood vessel—the blood "carries" away the heat. Normally one does not treat large vessels, but it is important to recognize that safe use of the laser depends not only on the appropriate settings but also on a predictable degree of heat transfer away from the laser spot. This can become clinically significant if one needs to use high powers with a short duration. In this case there may not be time for the heat to spread out, and the burn can be much hotter than would be expected if the response of the tissue were truly linear.

Heat transfer also explains why the center of a burn will become whiter before the periphery of the burn as the power is increased. The temperature in the center of the spot will increase faster than in the periphery because heat can easily escape from the periphery of the burn toward the adjacent untreated cooler tissue, but heat in the center of the burn has nowhere to spread and can only build up. This can be problematic if one is using burns that are hotter than necessary. For example, there is a danger that if there is even a slight increase in the energy uptake in the tissue (such as increased pigmentation), then the temperature at the center of the burn can rise so fast and high that the water in the tissue will boil. The result is an explosively expanding bubble of water vapor that can cause a hole, a hemorrhage, or both.

Spot Size

It is important to recognize that both irradiance and fluence are an inverse function of the *square* of the spot radius. In other words, a small change in spot size can make a big difference in the irradiance (and fluence) delivered to the retina—adjusting spot size must always be accompanied by adjusting the power to compensate. A lot of energy delivered into a small spot is another way to raise the temperature so fast that a destructive bubble of water vapor occurs. Even if the temperature is insufficient to cause vaporization, there can still be severe complications, such as damaging retinal or choroidal vessels and causing hemorrhage or vascular closure. Another example of a more insidious problem is burning through Bruch's membrane when treating macular edema. This can result in the late development of a choroidal neovascular membrane.

Putting the Variables Together

All of these variables—power, duration, spot size, tissue absorption, and heat transfer—come into play when performing a treatment. For example, it may be necessary to use high powers when treating through media opacities, and one needs to be very careful if the media clears—a dangerously hot burn can result. One might also choose to use shorter exposure duration to try to make the laser less painful for the patient—but one needs to be careful because a higher power (irradiance) must be used and there is less time for heat to escape during the shorter exposure. If the treatment moves into a more pigmented area, the burns may suddenly become too hot.

Another common technique is to decrease the spot size in order to get a better burn when the media is hazy. When this is done, it is crucial to cut back on the power and work it back up to determine the amount needed for a safe burn. Otherwise the irradiance and fluence will be increased by the square of the difference in spot size, and a dangerously hot burn will ensue. This concept should be internalized to the point that it is automatic: if the spot size is decreased then the power must be reduced and retitrated up to a new level that results in a safe burn.

It is also important to remember that the spot size is not exclusively determined by the setting chosen on the slit-lamp adapter. Each type of contact lens will minify or magnify the size of the actual spot projected on the retina—the lens manufacturer provides this information. If one changes to a different contact lens during a treatment, it is possible to markedly decrease the spot size delivered to the retina and, again, the power setting needs to be decreased and brought back to a safe level.

There are other ways the spot size can change unintentionally. In the retinal periphery, the spot sometimes shrinks when treating through the edge of the patient's lens. Or during a macular laser in an area of swollen retina, the thickened retina tends to diffuse the beam, and when the treatment moves to an area of thin retina, the spot effectively shrinks. It is important to anticipate these changes and alter your parameters accordingly.

The bottom line is that there are 3 variables that you can control from the front panel of your laser and slit-lamp adapter when performing retinal photocoagulation. The power and the duration are fairly forgiving if small adjustments are made to titrate the treatment effect. Spot size, however, is a variable with exponential quadratic effects, and when switching to a smaller spot, the surgeon must turn the power down and titrate back up for a safe burn. Alternatively, if the spot size is increased, it is necessary to increase the power and re-titrate to perform an effective treatment.

When "unpacked" into its various components, retinal photocoagulation may seem daunting. However, the process will rapidly become intuitive with experience. The best way to approach it is to simply remember what a laser spot is. The retina is normally a beautifully transparent structure. If the organization of the cells and proteins is disrupted, then it begins to lose its transparency and to scatter the light, in the same way the cornea begins to become cloudy when it swells. A mild burn means that, literally, the retinal proteins are gently cooked so that the retina becomes translucent—it gets a slight grayish color as light begins to be mildly scattered. Choroidal details can still be seen through a light gray burn. As the burn gets hotter there is more disruption of the protein matrix, more scattering of light, and the retina gets whiter and whiter—the opaque white retina masks the choroidal detail. If burns suddenly become very white, it is crucial to stop immediately and adjust the settings—the easiest thing to do is turn down the power—to avoid complications such as retinal holes or hemorrhage.

Laser Safety

In the United States, the American National Standards Institute has set forth voluntary safety standards for laser use. Although these guidelines are voluntary, they can have legal ramifications if there are complications related to the use of the laser. The standards require that, in a laser facility, one person be given the responsibility of safety oversight (the laser safety officer). The guidelines also suggest that a laser warning sign be placed at the entrance of the treatment room and that visitors and assistants wear laser eye protection within the range of potentially hazardous exposure (referred to as the *nominal hazard zone*). The nominal hazard zone is considered to be less than 1–2 meters from the contact lens being used to treat the patient, depending upon the laser system.

Additional considerations include placing the laser in such a way that neither the direct output of the laser nor secondary reflections from the contact lens are likely to point toward unprotected personnel. The foot switch for the laser activation should also be clearly marked and protected from the possibility of accidental firing. The treating surgeon needs to be protected by filters with high optical density at the laser wavelength built into the slit lamp or operating microscope, and if auxiliary viewing optics for an assistant are used, these must also be protected by a laser filter. The recommendation for appropriate protective eyewear is important for nonmedical observers, such as the patient's relatives, because they may inadvertently place themselves in a potentially hazardous location. This is especially true when using a laser that has an output in the ultraviolet or infrared wavelength that is not visible because the presence of scattered secondary beams will be unrecognized. Laser photocoagulation systems using an indirect ophthalmoscope pose more of a danger because the beam can be directed anywhere the surgeon happens to be looking, and laser eye protectors are mandatory for anyone else in the room.

These issues are of less concern for fixed delivery systems such as excimer lasers where there is a stable beam path and a hazard zone that is very limited. Furthermore, the 193-nm wavelength of an argon-fluoride excimer laser has very little thermal spread and limited tissue penetrance (hence its ability to only affect the surface of the tissue being treated). In this case, the need for eye protection for people in the treatment area is questionable, but from a medical-legal standpoint it may be reasonable to offer visitors clear plastic goggles.

Although much has been written about the need for protective eyewear for observers, it is also important to remember that the most vulnerable eye is the patient's fellow eye—it is only centimeters from the area being treated. Although eye protection is generally not used for the fellow eye because it is well off-axis from the treatment, one should take care to avoid accidentally pointing the activated laser toward the fellow eye. This is particularly important when doing procedures using an indirect ophthalmoscope delivery system. Finally, it is always important to be sure that the appropriate eye is being treated using all of the guidelines designed to avoid surgery on the wrong eye as discussed in Chapter 17.

Patient Issues

There are additional factors to consider concerning the use of lasers, often depending on the sophistication of the patient. For example, some patients may equate medical lasers with the type of destructive energy beams depicted in science fiction movies, or they may equate laser light to the type of radiation used to treat cancer. Both the patient and their family members may therefore be very frightened to be in the same room with the laser. It is reasonable to reassure them about the relative safety of medical lasers compared to these other modalities. It often helps for the treating physician to keep up calm and reassuring "chatter" to help alleviate the patient's anxiety.

It is crucial to spend as much time as necessary explaining the nature and rationale for the treatment as well as the risks, benefits, and alternatives. (The specifics of various laser procedures are covered in the companion book, *Basic Techniques of Ophthalmic Surgery.*) It is very helpful to have a family member or friend present both for this discussion and the treatment, if logistics allow. The patient may be too nervous to fully absorb all the information, and having someone else to share the experience can be very reassuring.

As part of this process, one should make sure that the patient has appropriate expectations, regardless of the type of laser being performed. For refractive laser treatment, or Nd:YAG capsulotomy, the immediate effect of treatment is visual improvement that patients can detect for themselves. In such cases it is still important to be sure they do not have unrealistic expectations that will leave them disappointed with the results. However, most lasers involving retinal photocoagulation—or glaucoma lasers such as laser trabeculoplasty or iridotomy—do not directly improve the patient's vision, and a careful discussion of outcomes is especially important with such treatments. Patients' expectations may be wildly unrealistic in this setting, often because their main exposure to the concept of laser treatment comes from advertising for refractive procedures. For example, even with a careful informed consent, patients with diabetes may still assume that a laser procedure for macular edema or proliferative disease will immediately improve their vision, and they can be very disappointed with an otherwise successful outcome. Such expectations may go unvoiced and it behooves the ophthalmologist to explore this with the patient and to be sure that the goals of the treatment are repeated frequently. A classic example involves a symptomatic retinal tear. The ophthalmologist may feel very good about having avoided the need for retinal detachment surgery, but patients can be very upset that the laser treatment did not immediately get rid of their flashing lights and floaters.

Another concern that may go unvoiced is that patients may have been told by friends or family about someone who was "blinded by the laser." They can therefore be very reluctant to undergo treatment that they may perceive as unnecessary, especially in the setting of diabetes where problems are ideally identified prior to the patient having symptoms. It is important to explore these feelings and reassure the patient as much as possible. Often such stories arise from situations where patients presented very late in the course of their retinopathy and laser was attempted with only partial success. In other words, their vision deteriorated not from the laser but rather from disease that was discovered too late. A scenario like this can be turned around and used to better educate both the patient and family about the need for early diagnosis and treatment to avoid such outcomes.

Some patients may have a profound ocular-cardiac response to the placement of a contact lens and/or the noxious stimulus caused by the laser. Although no demographic is free from this, it seems to be more common in younger males. Patients should be warned to report any lightheadedness, which may indicate an impending syncopal episode. The treating ophthalmologist should be ready to discontinue the treatment immediately and have the patient put his or her head between the knees or even lie down on the floor until the episode passes. It is usually possible to restart the treatment cautiously after several minutes. Fortunately, this reaction is unusual, but it helps to mention it prior to initiating any treatment so that no one is surprised by what can be a rather dramatic occurrence. It is equally important to remember that patients with multiple medical comorbidities may have other reasons for feeling lightheaded at the laser, including hypoglycemia or true cardiac or neurologic emergencies, and appropriate emergency measures should be undertaken if patients do not improve in a manner consistent with a simple vasovagal episode.

New Directions

Retinal laser treatment has been a mainstay of ophthalmic therapy for decades. As a result there have been constant efforts to improve the efficacy and safety of the various techniques. Newer delivery systems have been developed that can apply multiple spots over a brief period of time—proponents feel that this can facilitate treatments such as panretinal photocoagulation. There are systems that track the retinal vasculature, allowing physicians to indicate the lesions to be treated, which are then automatically targeted by the laser. Extensive research has also been done using subthreshold treatments that do not have an obvious clinical effect when the treatment is performed. The goal is to induce a favorable effect in retinal tissue without causing the scarring that occurs with typical retinal photocoagulation burns. Advances in anterior segment techniques are also occurring at a dramatic rate as more sophisticated algorithms are developed for optimizing refractive laser treatment and new indications are developed for the femtosecond laser. It is incumbent on the ophthalmologist to become familiar with the newest techniques to provide optimal patient care and, at the same time, to remember the fundamentals of laser treatment to ensure that these devices are used safely and effectively.

Key Points

- The nature of laser light makes it ideal for treating ophthalmic diseases. The wavelength of light generated by the laser, as well as whether it is pulsed or continuous wave, determines the type of tissue effect and allows the surgeon to optimize treatment depending on the pathology.
- Understanding the variables that can be controlled by the surgeon is crucial to performing a safe and effective treatment. This includes being familiar with the way different lasers interact with ocular structures and how the laser settings can be used to titrate the clinical effect. For example, with retinal photocoagulation it is important to understand the change in energy delivered to the retina caused by altering variables such as the power, duration, and spot size. The treating physician also needs to observe for variations in pigmentation that can dramatically change the uptake of laser energy by tissue.

- A complete discussion of both the rationale and the risks and benefits of a given procedure is required to ensure patient understanding and cooperation. The treating physician must also be prepared to address issues that may go unvoiced by the patient, such as fear of the laser and unrealistic expectations regarding the treatment.
- Safety issues should also be addressed, including appropriate location of the laser, ensuring treatment of the correct eye and correct settings, and the use of protective eyewear when appropriate.

American Academy of Ophthalmology. *Basic and Clinical Science Course, Section 3: Clinical Optics.* San Francisco: American Academy of Ophthalmology; 2014.

American Academy of Ophthalmology. "Charles R. and Judith G. Munnerlyn Laser Surgery Education Center." Available at http://one.aao.org/laser-surgery-education-center. Accessed October 10, 2014.

American Academy of Ophthalmology. *Basic and Clinical Science Course, Section 13: Refractive Surgery.* San Francisco: American Academy of Ophthalmology; 2014.

Barteselli G, Kozak I, El-Emam S, Chhablani J, Cortes MA, Freeman WR. 12-month results of the standardised combination therapy for diabetic macular oedema: intravitreal bevacizumab and navigated retinal photocoagulation. *Br J Ophthalmol.* 2014;98(8)1036–1041.

Folk JC, Pulido JS. *Laser Photocoagulation of the Retina and Choroid.* Ophthalmology Monograph 11. San Francisco: American Academy of Ophthalmology; 1997.

Hatch KM, Talamo JH. Laser-assisted cataract surgery: benefits and barriers. *Curr Opin Ophthalmol.* 2014;25(1):54–61.

Hausheer J, ed. *Basic Techniques of Ophthalmic Surgery.* 2nd ed. San Francisco: American Academy of Ophthalmology; 2015.

Mainster MA. Decreasing retinal photocoagulation damage: principles and techniques. *Semin Ophthalmol.* 1999;14:200–209.

Mainster MA. Wavelength selection in macular photocoagulation. Tissue optics, thermal effects, and laser systems. *Ophthalmology.* 1986;93(7):952–958.

Muqit MM, Marcellino GR, Henson DB, Young LB, Turner GS, Stanga PE. Pascal panretinal laser ablation and regression analysis in proliferative diabetic retinopathy: Manchester Pascal Study Report 4. *Eye (Lond).* 2011;25(11):1447–1456.

Sivaprasad S, Elagouz M, McHugh D, Shona O, Dorin G. Micropulsed diode laser therapy: evolution and clinical applications. *Surv Ophthalmol.* 2010;55(6):516–530.

Sliney DH. Ophthalmic laser safety. In: Fankhauser F, Kwasniewska S, eds. *Lasers in Ophthalmology: Basic, Diagnostic, and Surgical Aspects. A Review.* The Hague, Netherlands: Kugler Publications; 2003:1–10.

Walker J. *Diabetic Retinopathy for the Comprehensive Ophthalmologist.* Fort Wayne, IN: Deluma Medical Publishers; 2009.

Self-Assessment Test

1. When performing retinal photocoagulation, which of the following should be done if one decreases the spot size from 200 µm to 100 µm?
   a. Increase power to ensure effective treatment at the new spot size.
   b. Increase the duration given the slower uptake with the smaller spot.
   c. Turn down the power and re-titrate back up to obtain an appropriate burn.
   d. Switch to a different contact lens that is better suited to the smaller spot size.

2. Which of the following wavelengths is least absorbed by melanin?
   a. 647 nm/red
   b. 532 nm/green
   c. 577 nm/yellow
   d. 810 nm/infrared

3. Which of the following variables are used in the formula for determining the fluence of a laser spot? (Choose all that apply.)
   a. spot size
   b. duration
   c. contact lens type
   d. wavelength
   e. power

4. Which of the following preparations are important to perform prior to doing any laser? (Choose all that apply.)
   a. Ensure that visitors and staff are wearing appropriate protective eyewear.
   b. Ensure that the patient is aware of the risks, benefits, and alternatives of the procedure.
   c. Ensure that the patient has appropriate expectations regarding the visual outcome.
   d. Warn the patient about possible vasovagal response from the laser.

5. When performing an Nd:YAG capsulotomy, which of the following laser-tissue interactions are involved?
   a. photoablation
   b. photodisruption
   c. photocoagulation
   d. photochemical

For preferred responses to these questions, see Appendix A.

CHAPTER 11

ACGME Requirements for Surgical Training

Bryan J. Winn, MD

The Accreditation Council for Graduate Medical Education (ACGME) is a private, nonprofit organization that accredits residency programs and fellowships in 130 medical and surgical specialties. Residency programs must maintain ACGME accreditation in order to receive graduate medical education funds from the federal government. In order to be eligible to take board certification examination, residents must graduate from ACGME-accredited programs. In addition, states frequently require completion of an ACGME-accredited residency program for medical licensure.

In surgical specialties such as ophthalmology, the creation and maintenance of an accurate surgical case log by each resident is critical for his or her program's maintenance of accreditation. In addition, beginning in 2014, ophthalmology residency programs are required to report on specific milestones, some of which involving the development of both cognitive and technical skills required for surgical competency.

ACGME Case Logs

In order for residency programs to maintain accreditation, residents in ophthalmology must log their surgical procedures into the ACGME Case Log System that can be accessed at www.acgme.org. The ACGME has set a minimum number of cases required for the various surgical categories within ophthalmology. Graduating residents are currently required to meet minimums for all procedures (Table 11-1). The minimums were set at the twentieth percentile of surgical procedures performed by residents nationwide in 2006. The Residency Review Committee (RRC) for Ophthalmology periodically reviews these minimums and makes changes when deemed appropriate.

Meeting minimums, while required, is not an indicator of surgical competence but rather an indicator of experience. Residents may need to perform more than the minimum number of cases in an area before competence is attained. Residency programs must evaluate competence in these procedures to ensure that resident graduates of the program are able to perform these procedures competently without supervision.

Accurate surgical logs are important from a programmatic standpoint. Residency program directors and clinical competency committees use case log data to make sure

Table 11-1 **Required Minimum Number of Procedures for Graduating Residents in Ophthalmology (2014)**

Category[a]	Minimums
Cataract – total (S)	86
Laser surgery –YAG capsulotomy (S)	5
Laser surgery – laser trabeculoplasty (S)	5
Laser surgery – laser iridotomy (S)	4
Laser surgery – panretinal laser photocoagulation (S)	10
Corneal surgery	
Keratoplasty (S+A)	5
Pterygium/conjunctival and other cornea (S)	3
Keratorefractive surgery – total (S+A)	6
Strabismus – total (S)	10
Glaucoma – filtering/shunting procedures (S)	5
Retinal vitreous – total (S+A)	10
Intravitreal injection (S)	10
Oculoplastic and orbit – total (S)	28
Oculoplastic and orbit – eyelid laceration (S)	3
Oculoplastic and orbit – chalazia excision (S)	3
Oculoplastic and orbit – ptosis/blebpharoplasty (S)	3
Globe trauma – total (S)	4

[a]S = surgeon procedures only. S+A = surgeon and assistant procedures.

(Courtesy of the Accreditation Council for Graduate Medical Education.)

that all residents have an equivalent educational experience. They also make critical decisions regarding the curriculum and rotation changes based in part on the data collected in the surgical case logs. In addition, applicants for residency will often use the "surgical case numbers" when evaluating programs for desirability.

Residents are required to log each procedure in which they perform the role of first assistant or primary surgeon into the ACGME Resident Case Log System. As of this writing, at least 364 total procedures including both surgeon and assistant roles should be completed by graduation from the program. The system uses Current Procedural Terminology (CPT) codes to identify the specific types of procedures performed. While it is helpful and efficient if the resident knows the CPT codes for the individual cases he or she is logging, a search function included in the system allows the resident to scroll through procedures of a specific category. In addition, the date of service, patient's date of birth and unique identifier, attending physician, institution, and resident role are required as part of the log.

Resident Roles

When logging a case in the system, the resident must select the role of surgeon or assistant. In order to be considered the surgeon, the resident must be present for all of the critical portions of the case and must perform the majority of those critical portions under appropriate attending physician supervision. Critical portions of the case do include both the preoperative assessment and postoperative management. A resident may be considered the assistant only if he or she is the first assistant to either the attending surgeon performing the case or another resident or fellow performing the case under supervision of the attending surgeon.

Bilateral and Multi-Part Cases

In bilateral cases, if a resident performs the role of surgeon on one side, he can count that as 1 case. If he performs both sides of a bilateral case, he can still only count this as 1 case. However, if 2 residents participate in a case and one functions as the primary surgeon role on 1 side and the second resident performs the role of primary surgeon on the contralateral side, both residents can count that surgery as 1 case. For example, if a resident performs both sides of bilateral complex ectropion repair, she can only count this as 1 case. However, if she performs 1 side and another resident performs the other side, both can claim a primary surgeon role for that case.

In the situation of surgeries that involve multiple procedures, the resident may count the individual procedures as separate surgeries so long as these procedures are not part of the same category (eg, cataract, cornea, strabismus, glaucoma, retina/vitreous, oculoplastics/orbit, globe trauma). For example, if a resident performs both an eyelid laceration repair and a corneal laceration repair on the same patient as part of the same surgery, he can record both procedures as surgeon, since one falls under the category of oculoplastics/orbit and the other globe trauma. However, if a resident performs both a scleral buckle procedure and a pars plana vitrectomy to treat a retinal detachment, he can only record 1 procedure as surgeon. In the same example, if there were 2 residents operating and one performed the scleral buckle and the other performed the vitrectomy, each could record his procedure as primary surgeon as long as she performed the majority of the critical components of the case.

Common Pitfalls

There are several issues that can arise leading to inaccurate and incomplete surgical case logs:

1. *Procrastination.* It is very easy during a busy residency to put off logging in cases until "tomorrow." However, if one does not keep meticulous records in a physical notebook or a HIPAA-compliant electronic database, surgical logs are destined to become less accurate with time. The ACGME Case Log System is now optimized for use with mobile devices and smartphones (www.acgme.org/mobilercl). This should make logging cases in "real time" easier for the resident.
2. *Not starting on Day 1.* Surgical case logs are often the furthest things from the minds of new residents. However, even first-year residents may assist or perform

the role of surgeon on cases during the very first week of residency. If residents are not aware that they should be recording the details of each case, these records may be lost when it comes to logging them into the ACGME Resident Case Log System.

3. *Not knowing what to log.* While it is likely obvious that every case performed in the operating room should be logged, many in-office minor procedures have the potential to be overlooked for logging. All in-office procedures must be logged into the system. These include, but are not limited to,

   - chalazion incision and curettage
   - eyelid lesion removal
   - eyelid biopsy
   - paracentesis to release intraocular fluid
   - repair of a corneal leak or laceration with tissue glue
   - botulinum toxin injection (chemodenervation) to treat blepharospasm
   - intravitreal injection
   - tarsorrhaphy
   - canthotomy
   - eyelid laceration repair
   - closure of punctum via cautery
   - probing of lacrimal canaliculi, with or without irrigation
   - incision and drainage of lacrimal sac
   - all laser procedures

It is recommended that the resident become familiar with the CPT codes used in the ACGME Ophthalmology Case Log System. These codes can be found on the ACGME website (www.acgme.org). In addition, the resident should consult with the supervising attending physician regarding the specific procedures and CPT codes associated with each case performed or assisted on.

Tips on Maintaining an Accurate Surgical Log

1. Keep a secure notebook (digital or paper) on hand at all times, and create an entry with every procedure performed.
2. Keep track of the patient identifier, date of birth, actual procedure(s) performed, your role in the procedure(s), attending name, date of procedure, institution.
3. If unsure, discuss the surgery with the attending physician to make sure that you are accurately and completely listing all of the procedures performed.
4. Print out the ophthalmology CPT codes used by the ACGME. Keep this list with your notebook and use it for reference when coding your procedures.
5. Remember that all procedures, not only cases performed in the operating room, need to be recorded in the log. These include common in-office diagnostic and therapeutic procedures.
6. Do not forget about cases when you only assisted. These need to be logged, too.

7. Enter your cases into the ACGME Case Log System daily, if possible. The longer the interval between entries, the more time-consuming and unmanageable the process becomes.
8. Log via app. The ACGME mobile site (www.acgme.org/mobilercl) may save time when logging cases.

Beyond Residency and the ACGME

Maintenance of a surgical case log is helpful for practicing ophthalmologists even beyond residency. A surgical log is documentation of an ophthalmologist's professional experience. While the American Board of Ophthalmology (ABO) currently does not require documentation of a surgical case log for Maintenance of Certification (MOC), several other surgical specialty boards do and the ABO may follow suit in the future. Furthermore, hospitals, surgery centers, malpractice insurance carriers, and potential employers may require surgical logs from the most recent 12–36 months in order to be considered for privileges, insurance coverage, or employment.

Milestones

Beginning in 2014, ophthalmology residency programs are required to use and report on each resident's ophthalmology milestones. Akin to the developmental milestones used to help assess children as they progress socially, cognitively, and physically throughout childhood, the ophthalmology milestones were developed as a joint project of the ACGME and the ABO to provide structure for the assessment of the development of a resident's competency as a physician in the specialty of ophthalmology. The milestones were designed to be used by the program director and clinical competency committee in the semi-annual review of each resident's performance.

There are 24 milestones encompassing key knowledge, skills, attitudes, and other attributes of the ACGME core competencies. Each milestone is divided into 5 levels, with level 1 consistent with the expectations of a beginning resident who has some education in ophthalmology and level 5 consistent with the expectations of an ophthalmologist who has graduated residency and may have been in practice for several years. Level 4 is typically the target for residents in each of the 24 milestones by the time they graduate.

Patient care milestones 6 and 7 specifically address the subject of resident physician competency in both non-operating room based surgery and operating room based surgery, respectively.

The program director and clinical competency committee may use various assessment tools to determine the level of each resident with respect to these to milestones. These may include 360° global evaluations, chart audit or review, surgical case logs, oral and written examinations, chart-stimulated recall, focused skills assessment, Ophthalmic Clinical Evaluation Exercise (OCEX), operating room surgical skills assessment, Outcome and Assessment Information Set (OASIS), Global Rating Assessment of Skills in Intraocular Surgery (GRASIS, Fig 11-1), and surgical video review. It is, therefore, very

Global Rating Assessment of Skills in Intraocular Surgery (GRASIS): Global Rating Scale of Operative Performance

Resident: _____ Preceptor: _____

Circle Procedure: ClearCornea Extracap ScleralTunnel Trabeculectomy PPV PKP Other:

☐ Beginning ☐ Middle ☐ End of Rotation

Preoperative Planning/Knowledge of Patient				
1	2	3	4	5 N/A
Did not recognize or analyze potential ocular/non-ocular risk factors of case		Identified risk factors and had partially complete plan for them		Identified risk factors. Planned ahead appropriately
Knowledge of Procedure				
1	2	3	4	5 N/A
Required specific instructions at most steps		Demonstrated some forward planning		Familiar with all aspects of procedure
Microscope Use: Centration				
1	2	3	4	5 N/A
Constantly asked to re-center and/or re-focus the microscope or eye				Kept the eye centered. Maintained good view with microscope
Instrument Handling				
1	2	3	4	5 N/A
Repeatedly makes tentative, awkward, or inappropriate movements with instruments		Competent use of instruments but occasionally stiff or awkward		Fluid moves with instruments, no awkwardness
Treatment of Ocular Structures and Other Tissues				
1	2	3	4	5 N/A
Frequently used unnecessary force or caused damage by inappropriate use of instruments		Careful handling of tissues but occasionally caused inadvertent damage		Appropriate handling of tissues and structures. Produced no damage
Flow of Operation: Time and Motion				
1	2	3	4	5 N/A
Frequently seemed unsure of surgical plan. Many unnecessary movements. Entered and exited eye needlessly.		Knew most important steps of operation. Efficient time/motion/energy but some unnecessary movements		Progressed effortlessly. Maximum efficiency by conserving intraocular motion and energy
Use of Non-dominant Hand				
1	2	3	4	5 N/A
Does not use non-dominant hand or performs low, inappropriate movements		Performs few movements with dexterity at certain steps of procedure		Uses non-dominant hand with dexterity throughout the procedure
Knowledge of Phacoemulsification and Vitrector Equipment and Instruments				
1	2	3	4	5 N/A
Frequently asked/used wrong instrument. Unaware of proper equipment settings		Knew names of most instruments. Used appropriate settings/tools for task		Obviously familiar with instruments and equipment
Surgical Professionalism: Interaction with Assistants/Scrub Nurse/Surgical Preceptor				
1	2	3	4	5 N/A
Failed to request or use assistance when needed		Appropriate use of assistance most of the time		Strategically used assistant to the best advantage at all times
Handling of Unexpected Operative Events/Adverse Events				
1	2	3	4	5 N/A
Unable to recognize adverse events or inappropriate over reaction due to inability to request proper assistance		Professional and competent identification of event appropriate assistance		Superior independent management of event
Overall Performance				
1	2	3	4	5 N/A
Unable to perform operation independently		Competent, could perform operation with minimal assistance		Clearly superior, performed operation independently with confidence

Figure 11-1 The Global Rating Assessment of Skills in Intraocular Surgery (GRASIS). *(Reprinted, with permission, from Cremers SL. Global Rating Assessment of Skills in Intraocular Surgery [GRASIS], Ophthalmology. Volume 112, Issue 10, Pages 1655–1660, October 2005.)*

important for residents to comply with requests from the program director to participate in and complete any of these assessment tools. In addition to giving the program director and clinical competency committee the ability to better assess surgical competency, these can be directly useful to the resident in terms of better understanding his or her levels of performance and areas in need of improvement.

Key Points

- Residents must log each procedure that they perform or assist on throughout residency into the ACGME Case Log System.

- Accuracy and completeness of each resident's case log is critical for that residency program's maintenance of ACGME accreditation.
- Each resident is expected to have logged the required surgical minimums by the end of residency.
- Surgical case logs are measures of *experience,* whereas milestones are tools used to assess *competency.*
- Timely data entry into the ACGME Case Log System is the key to accurate and complete case log data.

Accreditation Council for Graduate Medical Education. Ophthalmology. Sub-site of www .acgme.org for ophthalmology-related documents, program requirements, milestones, deadlines, and other resources. Available at http://goo.gl/J28WJS. Accessed September 6, 2014.

Accreditation Council for Graduate Medical Education and the American Board of Ophthalmology. The Ophthalmology Milestone Project. Available at http://goo.gl/JIVP1F. Accessed September 6, 2014.

Cremers SL, Lora AN, Ferrufino-Ponce ZK. Global Rating Assessment of Skills in Intraocular Surgery (GRASIS). *Ophthalmology.* 2005;112(10):1655–1660.

Fisher JB, Binenbaum G, Tapino P, Volpe NJ. Development and face and content validity of an eye surgical skills assessment test for ophthalmology residents. *Ophthalmology.* 2006;113(12): 2364–2370. Epub 2006 Oct 23.

Taylor JB, Binenbaum G, Tapino P, Volpe NJ. Microsurgical lab testing is a reliable method for assessing ophthalmology residents' surgical skills. *Br J Ophthalmol.* 2007;91(12):1691–1694.

Self-Assessment Test

1. A resident is the primary surgeon under attending supervision for both sides of a bilateral upper blepharoplasty. The resident can log the case as which of the following?
   a. as 2 primary surgeon cases since the resident operated on both sides
   b. as 1 primary surgeon case since both procedures are in the area of oculoplastic/ orbital surgery
   c. as an assistant surgeon for 2 cases since there was an attending present who was billing for the case
   d. as an assistant for 1 case and as primary surgeon for 1 case
2. A resident is the primary surgeon for a combined cataract extraction via phaco-emulsification and trabeculectomy performed on the same patient on the same day. The resident can log the case as which of the following?
   a. 2 cases since one procedure is in the area of cataract and the other in the area of glaucoma
   b. 1 case since both procedures were performed by the same resident
   c. 1 case since both procedures were performed on the same day
   d. as an assistant for both since there was an attending present
3. Which of the following procedures should be logged into the ACGME Case Log System?
   a. extracapsular cataract extraction
   b. probing of canaliculi with or without irrigation

    c. gonioscopy

    d. all of the above

    e. A and B

4. What is required for a resident to claim the role of surgeon?

    a. The resident is present for and performs the majority of the critical portions of a surgical case.

    b. The resident participates in the preoperative assessment.

    c. The resident participates in the postoperative care.

    d. All of the above.

For preferred responses to these questions, see Appendix A.

PART **III**

Intraoperative Considerations

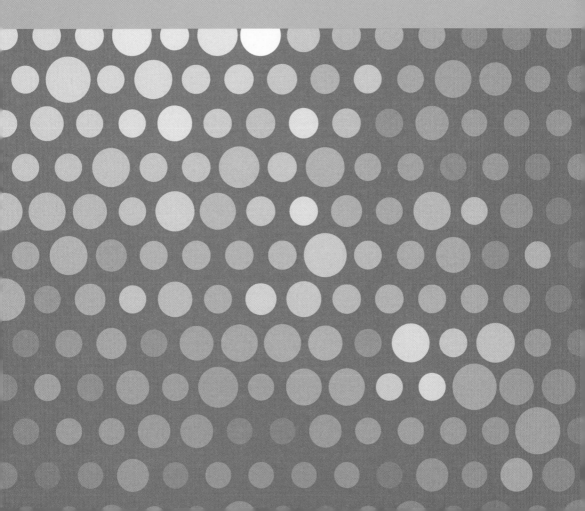

CHAPTER 12

Aseptic Technique and the Sterile Field in the Operating Room

Ensa K. Pillow, MD
Andrew A. Wilson, MD

Aseptic and sterile techniques have evolved tremendously since the medical profession officially accepted Joseph Lister's antiseptic principles of surgery in 1879. Often, the terms are used interchangeably.

Today, much time and care is taken to minimize the possibility of infection resulting from surgical procedures. According to the *Guideline for Prevention of Surgical Site Infection* published by the Centers for Disease Control and Prevention, the most common pathogens involved in postoperative eye infections are coagulase-negative *Staphylococcus, Staphylococcus aureus,* and gram-negative bacilli. This chapter introduces you to the agents, techniques, and practices used to reduce the infection rate following surgical procedures.

Skin Preparation

The most common antiseptic agents used in preoperative preparation of the surgical site are iodophors, alcohols, and chlorhexidine gluconate.

Iodophors, such as povidone-iodine (Betadine), are compounds based on a bactericidal complex of iodine and a nonionic surface-active agent. In ophthalmic surgery, iodophors are the agents used most frequently in prepping the skin around the eyes as well as the conjunctiva and cul-de-sac. They provide bactericidal effect as long as they are present on the skin, and they are effective against gram-positive and gram-negative bacteria, viruses, fungi, protozoa, and yeasts. Because they can cause skin irritation, iodophors should be avoided in patients with iodine sensitivity.

Alcohol (70% to 90% ethyl or isopropyl) works by denaturing proteins. It is effective against gram-positive and gram-negative bacteria, fungi, some viruses, and tuberculosis mycobacteria. Alcohol is readily available, inexpensive, and acts rapidly. Because it is easily ignited and burns rapidly, alcohol must be handled carefully in the operating room. (See Chapter 17 for discussion of preventing fire in the operating room.)

Chlorhexidine gluconate (Hibiclens), as with iodophors and alcohol, is effective on a broad spectrum of microbial activity including gram-positive and gram-negative bacteria, fungi, and spores but has less activity against viruses and tuberculosis mycobacteria. It works by disrupting the cell membrane of microorganisms. It is used for prepping the skin of the periocular area. In some countries the procedure is performed twice. Because residues tend to accumulate on skin with repeated use, chlorhexidine has a long duration of action (~6 hours). Toxicity can occur if the agent comes in contact with the middle ear or the cornea.

Application of Antiseptic Agents

In practice, if gross contamination is present from dirt, soil, or debris (as may occur in dirty lid lacerations), the skin should first be cleaned by irrigating the site with saline. The application of antiseptic begins with the eyelashes. Cotton swabs are soaked with the antiseptic and applied along upper and lower lash lines. Next, the surgical site is cleaned by applying the antiseptic using gauze sponges in concentric motions starting from the central operative site and moving peripherally. This process is repeated 3 times with new sponges/4 × 4s for each new application. Avoid moving from peripheral to central site because contamination can occur. All areas that will be exposed during the surgery should be covered with the antiseptic (Fig 12-1). For intraocular surgeries, drops of detergent-free povidone-iodine 5% are placed on the conjunctiva and fornices to reduce the risk of endophthalmitis.

For surgeries requiring local anesthetic, an alcohol swab is used to clean the injection site. Once the local anesthetic is injected, skin preparation begins as described above.

Hand Scrubbing

Scrubbing of the surgeon's hands and forearms involves antiseptic agents similar to those used in preparing the skin of the surgical site. Before scrubbing the hands, the surgeon dons a surgical mask and head cover. Any jewelry and artificial nails should be removed. Generally accepted practice for the first scrub of the day includes a total duration of 5-minutes; however, the optimum duration of scrubbing is not proven, with some studies suggesting that 2 minutes is effective. See also "Hand Preparation" in Chapter 3.

Here are the 4 basic steps in scrubbing the hands and forearms:

1. Begin by cleaning underneath the fingernails and then proceed proximally from the hand to the elbow (Fig 12-2A, 12-2B).
2. Elevate the tips of the fingers so the water and scrub solution drain down and off the elbow (Fig 12-3A, 12-2B).
3. Following the scrub, keep the hands up and away from the body with elbows bent.
4. When rinsing, take care to avoid allowing runoff to contaminate the opposite hand or forearm.

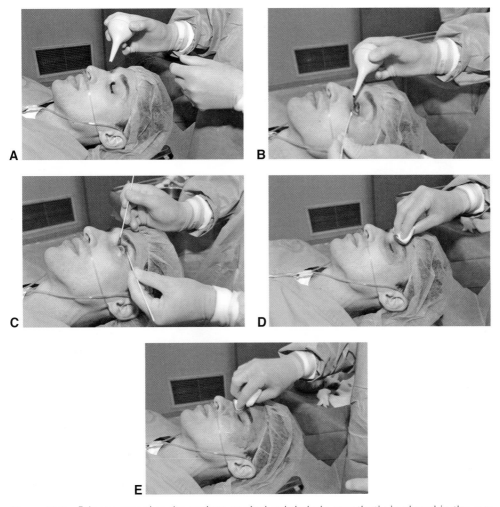

Figure 12-1 Prior to prepping the patient, topical ophthalmic anesthetic is placed in the eye to prevent irritation to the eye from the solution. **A, B,** For periocular or intraocular surgeries, 5% detergent-free Betadine is placed directly onto the conjunctiva and fornix using a bulb syringe or a soaked sponge/4 × 4. **C,** The lashes are cleaned with cotton-tipped swabs soaked in povidone-iodine 5%. **D, E,** The solution is wiped from central surgical site to peripheral in a circular motion. *(Courtesy of Scott C. Sigler, MD.)*

Hand scrubbing should be performed before the first case of the day and whenever the hands are contaminated (eg, after lunch, using the restroom). In addition, newer alcohol-based antiseptics are commonly used (eg, Avagard, Sterillium Rub). Prior to each gloving, the hands and fingers are massaged, paying particular attention to the fingers, cuticles, and interdigital spaces. If alcohol-based antiseptics are not used, massaging the hands with chlorhexidine solution for 2 minutes prior to each surgery is also acceptable.

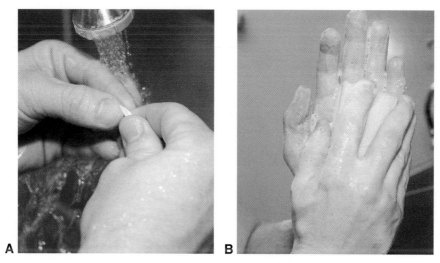

Figure 12-2 Hand scrubbing. **A,** The nails are addressed first with solution, water, and the nail pick. **B,** Note while scrubbing, the fingertips are pointed up. *(Courtesy of Scott C. Sigler, MD.)*

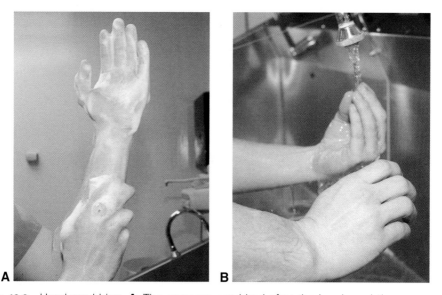

Figure 12-3 Hand scrubbing. **A,** The arms are scrubbed after the hands and the movement goes down to the elbows. **B,** The hands are rinsed first and followed by the forearms. The fingertips stay pointed up. *(Courtesy of Scott C. Sigler, MD.)*

Gowning and Gloving

Microorganisms are shed from hair, exposed skin, and mucous membranes. Surgical attire including scrubs, caps/hoods, masks, gowns, and gloves are used to minimize the exposure. In most operating rooms, a scrub technician is available for help with gowning and gloving. Informing the scrub tech of your gown and glove size is helpful. In situations where a technician is not available, you should be familiar with the technique of gowning and gloving yourself. This section discusses the procedures for doing so with or without an assistant.

Sterile towels are made available in the operating room for drying, usually placed on top of a gown. After a thorough scrub, the surgeon carefully grasps the towel, extending the arm and hand over the sterile field the least distance possible, without dripping water from the freshly scrubbed hands onto the field (see "Sterile Field" later in this chapter).

The towel is opened up with the right hand underneath the towel. The left hand is dried on the side of the towel opposite the right. Drying starts with the tips of the fingers and goes down to the elbows. Then the towel is flipped onto the left hand so the right hand can be dried on the opposite side. The towel is discarded away from the sterile field into the appropriate bin.

Gown and Glove Procedure With an Assistant

After you have dried your hands and forearms, the technician approaches, holding the gown open with the inside toward you. Insert your hands and arms into the arm holes, but do not extend your hands through the open end of the gown arms. The technician then offers one glove, typically fingers down. Extend the hand into the glove as it exits the open end of the gown arm, so that the glove may be pulled onto the hand and over the gown arm with minimal exposure of the hand. The same procedure is then performed with the other glove. The technician or scrub nurse ties the inside back of the gown and you rotate to wrap the gown around the back, which is also tied with the help of the technician or scrub nurse.

Gown and Glove Procedure Without an Assistant

The technician typically places the gown on the table with the back facing up. The goal is to touch anywhere within the interior of the gown without touching the outside surface. Carefully grasp the inside of the gown, near the top of the gown. With both hands and gravity, the gown is allowed to unfold and open up. Then carefully slide your hands and arms into the inside arm holes, keeping your hands within the sleeves. The scrub nurse or technician will tie the back of the gown. Fig 12-4 illustrates the steps of putting on sterile gloves without an assistant.

Draping

Draping refers to the positioning of sterile drapes around the surgical site to avoid contamination of the incision, instruments, and supplies. Depending on the procedure and the surgeon, draping can vary tremendously. The goal is to drape inside the previously prepped sterile field so that the drapes expose the sterile area to be operated, while covering the nonsterile surrounding areas. It is usually recommended that the edges of the drapes be adhesive material so there is a tight seal that prevents movement of the drapes during the procedure. The draping is performed after the antiseptic solution is used (Fig 12-5).

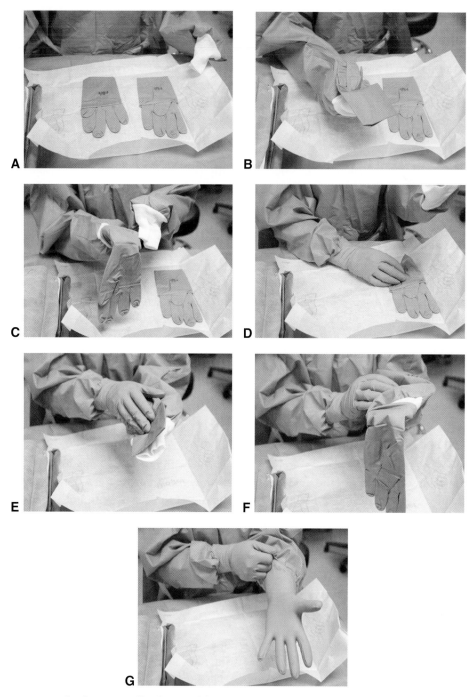

Figure 12-4 Putting on sterile gloves without an assistant. **A,** Placement of sterile gloves with right glove on right side. **B,** Using the unexposed left hand, place the right glove on top of the unexposed right hand thumb-to-thumb with fingers pointing proximally. **C,** Fold the unexposed right fingers into the glove. Using the unexposed left hand, grab the superior edge of the cuff and wrap it around the right hand. Pull the right sleeve and glove into place. **D–G,** Repeat the procedure for the left hand. *(Courtesy of Scott C. Sigler, MD.)*

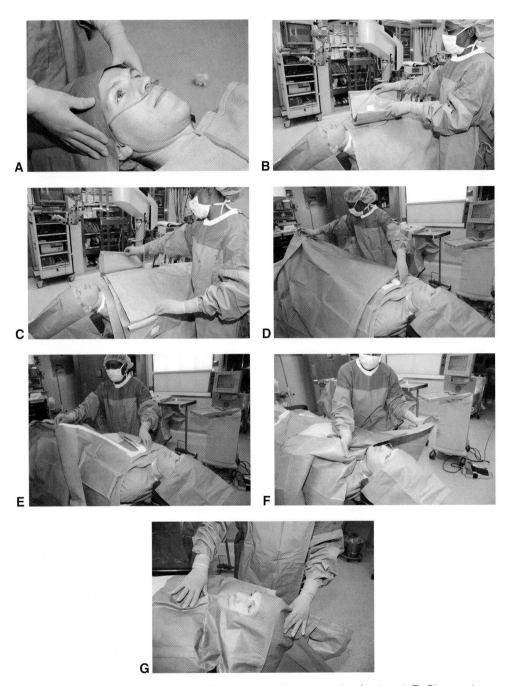

Figure 12-5 Example of draping. **A,** Place a head drape over the forehead. **B,** Place a drape on the patient's chest. Drapes will have labels indicating direction of the head. **C, D,** Fold out the drape toward the feet carefully without touching the nonsterile surroundings. **E,** Expose the drape adhesive by removing the paper tapes. **F, G,** When using nasal cannula, the full face must be prepped and exposed to avoid oxygen build up under the drape as this can cause ignition when the cautery is used. *(Courtesy of Scott C. Sigler, MD.)*

Sterile Field

The sterile field consists of the surgeon's gown in front of the chest to the level of surgical site, hands up to elbows, and the surface of the draped table. If there is any nonoperative time during the surgery (eg, waiting on proper instruments), hands should remain in the sterile field; they are usually clasped together in front of the chest or placed on the operating table. Arms should not be crossed with hands in axilla because the axillary region is considered nonsterile. Hands below the waist are considered no longer sterile. If an instrument falls below the level of the table, it is considered nonsterile and appropriately replaced. A nonsterile member of the surgical team should remove the instrument, not the surgeon or scrub technician. If the surgeon must cough or sneeze during the surgery, the correct technique is to back away from the table and cough or sneeze into the surgical mask. The surgeon should not turn his or her head since masks are not sealed to the face.

When using a surgical microscope, move it by the sterile handles; there are areas that are within reach that may not be sterile. If there is any question as to what is sterile or not within the field, it is best to ask before touching. If there is a question during the procedure whether an unsterile object touched an area, instrument, or part of the surgeon's gown or gloves, stop the procedure and cover the suspected area with a sterile towel if possible. If the surgeon's arm is contaminated, a sterile sleeve can be placed over it. A contaminated glove should be replaced.

When passing another gowned person, both people should pass face-to-face or back-to-back. The surgeon should never walk by the sterile field with his or her back to the sterile drapes or to the sterile surgical table.

Key Points

- The most commonly used skin preparation agents include iodophors, such as povidone-iodine (Betadine), alcohols, and chlorhexidine gluconate.
- The steps involved in the surgical hand scrub include cleaning the fingernails first, then scrubbing proximally from the hand to the elbow, elevating the tips of the fingers so the water and scrub solution drain down and off the elbow.
- Gowning and gloving involves maintaining the sterility of the outer (surgical field) surfaces, touching only the inner surfaces while donning.
- The sterile field consists of the surgeon's gown in front of the chest to the level of the surgical site, the hands up to the elbows, and the surface of the draped table.

Ahmed Y, Scott IU, Pathengay A, Bawdekar A, Flynn HW Jr. Povidone-iodine for endophthalmitis prophylaxis. *Am J Ophthalmol.* 2014;157(3):503–504.

Brunicardi CF, Andersen DK, Billiar TR, et al. *Schwartz's Principles of Surgery.* 9th ed. New York: McGraw-Hill Professional; 2009.

Buzard K, Liapis S. Prevention of endophthalmitis. *J Cataract Refract Surg.* 2004;30(9):1953–1959.

Centers for Disease Control and Prevention. "Surgical Site Infection." Available at www.cdc.gov/HAI/ssi/ssi.html. Accessed September 13, 2014.

Ciulla TA, Starr MB, Masket S. Bacterial endophthalmitis prophylaxis for cataract surgery: an evidence-based update. *Ophthalmology.* 2002;109:13–26.

Darouiche RO, Wall MJ Jr, Itani KM, et al. Chlorhexidine-alcohol versus povidone-iodine for surgical-site antisepsis. *N Engl J Med.* 2010;362(1):18–26.

Endophthalmitis Study Group (ESCRS). Prophylaxis of postoperative endophthalmitis following cataract surgery: results of the ESCRS multicenter study and identification of risk factors. *J Cataract Refract Surg.* 2007;33(6):978–988.

Phillips N. *Berry and Kohn's Operating Room Technique.* 11th ed. St Louis: Mosby; 2007.

Phippen MI, Wells MP. *Patient Care During Operative and Invasive Procedures.* Philadelphia: Saunders; 2000.

Speaker MG, Menikoff JA. Prophylaxis of endophthalmitis with topical povidone-iodine. *Ophthalmology.* 1991;98(12):1769–1775.

Self-Assessment Test

1. Which of the following is accurate regarding povidone-iodine? (Choose all that apply.)
   a. is bacteriostatic
   b. is effective against gram-positive and gram-negative bacteria
   c. is ineffective against fungi and yeast
   d. only rarely induces an allergic reaction
   e. is less effective than alcohol for antisepsis

2. Which of the following is true regarding the surgical hand scrub? (Choose all that apply.)
   a. is proven to require 5 minutes minimum
   b. proceeds from hand proximally to elbow
   c. always begins with the surgeon's dominant hand
   d. must include cleaning the fingernails

3. Which of the following is correct in the gown and glove procedure without an assistant? (Choose all that apply.)
   a. The surgeon exposes the hands through the end of the gown arms.
   b. The surgeon grasps only the inside surface of the gown.
   c. The surgeon must tie the back of the gown.
   d. Gloves are donned before the gown.

4. The sterile field typically includes which of the following? (Choose all that apply.)
   a. the area between the surgeon's waist and shoulders
   b. the microscope base
   c. the surgical field
   d. the underside of the operating table, if above the waist

5. In intraocular surgeries, what is the current accepted practice to reduce the rate of endophthalmitis?
   a. preoperative lash trimming
   b. preoperative saline irrigation
   c. preoperative topical antibiotics
   d. preoperative povidone-iodine

6. Which of the following is the most appropriate method to adjust surgical loupes on a gowned surgeon?
   a. Use one sterile hand to adjust the loupes and then replace that glove.
   b. Ask a nonsterile member of the team to adjust the loupes making sure not to contaminate the surgeon.
   c. Give the surgeon a towel originating off the surgical field to adjust the loupes.
   d. It is never appropriate to adjust surgical loupes during a case since the gowned surgeon is sterile.

For preferred responses to these questions, see Appendix A.

CHAPTER 13

Ophthalmic Anesthesia

Steven J. Gedde, MD
Yunhee Lee, MD, MPH

Adequate ophthalmic anesthesia is required for safe ocular surgery; it may be attained through local (topical, intraocular, regional) or general administration. Anesthesia techniques have evolved in recent years along with surgical procedures. Many intraocular surgeons utilize regional anesthesia by an orbital block, although topical anesthesia is growing in popularity, especially in small-incision cataract surgery. Typically, general anesthesia is typically reserved for patients who are not candidates for regional or topical anesthesia. This chapter reviews local and regional anesthetic agents in common use, techniques of ocular anesthesia, appropriate patient selection, and possible anesthesia complications. Discussion of inhaled general anesthetic gases is beyond the scope of this chapter.

Sedation

The goal of sedation is to achieve anxiolysis (minimal sedation), amnesia, or somnolence. The choice of sedative agents depends on the patient, the procedure, and the surgeon.

Often, patients undergoing ophthalmic surgery are elderly and may have multiple systemic illnesses that must be considered. In addition, surgical procedures differ in complexity, length, and degree of patient discomfort. In longer procedures patients may benefit from continuous sedation in order to tolerate lying quietly for a prolonged period. Some surgeons prefer that the patient be awake and cooperative, especially when topical anesthesia is used.

The desired level of sedation may be achieved with the intravenous administration of rapid-onset, short-duration drugs. For example, the benzodiazepine midazolam (Versed) can be titrated in 0.5–1.0 mg increments to a total dose of 2.0 mg. Alternatively the barbiturate methohexital (Brevital) or the sedative-hypnotic propofol (Diprivan) may be given in 15–20 mg increments to a total dose of 30–60 mg. The advantages of methohexital and propofol are rapid onset (45–90 seconds) and short duration (5–15 minutes) of sedation, compared with an onset of 3 minutes and duration of 1–3 hours for midazolam.

Patient safety always comes first. Oversedation or increased drug sensitivity may lead to hypoventilation, hypoxia, obstructed breathing, and disorientation. Oxygen and a manual resuscitator (eg, Ambu bag) for ventilation should always be readily available when sedation is given. Sedation must be attained while providing cardiopulmonary stability, good operating conditions, and a rapid return to the patient's preoperative mental and general physical status. Most ophthalmic surgery is performed on an outpatient basis, so a rapid return to full recovery is extremely important. In many cases, sedation is administered by anesthesia personnel who have experience with the medications and can focus solely on their management during the surgical procedure. (See also "Minimizing Medication Errors: Communication About Drug Orders" in Chapter 17.)

Local Anesthetic Agents

Local anesthetic agents may be delivered topically, intraocularly, or by orbital injection. It is important to be familiar with the onset and duration of action of the various agents, as the expected length of the surgical procedure influences the choice of agent. Local anesthetics administered by orbital injection are frequently combined to produce a rapid onset and long duration. Certain adjuvant drugs are also commonly used to augment their effect.

Topical Anesthetic Agents

Table 13-1 lists topical anesthetic agents in common use for ocular surgery. The onset of anesthesia following instillation of each of the commonly used agents is within 15–20 seconds and lasts 15–30 minutes. Superficial punctate keratopathy may result from all of the topical anesthetic agents due to epithelial toxicity and inhibition of epithelial cell division.

Cocaine

Cocaine was one of the first anesthetic agents used in ocular surgery. In addition to its anesthetic effect, cocaine is unique in that it produces vasoconstriction. Cocaine's use for topical anesthesia in ocular surgery has largely been abandoned because it produces corneal clouding due to epithelial toxicity. Its most common current use is for surface anesthesia of the upper respiratory tract in select oculoplastics procedures.

Proparacaine

Proparacaine 0.5% produces a rapid onset of corneal and conjunctival anesthesia with the least amount of discomfort. A single drop is adequate to anesthetize the eye for applanation

Table 13-1 Topical Anesthetic Agents

Generic Name	Trade Name	Concentration (%)	Duration of Action (min)
Cocaine		20	1–4
Proparacaine	AK-Taine	0.5	15
	Alcaine		
	Ophthaine		
	Ophthetic		
Tetracaine	Ak-T-Caine	0.5	15
	Pontocaine		
	Anethaine		
Lidocaine	Xylocaine	2–4	15
	Atken		

tonometry. However, 1 drop should be administered every 5 minutes for approximately 5 doses to produce deeper anesthesia for ocular surgery.

Tetracaine

Tetracaine 0.5% has a slower time of onset and invokes more discomfort than proparacaine. The deeper anesthesia it produces still makes it a very useful agent in ophthalmic procedures. Local vasodilation results from its direct action on blood vessels.

Lidocaine

Lidocaine 4% solution and 2% or 3.5% gel is often used topically in ophthalmology. Of all anesthetic agents for ocular use, it is the least toxic to the corneal epithelium. Topical lidocaine produces deep anesthesia with a relatively long duration of action, making it a popular anesthetic agent among cataract surgeons.

Intraocular Anesthetic Agents

Intraocular anesthesia may be administered as an adjunct to topical anesthesia. Benzalkonium chloride is known to be toxic to the corneal endothelium, so agents injected intraocularly should be free of this preservative. Nonpreserved lidocaine 1% is generally the anesthetic agent injected intracamerally, but the use of preservative-free tetracaine has been reported.

Regional Anesthetic Agents

Table 13-2 lists regional anesthetic agents in common use for ocular surgery. Combining local anesthetics is a common practice when providing regional ophthalmic anesthesia. Rapid-onset, short-acting agents like lidocaine or mepivacaine are frequently compounded with a long-acting, slow-onset agent like bupivacaine. The mixture combines the best properties of its constituents providing a fast onset of anesthesia and long duration of postoperative analgesia. When local anesthetics are mixed for injection, the final concentration of each constituent is diluted by the others. For example, a 1:1 mixture of lidocaine 4% and bupivacaine 0.75% produces a solution containing lidocaine 2% and bupivacaine 0.375%. The incidence of systemic toxicity with regional anesthesia relates to the drugs used, the total dosage administered, the vascularity of the injection site, and whether epinephrine was used as an adjuvant. Systemic toxicity with regional ophthalmic anesthesia is very rare, given the relatively small amount of anesthetic agent required for ophthalmic procedures.

Table 13-2 Regional Anesthetic Agents

Generic Name	Trade Name	Concentration (%)	Onset of Action (min)	Duration of Action (min)
Lidocaine	Xylocaine	1–4	4–6	40–60 120 (with epinephrine)
Mepivacaine	Carbocaine	1–2	3–5	120
Bupivacaine	Marcaine	0.25–0.75	5–11	480–720 (with epinephrine)
Etidocaine	Duranest	1–1.5	3	300–600

Lidocaine

Lidocaine (Xylocaine) is commonly used in concentrations of 2% and 4% for regional anesthesia. It has a rapid onset of action and superb tissue penetration. The relatively short duration of action of lidocaine may be disadvantageous with prolonged ocular surgery, but its action may be extended by 75% or more with the addition of epinephrine.

Mepivacaine

Mepivacaine (Carbocaine) is generally used in a concentration of 2%. It has a clinical activity similar to lidocaine, but the duration of action of mepivacaine is about twice that of lidocaine because it has fewer vasodilatory properties.

Bupivacaine

Bupivacaine (Marcaine) in a concentration of 0.75% is typically used for regional ophthalmic anesthesia. It is a modified form of mepivacaine with higher lipid solubility and protein-binding properties resulting in an increased potency and longer duration of action. The reduced tissue penetrance of bupivacaine delays its onset of action. Sodium bicarbonate will precipitate bupivacaine.

Etidocaine

Etidocaine (Duranest) is used in ophthalmic anesthesia typically in a 1.5% concentration. It is a modified form of lidocaine with a higher potency and a more prolonged duration of action. Unlike bupivacaine, etidocaine has a rapid onset of action. Because it couples fast onset and long duration of effect, etidocaine is a popular local anesthetic agent in many ophthalmic practices.

Adjuvant Agents

Epinephrine, hyaluronidase, and sodium bicarbonate are adjuvant drugs that are commonly used to enhance the effect of regional anesthesia. Table 13-3 lists the constituents of a solution commonly used for regional anesthesia administered in a retrobulbar or peribulbar block.

Epinephrine

Epinephrine causes vasoconstriction at the site of injection, thereby delaying the absorption of regional anesthetic agents. The duration of action is prolonged for all except the

Table 13-3 Anesthetic Solution Commonly Used for Regional Anesthesia

Amount	Generic Name
10 mL	Lidocaine 2%–4%
10 mL	Bupivacaine 0.75%
0.1 mL	Epinephrine 1:200,000
150 units	Hyaluronidase
0.1 mEq	Sodium bicarbonate

longest-acting agents, and the effectiveness of the block is improved. The addition of 0.1 mL of 1:1000 epinephrine (100 µg) to 20 mL of regional anesthetic solution is standard, producing a concentration of 5 µg/mL (1:200,000).

Hyaluronidase

Hyaluronidase promotes the spread of the anesthetic solution through tissue. The enzyme causes a reversible hydrolysis of extracellular hyaluronic acid, breaking down collagen bonds and allowing the anesthetic to spread across fine connective tissue barriers. Hyaluronidase is typically added to the regional anesthetic injectant in a concentration of 7.5 units/mL.

Sodium bicarbonate

Sodium bicarbonate augments the tissue penetrance and onset of action of local anesthetic agents by adjusting the pH of the solution toward the un-ionized basic form.

Local Anesthesia

The use of topical and intraocular anesthesia involves appropriate patient selection and modification in surgical techniques.

Topical Anesthesia

With the advent of small-incision phacoemulsification cataract surgery, topical anesthesia has grown in popularity. Topical anesthesia provides anesthesia to the cornea, conjunctiva, and anterior sclera, but sensation is maintained in the eyelids, posterior sclera, intraocular tissues, and extraocular muscles. Therefore, when using topical anesthesia it is important to avoid excessive cautery, placement of a bridle suture, or manipulation of the iris. A modification in surgical technique is required when using topical anesthesia because sudden eye movements may be dangerous when instrumenting the eye. The surgeon may choose to immobilize the globe using his or her nondominant hand whenever instruments are being used.

Appropriate patient selection is critical when considering topical anesthesia. A cooperative patient who is able to follow instructions during surgery is required. The patient's response to tonometry and A-scan ultrasonography appears to be a good predictor of how he or she will tolerate ocular surgery with this technique. Monocular patients may benefit from topical anesthesia because of their unique need for quick recovery of vision from the operated eye. Inappropriate candidates include patients who are very young, have a strong blink reflex, are unable to fixate (eg, because of macular degeneration), or have difficulty following commands (eg, because of dementia, deafness, language barriers). Patients for whom surgery will be longer (more than 30–40 minutes) or difficult (eg, dense cataracts, small pupils, weak zonules) are best managed with other forms of anesthesia.

Table 13-4 lists the advantages and disadvantages of topical anesthesia. The obvious advantage is avoidance of complications associated with injection into the orbit. Additionally, topical anesthesia eliminates the need to patch the eye after surgery because it avoids the temporary visual loss from the eye undergoing surgery as well as the risk of exposure keratopathy from lagophthalmos resulting from a block. Furthermore, there is no need to

Table 13-4 Advantages and Disadvantages of Topical Anesthesia

Advantages	Avoids complications associated with orbital injection of anesthesia
	Eliminates the need to patch the eye after surgery
	Avoids the temporary loss of vision in the eye undergoing surgery
	No need to interrupt anticoagulant or antiplatelet therapy
Disadvantages	Patients are aware of surgical procedure
	Discomfort with the eyelid speculum and microscope light
	Pain associated with intraocular manipulation or IOP fluctuations
	Lack of akinesia

consider interrupting anticoagulant or antiplatelet therapy. Disadvantages include patient awareness during the surgical procedure, discomfort with the eyelid speculum and microscope light, pain associated with intraocular manipulation or intraocular pressure (IOP) fluctuation, lack of akinesia, and reliance on patient cooperation.

Delivery of topical anesthesia

An anesthetic agent is instilled topically onto the eye just before prepping the eye. The patient is instructed to fixate on the microscope light during the surgery to keep the eye stationary. Anesthetic drops are administered during the surgical procedure as needed. A variation of the technique involves placing pieces of ophthalmic cellulose sponge (eg, Weck-Cel) or instrument wipe sponges (pledgets) saturated with anesthetic in the superior and inferior fornices. The pledgets are removed at the beginning or conclusion of the surgery. Sedative drugs can be helpful but are generally used minimally with topical anesthesia to allow retention of patient cooperation.

Intraocular Anesthesia

Intraocular anesthesia may be used in conjunction with topical anesthesia. The combination allows anesthesia of the cornea, conjunctiva, anterior sclera, iris, and ciliary body. The benefit of intraocular anesthesia is a reduction in pain associated with IOP fluctuation and manipulation of the iris, ciliary body, and lens. Patient selection is the same as for surgery performed under topical anesthesia alone.

Delivery of intraocular anesthesia

Nonpreserved lidocaine 1% is irrigated into the anterior chamber through a paracentesis or side-port incision. Directing the drug posterior to the iris during injection may provide a maximal effect on the iris and ciliary body. After 15–30 seconds, the anesthetic is washed out by irrigation of balanced salt solution or viscoelastic. (See the review of intraocular fluids in Chapter 16.) A transient decrease in vision may occur if the anesthetic reaches the retina.

Regional Anesthesia

Regional anesthesia for intraocular surgery involves the injection of anesthetic agents into the orbit to provide anesthesia to the cornea, conjunctiva, sclera, intraocular structures, and extraocular muscles. Retrobulbar, peribulbar, and parabulbar blocks are the common methods to deliver regional anesthesia. There is little or no patient sensitivity to IOP fluctuations and to the microscope light with regional anesthesia. Extraocular motility is eliminated, so there is less need for patient cooperation to control eye movements. Surgical procedures that require extensive intraocular manipulation or are expected to be lengthy (more than 30–40 minutes in duration) are best performed with regional anesthesia.

Table 13-5 lists the advantages and disadvantages of regional anesthesia. Regional anesthesia offers the advantages of full anesthesia and akinesia of the eye, reduced reliance on patient cooperation as compared with topical anesthesia, and suitability for surgical procedures of relatively greater complexity and longer duration. Disadvantages of this technique for ocular anesthesia include the need to patch the eye during the postoperative period of recovery from anesthesia, advisability of interrupting anticoagulant or antiplatelet therapy, and potential complications associated with the orbital injection of anesthesia.

Retrobulbar Block

In a retrobulbar block, anesthetic solution is injected into the space behind the globe within the muscle cone of the 4 rectus muscles. A 1.25-inch, 25- or 27-gauge needle is inserted transcutaneously or transconjunctivally just above the inferior orbital rim at a point in line with the lateral limbus (Fig 13-1). A short-beveled, blunt needle (Atkinson) can be used to reduce the risk of scleral perforation and retrobulbar hemorrhage. A sharp disposable needle produces less injection pain and is safe when proper injection technique is employed. The patient should be in primary gaze; an upward and inward gaze should be avoided because it places the optic nerve in a more vulnerable position. During entry of the needle, an index fingertip may be positioned between the globe and orbital rim to elevate the eye. The needle is advanced tangential to the globe and parallel to the bony floor of the orbit.

Once the equator of the globe is passed, the needle is redirected upward and medially into the muscle cone. Increased resistance or globe rotation during needle advancement could indicate engagement of the sclera; if either is detected, the needle should be repositioned. It has been suggested that the needle should not be inserted more than 31 mm from the orbital rim, and the midsagittal plane of the eye should not be crossed because the optic nerve lies on the nasal side of this plane. After aspiration to ensure that the needle tip is not in a blood vessel, 3–4 mL of anesthetic solution is injected slowly. As the needle is withdrawn, orbicularis oculi muscle akinesia may be achieved by injecting 1–2 mL of anesthetic anterior to the orbital septum.

Table 13-5 Advantages and Disadvantages of Regional Anesthesia

Advantages	Full anesthesia and akinesia of the eye
	Reduced reliance on patient cooperation
	Suitable for surgical procedures of relatively greater complexity and longer duration
Disadvantages	Need to patch the eye during postoperative period of recovery from anesthesia
	Advisable to interrupt anticoagulant and antiplatelet therapy
	Complications associated with orbital injection of anesthesia

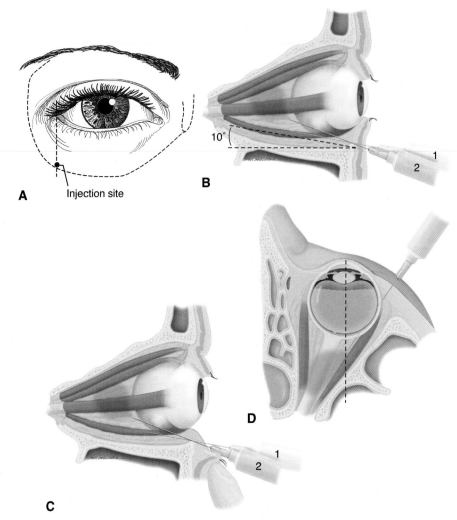

Figure 13-1 Retrobulbar block. A 1.25-inch, 25- or 27-gauge needle is inserted at the inferotemporal orbital rim at a point in line with the lateral limbus **(A)**. The needle is advanced tangential to the globe and parallel to the bony floor of the orbit, which inclines at an angle of 10° from the transverse plane **(B1)**. Once the equator of the globe is passed, the needle is redirected upward and medially into the muscle cone **(B2)**. Either a transcutaneous **(B)** or transconjunctival **(C)** approach may be used. **(D)** The midsagittal plane of the eye should not be crossed because the optic nerve lies on the nasal side of this plane. *(Illustration by Mark M. Miller.)*

After injection, orbital compression is maintained for several minutes using manual compression or a mechanical compression device (eg, Honan balloon) to assist in the spread of anesthesia. While orbital compression has been used safely for many years, it has been implicated as a cause of ptosis and impaired retinal circulation in case reports.

After about 5 minutes, an assessment of globe movement and orbicularis function is made. If akinesia is inadequate, a supplemental injection may be given. Small rotational movements of the globe are commonly seen. The motor nerves to the 4 rectus muscles and inferior oblique access their respective muscle bellies within the muscle cone, whereas the trochlear nerve remains outside the cone and enters the superior oblique at its superolateral edge. This anatomic difference explains the limited akinesia of the superior oblique after a retrobulbar block.

Peribulbar Block

A peribulbar block involves injection of anesthetic solution within the orbit, but outside the muscle cone. A 1-inch, 25- or 27-gauge, blunt-tipped (Atkinson) or sharp disposable needle is inserted in the same transcutaneous or transconjunctival location as described for a retrobulbar block (Fig 13-2). The needle is advanced tangential to the eye with penetration 3–4 mm posterior to the equator of the globe. After aspiration, 4–8 mL of anesthetic solution is injected slowly. Akinesia of the orbicularis muscle can

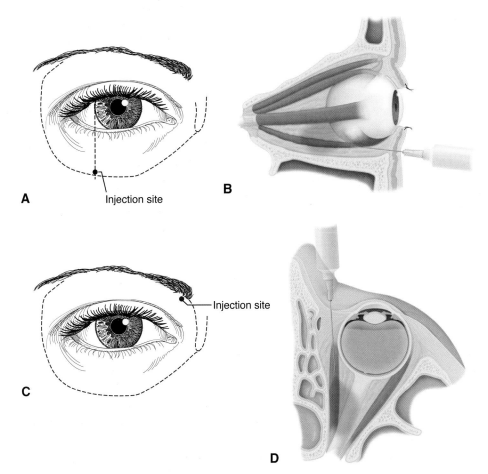

Figure 13-2   Peribulbar block. A 1-inch, 25- or 27-gauge needle is inserted at the inferotemporal orbital rim at a point in line with the lateral limbus **(A). B,** The needle is advanced tangential to the globe and parallel to the orbital floor with penetration 3–4 mm posterior to the equator. **C,** If necessary, an additional injection may be made in the upper eyelid at a point midway between the medial canthus and supraorbital notch. **D,** The needle is advanced tangential to the globe to the equator. *(Illustration by Mark M. Miller.)*

be achieved by injecting 1–2 mL of anesthetic into the lower lid anterior to the orbital septum. Pressure is applied to the eye using manual compression or a mechanical compression device (eg, Honan balloon). Globe motility and eyelid function are evaluated after 10–20 minutes.

If necessary, an additional injection may be made in the upper eyelid at a point midway between the medial canthus and supraorbital notch at a point in line with the medial limbus. The needle is advanced tangential to the globe to the equator, and an additional 2–3 mL of anesthetic solution is injected after aspiration. Only 15%–20% of peribulbar blocks require an upper lid injection to supplement a lower lid injection. There is a greater risk of ptosis and scleral perforation with upper lid injections.

Many surgeons have abandoned the retrobulbar block in favor of the peribulbar block. The major advantage of the peribulbar block over the retrobulbar block is the reduced risk of rare, yet serious complications such as retrobulbar hemorrhage, scleral perforation, central nervous system anesthesia, and optic nerve damage. In patients with high myopia and a long axial length, which may increase the risk of globe perforation with more posterior injection, it is prudent to use a peribulbar block or general anesthesia rather than a retrobulbar block. The disadvantage of the peribulbar technique is a slower onset of anesthesia, the need for a larger total volume of injected anesthetic solution, and the frequent requirement for supplemental injections.

Parabulbar Block

A parabulbar block entails injection of anesthetic solution into the anterior intraconal space using a blunt cannula after dissection into the sub-Tenon space. After administration of topical anesthesia, an incision is made through conjunctiva and Tenon capsule. A blunt metal or flexible cannula is introduced into the sub-Tenon space, and the tip is passed posteriorly beyond the equator of the globe (Fig 13-3). Local anesthetic solution is injected; the degree of akinesia and anesthesia is proportional to the volume of anesthetic used. Disadvantages of this technique include an increased incidence of conjunctival chemosis and hemorrhage, risk of damage to the vortex veins, and a frequent need for supplementation.

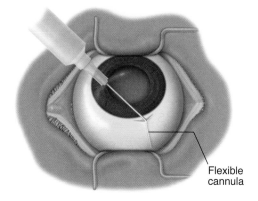

Figure 13-3 Parabulbar block. A blunt metal or flexible cannula is introduced into the sub-Tenon space and passed posteriorly beyond the equator of the globe. *(Illustration by Mark M. Miller.)*

Flexible cannula

General Anesthesia

In the elderly population, the advantages of regional anesthesia usually outweigh those of general anesthesia for the performance of safe and comfortable surgery in a cost-effective manner. While the incidences of death and major complications are similar between general and regional anesthesia, general anesthesia has been reported to produce more postoperative nausea and vomiting, intraoperative oxygen desaturation and hemodynamic fluctuation, and initial postoperative pain. Therefore, it is prudent to avoid general anesthesia in patients with severe cardiovascular or pulmonary disease if possible.

General anesthesia in ophthalmology is typically used in pediatric strabismus surgery and lengthy vitreoretinal procedures. Additionally, patients who cannot cooperate adequately (eg, children or people with tremor, inability to lie supine, or severe mental or psychological impairment) may not be candidates for regional anesthesia in any surgical procedure. Patients who have experienced a prior complication with regional anesthesia (eg, retrobulbar hemorrhage, inadvertent intrathecal injection of anesthetic) should have subsequent ocular surgery under general anesthesia. Lengthy ocular procedures (more than 3 or 4 hours) may require general anesthesia or may benefit from the use of low-dose propofol, dexmedetomidine, or remifentanil.

Table 13-6 lists advantages and disadvantages of general anesthesia. General anesthesia offers the advantages of complete control of the patient, avoidance of complications associated with orbital injection, and application to patients in all age groups. Disadvantages of general anesthesia include absence of postoperative analgesia, an increased incidence of postoperative nausea and vomiting, greater intraoperative cardiovascular and pulmonary stress, a risk of malignant hyperthermia, slower immediate postoperative recovery, and greater cost.

The main requirements for general anesthesia in ocular surgery are anesthesia and akinesia of the globe and eyelids and control of the IOP (to protect against extrusion of intraocular contents). A variety of inhalation and intravenous agents may be used to accomplish these goals. Following a smooth induction, a deep level of anesthesia is maintained until the wound has been closed. A depolarizing muscle relaxant is commonly administered while the eye is open. Intraoperative use of antiemetics decreases the incidence of postoperative nausea and vomiting.

Table 13-6 Advantages and Disadvantages of General Anesthesia

Advantages	Complete control of patient
	Avoids complications associated with orbital injection
	Applicable to all ages
Disadvantages	Absence of postoperative analgesia
	More postoperative nausea and vomiting
	Greater cardiovascular and pulmonary stress
	Risk of malignant hyperthermia
	Slower immediate postoperative recovery
	More expensive

Ocular complications associated with general anesthesia for eye surgery are usually related to coughing and straining during surgery or nausea and vomiting in the postoperative period. Sudden changes in IOP may lead to suprachoroidal hemorrhage, wound dehiscence, or vitreous loss. Most intravenous and inhalation anesthetics used in general anesthesia produce a reduction in IOP. The use of nitrous oxide gas should be discontinued at least 20 minutes before intravitreal gas injection (SF_6, C_3F_8) during vitreoretinal procedures. Nitrous oxide rapidly enters the gas bubble, producing an increase in its size and IOP elevation.

Facial Nerve Blocks

Contraction of the orbicularis oculi muscle (innervated by branches of the facial nerve) causes eyelid closure. Following orbital injection of an anesthetic agent and hyaluronidase, spread of the agent anteriorly through the orbital septum typically produces akinesia of the orbicularis oculi muscle. Therefore, facial nerve blocks are generally not required when a retrobulbar or peribulbar block is administered. In the rare cases when eyelid squeezing is still present, a facial nerve block may prove useful. Various techniques for facial nerve blocks (including the Van Lint block, O'Brien block, and Nadbath-Ellis block) have been developed.

Van Lint Block

The Van Lint block involves infiltrating anesthesia in the region of the terminal branches of the facial nerve. A 1.5-inch, 25-gauge disposable needle is inserted 1 cm lateral to the lateral orbital rim (Fig 13-4A). After aspiration, 1–2 mL of anesthetic solution is injected

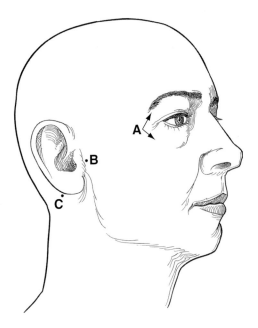

Figure 13-4 Facial nerve blocks. **A,** Van Lint block. **B,** O'Brien block. **C,** Nadbath-Ellis block. *(Illustration by Mark M. Miller.)*

deeply on the periosteum. The needle is withdrawn slightly and redirected along the inferior orbital margin injecting 1–2 mL of anesthetic outside the orbital rim. The needle is withdrawn to the original entry site and redirected along the superior orbital margin injecting an additional 1–2 mL of anesthetic solution.

O'Brien Block

The O'Brien block produces akinesia of the orbicularis oculi muscle by anesthetizing the facial nerve at its proximal trunk. The condyloid process of the mandible is palpated in front of the tragus. By asking the patient to open and close his or her mouth, the condyloid process may be felt moving forward under the finger. A 1-inch, 27-gauge disposable needle is inserted at the center of the condyloid process to the periosteum (Fig 13-4B). After aspiration, 3 mL of anesthetic solution is injected.

Nadbath-Ellis Block

The Nadbath-Ellis block involves injection of anesthetic solution in the region where the facial nerve emerges from the stylomastoid foramen. The tympanomastoid fissure is palpated at the anterosuperior border of the mastoid process, where it fuses with the tympanic portion of the temporal bone. The area may be felt as a convexity below the external auditory meatus and behind the pinna. A 5/8-inch, 25- or 26-gauge disposable needle is inserted into the tympanomastoid fissure (Fig 13-4C). After aspiration, 1–2 mL of anesthetic solution is injected. The injection should be made with the head turned to the opposite side to pull the sternocleidomastoid muscle out of the area, and with the mouth closed to widen the space between the mandible and mastoid process.

Complications of Ophthalmic Anesthesia

Possible complications of ophthalmic anesthesia include those associated with orbital injection, the oculocardiac reflex, and malignant hyperthermia.

Complications of Orbital Injection

Complications as a result of injection of anesthesia into the orbit include retrobulbar hemorrhage, scleral perforation, spread of anesthetic into the central nervous system, and strabismus.

Retrobulbar hemorrhage

Retrobulbar hemorrhages vary in severity but generally present with subconjunctival hemorrhage, eyelid ecchymosis, proptosis, and elevated IOP. Venous hemorrhages usually spread slowly and are limited, while arterial hemorrhages develop rapidly and can be massive. Vascular compromise to the optic nerve and retina may result. The incidence of serious retrobulbar bleeding has been reported as 0.1%–3%. The IOP should be monitored after a retrobulbar hemorrhage. Treatment should be instituted with aqueous suppressants, a hyperosmotic agent, and lateral canthotomy and cantholysis as needed.

The surgical procedure should be cancelled when a serious retrobulbar hemorrhage has occurred.

Scleral perforation

It is imperative that proper technique be used when administering regional anesthetic blocks to minimize the risk of scleral perforation. There is a greater risk of globe perforation in myopic eyes, a superior injection, improper needle insertion, and use of long (1.5-inch), sharp needles. Scleral perforation is a complication occurring in 1 in 1,300 to 12,000 retrobulbar and peribulbar blocks. It may manifest with immediate ocular pain with injection, hypotony, poor red reflex, and vitreous hemorrhage. The planned surgery should be cancelled if this complication occurs, and immediate consultation with a vitreo-retinal specialist arranged, to evaluate the retina for tears and detachment.

Central nervous system spread of anesthesia

A potentially lethal complication of regional anesthetic blocks is the central nervous system (CNS) spread of anesthetic along the optic nerve dural sheath into the subarachnoid space, pons, and midbrain. The incidence of this complication is 1 in 350 to 500 patients. CNS spread of anesthesia should be suspected with symptoms of mental confusion, shivering, seizures, nausea or vomiting, dysphagia, sudden swings in cardiovascular vital signs, or respiratory depression. There may be amaurosis, extraocular muscle paresis, and pupillary dilation in the contralateral eye.

Symptoms of brainstem anesthesia usually develop within 2–30 minutes of retrobulbar injection, and they may last for 30 minutes or several hours. This complication emphasizes the need for a standby anesthesiologist when administering regional ocular anesthesia and a favorable outcome is usually observed when immediate support is provided. To prevent the CNS spread of anesthesia, deep orbital injection should be avoided and the eye should be maintained in primary gaze during the block. When the eye is turned upward and inward, the optic nerve and nerve sheath are in a more vulnerable position to the retrobulbar needle.

Strabismus

Strabismus may develop after injection of regional anesthesia into the orbit. Persistent extraocular muscle dysfunction and diplopia is common during the first 24–48 hours postoperatively, especially when large volumes of long-acting anesthetic agents are used. Permanent strabismus may occur if fusion cannot be recovered after disruption by the anesthesia, due to pre-existing conditions such as thyroid eye disease, myasthenia gravis, cranial nerve palsies, or prolonged visual deprivation from a cataract. Animal and human studies have demonstrated myotoxicity of local anesthetic agents, particularly when injected into muscle bellies. The inferior rectus muscle is most often affected. Persistent diplopia may be treated with prism or strabismus surgery.

Oculocardiac Reflex

The oculocardiac reflex (OCR) is stimulated when traction on extraocular muscles produces vagal effects on the heart via a trigeminal-vagal reflex. Direct pressure on the globe, orbital anesthetic injection, and elevation of IOP may also elicit this reflex. Cardiac manifestations of the OCR include bradycardia, ectopic beats, nodal rhythms, atrioventricular block, and even cardiac arrest. The OCR is most commonly observed with strabismus surgery, but it may occur with other ocular procedures (eg, enucleation, retinal surgery) under either local or general anesthesia. Therefore, EKG monitoring should be performed continuously during all ophthalmic surgeries. The surgeon should immediately stop manipulating the eye or its muscles when an arrhythmia occurs. The OCR fatigues easily, and usually there is little or no activity after a brief pause in surgical stimuli. When OCR is severe, it may be treated with intravenous atropine.

Malignant Hyperthermia

Malignant hyperthermia is a rare disorder of skeletal muscle metabolism that can be triggered by succinylcholine and the inhalation anesthetics halothane, enflurane, and isoflurane. Its incidence has been estimated as 1 in 15,000, and patients with muscle abnormalities like strabismus and ptosis are thought to be at greater risk for developing it. The disorder is inherited in an autosomal dominant pattern. Before strabismus surgery, it is important to inquire about previous anesthetic problems in both parents and their families.

Malignant hyperthermia presents with tachycardia, tachypnea, hypercarbia, muscle spasm, severe acidosis, and a rapid rise in body temperature, The ophthalmic surgeon should be aware of these early manifestations, as early recognition may be life-saving. Upon recognition of malignant hyperthermia, anesthetic agents should be discontinued, hyperventilation with oxygen started, and treatment with dantrolene begun. Surgery should be terminated as soon as possible, even if the procedure is not complete.

Key Points

- The most commonly used topical ophthalmic anesthetic agents are proparacaine 0.5%, tetracaine 0.5%, and lidocaine 2%–4%.
- The most commonly used regional ophthalmic anesthetic agents are lidocaine (Xylocaine) 2%–4%, mepivacaine (Carbocaine) 2%, bupivacaine (Marcaine) 0.75%, and etidocaine (Duranest) 1.5%.
- Epinephrine (1:1000) and hyaluronidase are often added to regional anesthesia solutions to enhance activity.
- Common regional ophthalmic anesthetic techniques include retrobulbar or peribulbar injection and facial nerve blocks.
- Potential complications from orbital injection include orbital hemorrhage, scleral perforation, CNS spread of anesthesia, and strabismus.
- General anesthesia in ophthalmology is typically used in pediatric strabismus surgery and lengthy vitreoretinal procedures, and in patients who cannot cooperate adequately for local anesthesia.

Ahn JC, Stanley JA. Subarachnoid injection as a complication of retrobulbar anesthesia. *Am J Ophthalmol.* 1987;103(2):225–230.

Britton B, Hervey R, Kasten K, Gregg S, McDonald T. Intraocular irritation evaluation of benzalkonium chloride in rabbits. *Ophthalmic Surg.* 1976;7(3):46–55.

Cyriac IC, Pineda R. Postoperative complications of periocular anesthesia. *Int Ophthalmol Clin.* 2000;40(1):85–91.

Donlon JV. Anesthesia for ophthalmic surgery. In: Albert DM, Jakobiec FA, et al, eds. *Principles and Practice of Ophthalmology.* Philadelphia: Saunders; 1994: vol 5.

Duker JS, Belmont JB, Benson WE, et al. Inadvertent globe perforations during retrobulbar and peribulbar anesthesia. Patient characteristics, surgical management, and visual outcome. *Ophthalmology.* 1991;98(4):519–526.

Fanning GL. Monitored sedation for ophthalmic surgery. In: Kumar CM, Dodds C, Fanning GL, eds. *Ophthalmic Anesthesia.* Lisse, Netherlands: Swets & Zeitlinger; 2002: chap 8.

Fraser SG, Siriwadena D, Jamieson H, Girault J, Bryan SJ. Indicators of patient suitability for topical anesthesia. *J Cataract Refract Surg.* 1997;23(5):781–783.

Hamilton RC, Gimbel HV, Strunin L. Regional anaesthesia for 12,000 cataract extraction and intraocular lens implantation procedures. *Can J Anaesth.* 1988;35(6):615–623.

Katsev DA, Drews RC, Rose BT. An anatomic study of retrobulbar needle path length. *Ophthalmology.* 1989;96(8):1221–1224.

Kumar CM, Dowd TC. Complications of ophthalmic regional blocks: their treatment and prevention. *Ophthalmologica.* 2006;220(2):73–82.

Lynch S, Wolf GL, Berlin I. General anesthesia for cataract surgery: a comparative review of 2217 consecutive cases. *Anesth Analg.* 1974;53(6):909–913.

Morgan CM, Schatz H, Vine AK, et al. Ocular complications associated with retrobulbar injections. *Ophthalmology.* 1988;95(5):660–665.

Navaleza JS, Pendse SJ, Blecher MH. Choosing anesthesia for cataract surgery. *Ophthalmol Clin N Am.* 2006;19(2):233–237.

Nicoll JM, Acharya PA, Ahlen K, Baguneid S, Edge KR. Central nervous system complications after 6000 retrobulbar blocks. *Anesth Analg.* 1987;66(12):1298–1302.

Rainin EA, Carlson BM. Postoperative diplopia and ptosis. A clinical hypothesis based on the myotoxicity of local anesthetics. *Arch Ophthalmol.* 1985;103(9):1337–1339.

Rosenthal KJ. Deep, topical, nerve-block anesthesia. *J Cataract Refract Surg.* 1995;21(5): 499–503.

Stead SW, Miller KM. Anesthesia for ophthalmic surgery. In: Spaeth GL, ed. *Ophthalmic Surgery: Principles and Practice.* Philadelphia: Saunders; 2003: chap 2.

Unsold R, Stanley JA, DeGroot J. The CT-topography of retrobulbar anesthesia. Anatomic-clinical correlation of complications and suggestion of a modified technique. *Albrecht von Graefes Arch Klin Exp Ophthalmol.* 1981;217(2):125–136.

Self-Assessment Test

1. A rapid-onset, short-acting anesthetic agent like lidocaine is frequently combined with a long-acting, slow-onset agent like bupivacaine for regional anesthesia by orbital injection. (true or false)

2. Which agent is routinely added to anesthetic solution to enhance regional anesthesia?

   a. hyaluronidase

   b. sodium chloride

   c. atropine

   d. cocaine

3. When administering a retrobulbar block, the patient should be instructed to look upward and inward. (true or false)
4. Which of the following would make a patient a poor candidate for topical anesthesia? (Choose all that apply.)
    a. demented person
    b. deaf person
    c. person with a strong blink reflex
    d. all of the above
5. Which patient should have his or her ocular procedure performed under general anesthesia? (Choose all that apply.)
    a. 6-month-old infant undergoing strabismus surgery
    b. 50-year-old man undergoing a lengthy vitreoretinal procedure
    c. 72-year-old woman undergoing cataract surgery after her prior surgery was cancelled due to a retrobulbar hemorrhage during the retrobulbar block
    d. all of the above
6. During general anesthesia, nitrous oxide should be discontinued at least 20 minutes before injection of C_3F_8 or SF_6 gas into the vitreous cavity. (true or false)
7. It is best to avoid a retrobulbar block in highly myopic eyes with a long axial length. (true or false)

For preferred responses to these questions, see Appendix A.

CHAPTER 14

Hemostasis

J. Paul Dieckert, MD, MBA

Hemostasis in ocular surgery is vital to achieving surgical objectives, visualizing important structures, increasing operative safety, and minimizing surgical complications. This chapter organizes the subject into 6 key areas: prevention, heating, vasoconstriction, biochemical enhancement of hemostasis, mechanical tamponade, and embolization.

Prevention

In ophthalmic plastic surgery, preoperative control of hypertension and avoidance of aspirin 2 weeks prior to surgery are important measures to diminish risk of excessive intraoperative and postoperative bleeding. The reverse Trendelenburg position reduces venous congestion and may lessen the risk of hemorrhage associated with anesthetic injection. Hypotensive anesthesia can be an important intraoperative preventative measure. In patients with classic hemophilia, intravenous (IV) cryoprecipitate factor VIII has been used effectively to prevent hemorrhage during retrobulbar anesthesia and peripheral iridectomy in patients with classic hemophilia. As citric acid in balanced salt solution causes a 50% increase in bleeding times, avoidance of irrigating solutions containing citric acid is recommended in trauma and other cases prone to heavy bleeding.

Heating

Cautery, diathermy, and photocoagulation are thermal methods used to achieve homeostasis.

Cautery

Cautery, once common in eyelid procedures, involves the application of an electrically heated wire to bleeding vessels. The heating induces coagulation of tissue proteins. The coagulum then acts as a barrier to further blood flow, followed by blanching, charring, and tissue contraction.

Diathermy

Diathermy, either monopolar or bipolar, achieves heating by passing an electric current through the target tissue (Figs 14-1, 14-2, and 14-3). Monopolar diathermy occurs when

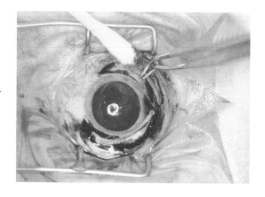

Figure 14-1 Bipolar diathermy forceps. *(Courtesy of J. Paul Dieckert, MD.)*

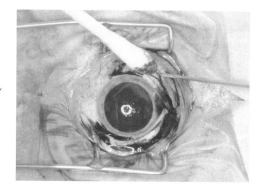

Figure 14-2 Bipolar diathermy probe. *(Courtesy of J. Paul Dieckert, MD.)*

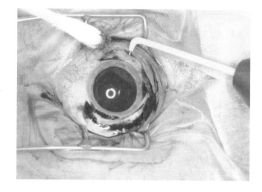

Figure 14-3 Monopolar diathermy probe. *(Courtesy of J. Paul Dieckert, MD.)*

electrical current is passed from an electrode near the tissue to be treated to an electrode elsewhere in the body. Bipolar diathermy occurs when both electrodes are mounted on the same device and electrical current passes only through the target tissue. The resistance of the tissue to the electrical current results in heating of the tissue with subsequent co-agulation of proteins and the formation of a coagulum that prevents further blood flow.

Bipolar diathermy is preferred because it restricts the current to an elliptical field between 2 electrodes and avoids passage of current with inadvertent heating injury to nontarget tissues. Bipolar diathermy is useful for intraocular hemostasis. Monopolar diathermy is used to achieve skin hemostasis and to create full-thickness thermal reaction in the choroid and retina during retinopexy.

Diathermy requires direct visualization of the bleeding vessel and is difficult to achieve if diffuse bleeding is present. Excessive diathermy leads to tissue destruction and necrosis. Multifunction instruments with combined bipolar diathermy, aspiration, and reflux are useful in controlling intraocular bleeding during vitrectomy by minimizing the need for multiple instrument exchange. Bipolar diathermy instruments with a tapered blunt tip and 23-gauge diameter are useful in trabeculectomy.

Laser Photocoagulation

Laser photocoagulation achieves heating by application of laser energy to the target tissue. Absorption of the laser energy by the target tissue results in localized heating that creates a coagulum and a secondary barrier to blood flow. Endophotocoagulation is applied via a handheld intraocular probe. The probe contains a fiber-optic line that directly carries the laser energy from a diode or argon laser to the intraocular target tissue. Laser photocoagulation does not require direct contact with bleeding tissue. By aspirating blood, raising intraocular pressure (IOP), and applying photocoagulation to the hemoglobin within the bleeding vessels, hemostasis can be achieved. The carbon dioxide laser has been found to be useful in orbital surgery for hemostasis. The carbon dioxide laser has been used effectively to prevent bleeding during excision of lymphangiomatous tissue involving the ocular adnexa by flash boiling intracellular water at extremely high temperature and creating a thin layer of heat-coagulated tissue in which blood vessels smaller than 1 mm are sealed. High-frequency electrical current similarly cuts and fulgurates tissue, achieving good hemostasis while simultaneously creating a surgical incision.

Vasoconstriction

Vasoconstriction is achieved through the application of epinephrine to the target tissue. The vasoconstriction induced by the epinephrine diminishes blood flow and allows hemostasis to occur. Epinephrine-induced vasoconstriction is restricted to extraocular adnexal surgery in the eyelids and orbit and is available in a premixed proprietary preparation of lidocaine and epinephrine diluted at 1:100,000 for use in local infiltrative anesthesia. Phenylephrine is added to intraocular irrigating solutions primarily to maintain mydriasis.

Biochemical Enhancement of Hemostasis

Thrombin is the mainstay of biochemical enhancement of hemostasis. It can be used in both intra- and extraocular surgery. Thrombin converts fibrinogen to fibrin, induces platelet aggregation, and is nontoxic to the corneal endothelium. It can be used topically or intraocularly. A sterile absorbable gelatin sponge (Gelfoam) soaked with thrombin and used as a stent in dacryocystorhinostomy is useful for hemostasis and does not have to be removed.

Intraocular thrombin is very useful in treatment of penetrating ocular injuries. Thrombin at 100 units/mL is infused intraocularly via the infusion line when bleeding is encountered. In diabetic patients, thrombin can cause excessive postoperative inflammation and sometimes sterile hypopyon.

Surgeons using thrombin intraoperatively should be aware of the dangers of inadvertent intravenous administration. Many surgeons are unaware of the potentially lethal effect of inadvertent IV injection of thrombin. Wesley reported rapid death in an animal model using a dosage similar to that used in ocular surgery. Care should be taken to label or color code containers containing thrombin to avoid accidental IV injection. Heparin injection prior to and after thrombin injection has been shown to prevent the lethal effect in an animal model.

Mechanical Tamponade

Mechanical tamponade refers to the direct application of physical force to staunch blood flow from a bleeding vessel. Raising IOP is the most common and effective way to mechanically control intraocular bleeding. Increased IOP is translated into increased transmural pressure of the blood vessel wall that causes collapse or slowing down of blood flow. This is readily accomplished by raising the level of the infusion bottle. Elevating the IOP risks ocular ischemia and stress to surgical repair of surgical wounds.

Fluid–gas exchange mechanically achieves hemostasis by elevating IOP via control of pump pressure. Intraocular gas has a higher surface tension than intraocular saline and impedes blood flow. Fluid trapped behind a gas bubble has higher concentration of coagulation factors, which contributes to hemostasis. Unfortunately, intraocular gases can impede visibility during surgery, and this technique is usually reserved for the last minutes of the operation.

Other intraocular substances can help control intraoperative bleeding. Perfluorooctane may control intraocular bleeding during vitreoretinal surgery by direct compression or concentration of clotting factors near the bleeding site. Silicone oil controls bleeding by 2 mechanisms: by physical compression and by concentrating clotting factors in a smaller space. Silicone oil interferes with other intraocular maneuvers and is used typically at the end of surgery. Sodium hyaluronate mechanically confines blood and enhances visualization. Unfortunately, it also has mild antiplatelet and anticoagulation properties.

Gelfoam (absorbable gelatin sponge), Surgicel (oxidized regenerated cellulose), and Avitene (microfibrillar collagen) are useful mechanical measures to control and confine intraoperative bleeding in ocular adnexal surgery.

Wound closure is a straightforward technique of mechanically controlling intraoperative bleeding. Direct compression to bleeding vortex veins is useful in strabismus and retinal surgery where vortex vein injury can occur.

Embolization

Preoperative arteriography and embolization with polyvinyl alcohol foam, metrizamide dissolved in dimethyl sulfoxide, steel coils, gel foam particles, and n–butyl cyanoacrylate have been found to be useful preoperatively in minimizing hemorrhage during excision of orbital lymphangiomas and arteriovenous malformations. Inadvertent unintended injury to the optic nerve and retina and spasm of the ophthalmic artery may occur during embolization therapy.

Key Points

- The ophthalmic surgeon has a wide array of preventative, mechanical, and pharmacologic techniques to control surgical bleeding.
- The experienced surgeon applies appropriate measures in a timely fashion to enhance surgical results and surgical efficiency in ophthalmic surgery.

de Bustros S. Intraoperative control of hemorrhage in penetrating ocular injuries. *Retina.* 1990; 10S 1:S55–58.

Fleischman J, Lerner BC, Reimels H. A new intraocular aspiration probe with bipolar cautery and reflux capabilities. *Arch Ophthalmol.* 1989;107(2):283.

Jordan DR, Anderson RL. Carbon dioxide (CO2) laser therapy for conjunctival lymphangioma. *Ophthalmic Surg.* 1987;18(10):728–730.

Kim SH, Cho YS, Choi YJ. Intraocular hemocoagulase in human vitrectomy. *Jpn J Ophthalmol.* 1994;38(1):49–55.

Leone CR Jr. Gelfoam-thrombin dacryocystorhinostomy stent. *Am J Ophthalmol.* 1982;94(3): 412–413.

Mannis MJ, Sweet E, Landers MB 3rd, Lewis RA. Uses of thrombin in ocular surgery. *Arch Ophthalmol.* 1988;106(2):251–253.

Maxwell DP Jr, Orlick ME, Diamond JG. Intermittent intraocular thrombin as an adjunct to vitrectomy. *Ophthalmic Surg.* 1989;20(2):108–111.

Rothkoff L, Biedner B, Shoham K. Bilateral cataract extraction in classic haemophilia with retrobulbar anaesthesia and peripheral iridectomy. *Br J Ophthalmol.* 1977;61(12):765–766.

Shields BM. Evaluation of a tapered, blunt, bipolar cautery tip for trabeculectomy. *Ophthalmic Surg.* 1994;25(1):54–56.

Verdoorn C, Hendrikse F. Intraocular human thrombin infusion in diabetic vitrectomies. *Ophthalmic Surg.* 1989;20(4):278–279.

Wesley JR, Wesley RE. A study of the lethal effects of intravenous injection of thrombin in rabbits. *Ann Ophthalmol.* 1990;22(12):457–459.

Wesley RE. *Techniques in Ophthalmic Plastic Surgery.* New York: John Wiley & Sons; 1986:231.

Self-Assessment Test

1. Which measures prevent excessive bleeding? (Choose all that apply.)
   a. discontinuance of aspirin
   b. avoidance of nitric oxide in irrigating fluids
   c. hypotensive anesthesia
   d. control of hypertension
2. What is the major advantage of bipolar diathermy?
   a. focus of heating energy on target area
   b. lack of coagulum production
   c. increased tissue destruction
   d. simultaneous tamponade

3. Which of the following accurately describes the use of epinephrine in achieving hemostasis? (Choose all that apply.)
    a. may be used in intraocular solutions
    b. shortens duration of infiltrative anesthesia
    c. reduces bleeding by its biochemical enhancement of hemostasis
    d. is a potent vasoconstrictor
4. What are 2 risks of use of thrombin for hemostasis?
5. What are 2 methods of creating tamponade in intraocular surgery?

For preferred responses to these questions, see Appendix A.

CHAPTER 15

Suturing and Knot Tying

Edward J. Wladis, MD
Paul D. Langer, MD

Optimal wound closure apposes the separate edges of the wound, thereby providing critical physical support to the tissue during the early phases of healing. Meticulous surgical technique and proper knot tying enable the clinician to achieve the functional aspects of wound closure without distortion of the tissue.

This chapter describes techniques of simple wound closure, starting with placement of a square surgical knot; reviews basic principles for needle handling in suture placement; and covers techniques for placement of interrupted, continuous, and mattress sutures. (See Chapter 9 for the overview of surgical instrumentation and materials, including suture characteristics and sutures commonly used in ophthalmic surgery.)

Simple Square Knot (Instrument Tie)

Tying a square knot is a basic skill in suturing; success in placing more complex sutures largely depends upon mastering this technique. Placing a square knot involves the following steps.

1. The needle is passed through both sides of the wound and pulled until the opposite end of the suture is sufficiently short (Fig 15-1A). At that point, the needle is released, and forceps are used to grasp the long end of the suture approximately 3 cm from the wound. The needle holder is then held in the center of the wound just to the right of the suture (for a right-handed surgeon) with the jaws closed and pointing away from the surgeon (Fig 15-1B). The first loop of the knot is then wrapped around the tip of the waiting needle holder (Fig 15-1C).

2. A second and even third loop can be wrapped around the needle holder, depending on the tension of the wound and size of the suture, in order to prevent the wound from gaping after the first loops are tied down. (For example, 3 loops may be required for 10-0 nylon sutures in the cornea, but only 1 loop is necessary for skin closure in the eyelids.) The jaws of the needle holder are then opened and the opposite, short end of the suture is grasped (Fig 15-1D).

This chapter includes a related video, which can be accessed by scanning the QR code provided in the text or going to www.aao.org/bposvideo.

3. The short end of the suture is pulled toward the surgeon and the long end away from the surgeon, with sufficient tension to approximate the walls of the wound with only slight eversion (Fig 15-1E). Care should be taken to avoid excessive tension, as this may result in excessive tissue eversion after healing or in strangulation of the tissue with subsequent ischemia and tissue necrosis. When 1 or more loops are tied down, it is referred to as a *throw*.

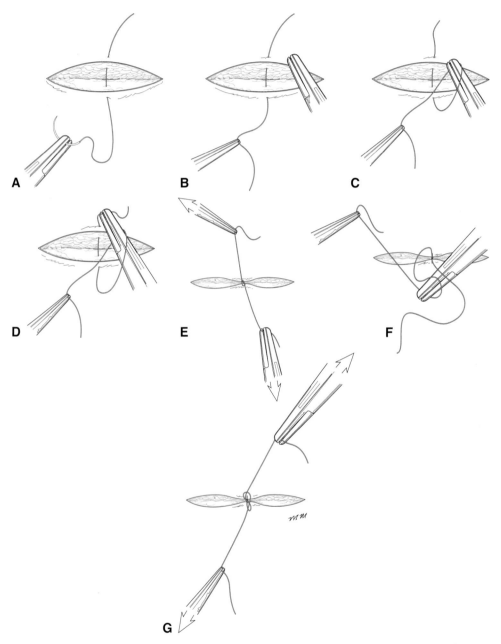

Figure 15-1 Simple square knot. Refer to the text for a description of each part. *(Illustration by Mark M. Miller.)*

4. At this point, the surgeon releases the end of the suture held by the needle holder and repositions the closed needle holder in the center of the wound, again to the right of the suture (for a right-handed surgeon), but now pointing toward the surgeon and the short end of the suture. The long end of the suture is then looped over the closed tips of the needle holder (Fig 15-1F).

5. Again, the jaws of the forceps are opened and the short end of the suture is grasped; however, this time the short end of the suture grasped by the needle holder is pulled *away* from the surgeon while the longer suture end grasped by the forceps is pulled *toward* the surgeon, tightening the knot (Fig 15-1G).

The result of this sequence, in which 2 throws are tied down in opposite directions, is 1 *square knot*. When the first throw of a knot consists of 2 loops, the result is termed a *surgeon's knot*; this technique is used when the wound tension would cause the first throw of a square knot to loosen. In ophthalmology it is customary to place 3 loops in the first throw of the knot when using 10-0 nylon because of the tendency for 10-0 suture to loosen.

Typically, an additional throw is placed over a square knot or a surgeon's knot to complete the tie, although in some circumstances, 2 knots (4 throws) or more can be placed if unraveling of the knot is a concern. Regardless of the number of knots placed, it is critical that each consecutive throw result in the 2 ends of the suture each being pulled from 1 side of the wound to the opposite side; only in this fashion will the knot be "square."

Basic Suturing Principles

When placing sutures, the surgeon grasps the needle near the tip of the needle holder, at a point on the needle approximately two-thirds the distance from the needle tip to the swaged end (where the suture is attached). The needle should enter the tissue *perpendicular to the tissue* (Fig 15-2); such positioning frequently requires slight pronation of the wrist. In the case of a highly curved (such as a half-circle) needle, considerable wrist pronation may be necessary. The needle is then passed through the tissue by gently rotating the wrist in a motion that allows the suture to "follow the curvature of the needle" and slide easily through the tissue; the needle should not be "pushed" or forced through the tissue. At the same time, the edge of the wound where the needle is to be passed is grasped with forceps in the nondominant hand; the tissue in the forceps is not released until the

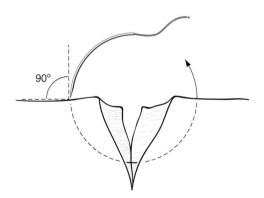

Figure 15-2 Position of entry for a highly curved needle. *(Illustration by Mark M. Miller.)*

needle is re-grasped with the needle holder after the needle emerges from the wound. The forceps should not grasp the needle as it emerges from the wound, as this will dull the needle unnecessarily.

While the underlying principles governing suture placement are identical for all procedures, the requirements of specific types of surgery deserve special mention.

Corneal Suturing

In cases requiring corneal suturing (as in penetrating keratoplasty), fine forceps (Castroviejo 0.12 mm forceps) should be used to firmly grasp the tissue but without damaging it. The 10-0 suture can then be driven beneath the forceps. Optimal technique requires radial placement of the needle in the case of a penetrating keratoplasty, or placement perpendicular to the wound when repairing corneal lacerations.

The tension on the corneal sutures determines the ultimate astigmatism found in corneal transplants and in repair of lacerations. As a result, these procedures require technique that creates enough suture tension necessary for sufficient closure but that avoids excess tension, which leads to significant astigmatism. Thus, sutures should be tied in a fashion that closes the wound with uniform tension but does not create lines of tension on the graft (or in a lacerated cornea). All suture sites should be checked with fluorescein (ie, Seidel) testing to be sure that there is no leakage from the wound.

Suturing in Strabismus Surgery

In strabismus surgery, the goal is to suture a surgically detached muscle back to the underlying sclera. Special care must be taken in these cases to avoid needle penetration of the sclera, which in turn might lead to a retinal hole. The potential for this serious complication is minimized by the use of a spatula needle. A spatula needle is flat on its underside and sharp on its outer edges; this design promotes a needle pass that maintains a steady depth during its passage through tissue, since the bottom surface of the needle is smooth. The needle is passed carefully through the sclera with attention directed to a "flat" needle approach and constant needle depth.

Common Suturing Techniques

In ophthalmology, several types of sutures are commonly used in wound closure:

- simple interrupted suture: basic tool
- vertical mattress suture: greater support
- near–far vertical mattress suture: raising subcutaneous tissue
- horizontal mattress suture: minimizing tension
- simple continuous (running) suture: rapid closure
- running horizontal mattress suture: speed and tension dispersion
- buried interrupted subcutaneous suture: minimizing closure tension subcutaneously
- running subcuticular suture: closing the skin without penetrating the epidermis

Simple Interrupted Suture

The interrupted suture is the basic tool of wound closure. To place an interrupted suture, the surgeon drives the needle from 1 edge of the wound through the underlying deep tissue, across the wound, and then through and out the tissue at the opposite side of the wound. Care should be taken to pass the needle at equal depths on both sides of the wound and equidistant from both sides of the wound edge (Fig 15-3). The needle can be passed across the wound in 1 bite or, if the pass is difficult, the needle can be re-grasped after passing through the initial side of the wound and passed through the opposite side of the wound in a second bite. Square knots are then placed and the ends of the suture are cut; when wound closure is complete, the knots are rotated to the same side of the wound.

Enough interrupted sutures are placed to create adequate strength for secure wound closure. Generally, the first suture is placed in the center of the wound, and each subsequent suture splits the remaining open portion of the wound in half until closure is achieved.

Vertical Mattress Suture

When greater support is needed to close a wound, vertical mattress sutures may be employed (Fig 15-4). The needle should be inserted a short distance from the wound edge and driven across the subcutaneous tissue, exiting on the contralateral side at an equally short distance from the wound edge. A wider site of needle insertion creates greater tension. The surgeon should then reload the needle so that it faces the opposite direction and the needle should be inserted on the side from which it just exited. However, the insertion should now be more distal to the wound edge than the previous site of exit. The surgeon

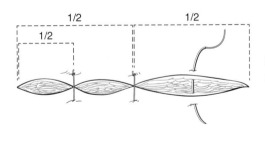

Figure 15-3 Simple interrupted suture. *(Illustration by Mark M. Miller.)*

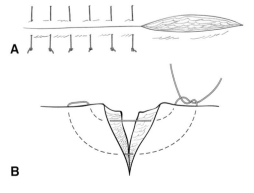

Figure 15-4 Vertical mattress suture. **A,** Vertical mattress sutures may be used to close a wound when greater support is needed. **B,** The suture ends are tied on the same side of the wound. *(Illustration by Mark M. Miller.)*

then drives the needle through the wound so that it exits farther from the wound edge on the initial side than the initial entry point. The distance between the 2 suture penetrations on each side of the wound should be identical. The suture ends are then tied on the same side of the wound.

The vertical mattress suture has a strong tendency to evert wound edges, so care should be taken not to overtighten the knots, in order to avoid excess eversion and a poorly healing wound. In ophthalmology, the vertical mattress suture is most frequently used when closing a lacerated (or incised) eyelid margin, where it provides strength as well as an everting tendency, preventing an eyelid margin "notch."

Near–Far Vertical Mattress Suture

In cases where one wishes to raise the subcutaneous tissue, the near–far mattress suture is a useful variation (Fig 15-5). The technique is largely the same as the standard vertical mattress, but the needle initially is driven distal to the wound and exits proximal to the edge on the contralateral side. It then enters on the initial side near the wound edge and exits on the second side far from the wound edge, in a "figure eight" pattern.

Horizontal Mattress Suture

The horizontal mattress suture is largely used to minimize wound tension by displacing tension away from the wound edge (Fig 15-6). To place a horizontal mattress suture, the surgeon enters on 1 side of the wound, drives the needle across the underlying tissue, and exits on the opposite side of the wound an equally short distance from the insertion. The surgeon then re-enters on the second side laterally, again equidistant from the wound edge, and drives the needle back through and out the first side, creating a "rectangle" out of the suture. The ends of the suture are then tied on the same side of the wound.

Figure 15-5 Near–far vertical mattress suture. *(Illustration by Mark M. Miller.)*

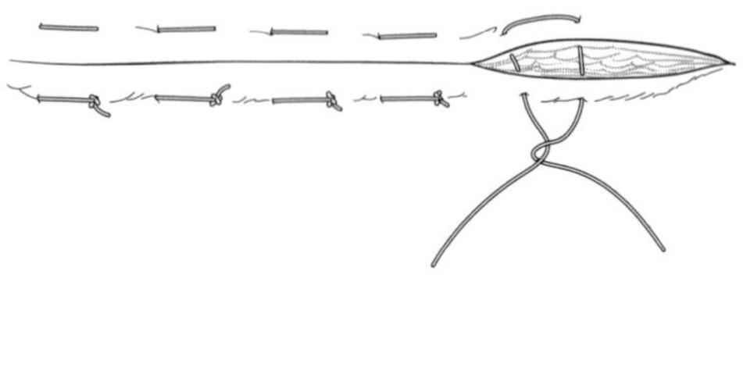

Figure 15-6 Horizontal mattress suture. *(Illustration by Mark M. Miller.)*

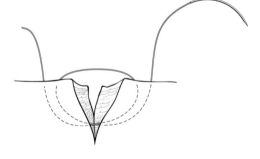

In ophthalmology, horizontal mattress sutures are frequently used when tying bolsters across the upper and lower eyelids to close the palpebral aperture temporarily. They are also sometimes employed to close scleral tunnel incisions after cataract surgery.

Simple Continuous (Running) Suture

Running sutures permit the surgeon to close wounds much more rapidly than other techniques (Fig 15-7A). Essentially, a simple suture is placed in the same fashion as an interrupted suture at 1 end of the wound, but in the case of running sutures, the thread attached to the needle is not cut. The surgeon places another simple suture by returning to the initial side and driving the needle to the contralateral side. No knot is tied until the surgeon reaches the termination of the length of the wound. A single knot is then placed, using the last loop tied as a suture end. Alternatively, in order to avoid distorting the end of the wound, a final bite can be taken in tissue just outside the end of the wound and this loop tied as a suture end (Fig 15-7B). Proper technique necessitates evenly spaced bites and the adjustment of suture tension prior to tying the final knot to ensure an even distribution of wound tension.

While running sutures save time (as well as suture), they have a greater tendency to strangulate or pucker the wound edges. Furthermore, any break along the string (or in a knot) can weaken the entire closure, whereas in an interrupted closure only a localized weakness would develop after a break.

Running Horizontal Mattress Suture

The running horizontal mattress suture affords the surgeon the benefits of speed and dispersion of tension (Fig 15-8). The surgeon enters on 1 side of the wound, passes the needle through the underlying deep tissue, and exits on the contralateral side an equally short distance from the point of insertion. The suture is then passed laterally on the second

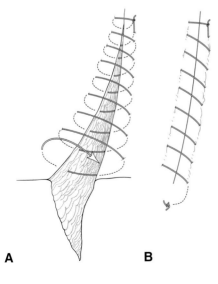

Figure 15-7 Running suture. **A,** Simple continuous (running) suture. **B,** Alternate final knot. *(Illustration by Mark M. Miller.)*

A   B

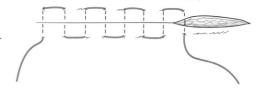

Figure 15-8 Running horizontal mattress suture. *(Illustration by Mark M. Miller.)*

side before passage back across the subcutaneous tissue to the first side. This process is repeated until the surgeon reaches the end of the wound, and a knot is then tied to the final suture loop.

Buried Interrupted Subcutaneous Suture

In many cases, subcutaneous sutures are needed to minimize the tension of closure (Fig 15-9). To place a subcutaneous suture such that the knot is buried, the surgeon should evert the wound edge mildly, and should enter the wound in the dermis as close to the base as possible. The needle is then passed to exit through the dermis superiorly on the same side, and is passed through the superior dermal edge of the contralateral side, at a depth equal to the depth where the needle emerged from the initial side. The suture should then travel to the base of the wound, where it should exit at a depth equal to the depth of the initial needle entry. When the knot is tied, it will lie deep to the tissue closed by the suture.

Running Subcuticular Suture

A skin incision can be closed without penetrating the epidermis across the wound by means of a running subcuticular suture. The advantage of such a suture is a less conspicuous scar.

A running subcuticular suture is placed by first entering the skin at a point outside the termination of the wound and perpendicular to it, passing the needle toward the wound edge. The needle emerges just under the skin from 1 side of the wound. The needle then enters the opposite side of the wound, just below the skin at the edge of the wound, is passed subcutaneously parallel to the skin surface, and exits just below the skin edge (Fig 15-10A). The needle is placed again at the initial side of the wound, just below the skin, at a point directly opposite where it exited. A subcutaneous bite of identical length is then taken, parallel to the skin surface, again exiting just below the skin. In this fashion, successive bites are taken on alternate sides of the wound, always just beneath the skin, with the bites "staggered" on each side by a distance of 1 length of a "bite."

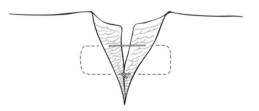

Figure 15-9 Buried interrupted subcutaneous suture. *(Illustration by Mark M. Miller.)*

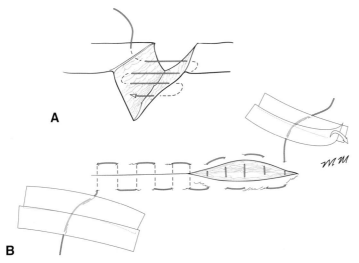

Figure 15-10 Running subcuticular suture. **A,** Subcutaneous bites parallel to the skin surface. **B,** Ends affixed with reinforced skin closures (Steri-Strips). *(Illustration by Mark M. Miller.)*

At the completion of the wound closure, the final needle bite on 1 side should be passed subcutaneously through the wound on the opposite side and then out onto the skin. The 2 ends of the suture are not tied but simply affixed to the skin with Steri-Strips (Fig 15-10B). The suture is pulled out of the wound from 1 end 5–7 days after placement.

Video 15-1 demonstrates basic surgical suturing technique in managing oculofacial disorders. Details of interrupted, running, mattress, and deep buried-knot sutures are shown.

 VIDEO 15-1 Basic Suturing Technique (07:41)
Courtesy of Richard Caesar, MPPB, FCOphth

Key Points

- Proper suture technique supports incisional edges during the early healing phases to facilitate more rapid healing with less scarring.
- The square knot may be placed with additional loops in the first throw (surgeon's knot) to allow stability against wound tension and the tendency of microscopic suture to slip with only 1 loop.
- Correct suturing technique includes avoiding grasp of the needle tip, entering tissue perpendicularly, and following the curve of the needle.
- Excessive suture tension may result in wound edge eversion, tissue strangulation, and, for corneoscleral incisions, increased astigmatism.

Dunn DL, cont ed. *Wound Closure Manual.* Somerville, NJ: Ethicon; undated.
Ethicon. *Knot Tying Manual.* Somerville, NJ: Ethicon; 2005.

Self-Assessment Test

1. Under which circumstances should a surgeon place 2 loops in the first throw of a surgical knot? (Choose all that apply.)
   a. always
   b. to prevent loosening of the knot while tying
   c. only in mattress sutures
   d. in a "surgeon's knot"

2. Which of the following statements are true regarding correct suturing technique? (Choose all that apply.)
   a. The needle is grasped at its blunt end to avoid damaging the tip.
   b. The needle should enter the tissue perpendicular to the tissue.
   c. The surgeon should follow the curvature of the needle in passing the suture.
   d. As the needle emerges from the tissue, it should be grasped at its tip to avoid tissue damage.

3. Which of the following statements regarding excessive tension on a corneal suture is correct?
   a. may produce astigmatism
   b. may induce wound leakage
   c. may be avoided by placing the suture in a radial fashion
   d. does not occur with 10-0 nylon

4. Which of the following statements regarding the continuous ("running") suture technique are correct? (Choose all that apply.)
   a. requires less time than interrupted sutures
   b. may produce greater wound dehiscence than interrupted sutures if the suture breaks
   c. is reserved for subcuticular closures
   d. may produce uneven wound tension and "puckering"
   e. requires more suture material than interrupted suture technique

For preferred responses to these questions, see Appendix A.

CHAPTER 16

Intraocular Fluids

James P. Dunn, MD

The use of intraocular fluids in anterior segment surgery is essential in providing effective working space, control of tissue, appropriate pupil size, and control of surgical instruments for the surgeon. This chapter helps the beginning resident understand when, how, and why to use these fluids in order to make cataract and glaucoma surgery safer and more effective. Additionally, the development of intraocular drugs has revolutionized the medical therapy in diseases such as macular degeneration and diabetic retinopathy, but has increased the potential for post-injection endophthalmitis or errors in compounding of these drugs.

Intraocular fluids can be classified into 7 categories: ophthalmic viscosurgical devices; irrigating fluids; mydriatics and miotics; anesthetics; corticosteroids, antibiotics, and antifungals; capsular staining agents; and biologic agents, including vascular endothelial growth factor (VEGF) antagonists.

Ophthalmic Viscosurgical Devices

Viscoelastics, or more specifically referred to as *ophthalmic viscosurgical devices* (OVDs), are gel-like materials that protect delicate intraocular structures, maintain space, and allow manipulation of crystalline and intraocular lenses. All OVDs share the desirable property of pseudoplasticity; that is, they assume a gel-like configuration at low shear rates (such as occurs during capsulorrhexis or lens cracking) but change to a more liquid solution at high shear rates (as occurs during phacoemulsification and aspiration). These materials are commonly classified as either *cohesive* or *dispersive*. Most OVDs are composed of hyaluronic acid of varying molecular weight (cohesive) or a combination of hyaluronic acid and chondroitin sulfate (dispersive). Hydroxypropyl methylcellulose 2% is another dispersive viscoelastic.

In general, cohesive OVDs are better at maintaining space and are more easily removed at the end of surgery. However, they are also more easily removed during phacoemulsification itself, thereby possibly jeopardizing endothelial cell protection in prolonged surgery or in eyes with small anterior chambers (as in hyperopia). Dispersive OVDs are

---

This chapter includes a related video, which can be accessed by scanning the QR code provided in the text or going to www.aao.org/bposvideo.

better at coating tissue and may provide more prolonged endothelial cell protection. However, they are less easily removed than cohesive OVDs, because they tend to "fragment" upon removal. Consequently, they may be more likely to induce elevated intraocular pressure (IOP) in the first 24 hours after cataract surgery. They are also more likely to produce bubbles when injected into the eye, which can compromise the surgeon's view.

There is no "perfect" viscoelastic, and the beginning surgeon should try to gain experience with both cohesive and dispersive types. Indeed, some surgeons prefer to use both types for "high-risk" eyes, such as those with borderline endothelial functioning, dense nuclei requiring high amounts of phaco energy for removal, or weak zonules. The so-called *soft shell technique* involves first injecting a dispersive viscoelastic into the anterior chamber (Fig 16-1), followed by a more posterior injection of a cohesive viscoelastic. The cohesive viscoelastic pushes the dispersive viscoelastic up against the corneal endothelium, where it theoretically remains during surgery.

OVDs are injected into the eye through a small-bore cannula, usually just prior to the creation of the corneal or scleral wound. The tip of the cannula should be placed opposite the site of entry, injecting the viscoelastic so that it fills the anterior chamber and forces aqueous out of the eye (Fig 16-2). Underfilling the anterior chamber prior to the phaco-emulsification incision results in a soft eye that tends to collapse and can result in a wound length longer than is desired. Overfilling the anterior chamber steepens the corneal curvature and can result in an incision length shorter than is desired; it may also worsen pre-existing zonular dehiscence by stretching weak or damaged zonules. Hydroxypropyl

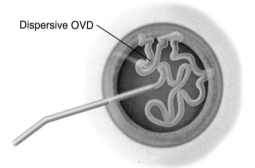

Dispersive OVD

Figure 16-1 Ring of dispersive ophthalmic viscosurgical device (OVD) pushed up against endothelium by injection of cohesive viscoelastic. *(Illustration by Mark M. Miller.)*

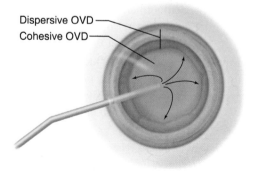

Dispersive OVD
Cohesive OVD

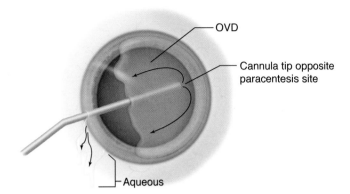

Figure 16-2 Injection of ophthalmic viscosurgical device (OVD) into the eye through a small-bore cannula. Note placement of the cannula tip opposite the site of entry, injecting the viscoelastic so that it fills the anterior chamber and forces aqueous out of the eye. *(Illustration by Mark M. Miller.)*

methylcellulose can also be used to coat the corneal surface, obviating the need for frequent irrigation by the assistant during surgery.

Cohesive OVDs

Cohesive OVDs are most useful in maintaining anterior chamber space. They can help maximally flatten the anterior lens capsule, which reduces the tendency for the capsular tear to "run downhill" and extend peripherally during capsulorrhexis, and should be used liberally in this stage of cataract surgery. They can also push away and flatten the capsule, which can sometimes fold up accordion-like and impair the surgeon's view of the leading edge of the capsulorrhexis (Fig 16-3). When a bent needle is used to perform capsulorrhexis (as opposed to Utrata forceps), it is highly recommended that the needle be attached to a cohesive viscoelastic syringe. Cohesive OVDs are also helpful in dilating a small pupil (often in combination with various mechanical pupil-stretching techniques), in maintaining maximal separation of nuclear sections to facilitate lens cracking, in manipulating lens fragments out of the capsular bag for phacoemulsification in the iris plane, and in expanding the capsular bag prior to intraocular lens placement. Another useful role of cohesive OVDs is in "viscodissection." In this technique, subincisional cortex which is difficult to remove can be separated from the posterior capsule and pushed into the peripheral capsular bag (Fig 16-4), where it can be more safely and easily aspirated after placement of the intraocular lens. The use of ultra-high viscosity cohesive OVDs such as hyaluronic acid 2.3% (Healon5, Abbott Medical Optics, Santa Ana, CA) may be helpful in maintaining intraoperative mydriasis but requires special care when being removed so as to prevent phacoemulsification wound burns or severe postoperative glaucoma.

Dispersive OVDs

On the other hand, the tendency of a dispersive viscoelastic to fragment upon removal can be used to the surgeon's advantage if there is a capsular tear or zonular dehiscence;

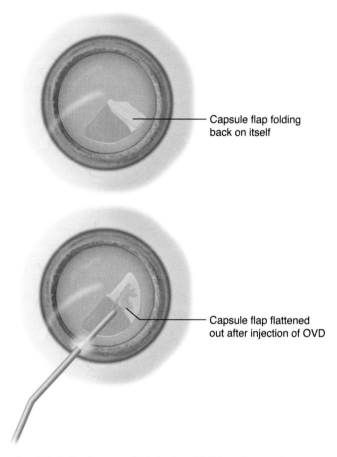

Capsule flap folding
back on itself

Capsule flap flattened
out after injection of OVD

Figure 16-3 Use of ophthalmic viscosurgical device (OVD) to flatten the capsulorrhexis flap. *(Illustration by Mark M. Miller.)*

tamponading the area with a dispersive viscoelastic may allow the surgeon to remove adjacent cortex without dragging vitreous into the aspiration tip.

Dispersive OVDs may provide more prolonged corneal endothelial cell protection than cohesive OVDs, and they are often recommended for cases in which the lens nucleus is especially dense (requiring higher phaco energy for removal), the anterior chamber is shallow (reducing the space between the phaco tip and the corneal endothelium), or there is preexisting compromise of the corneal endothelium.

Removing OVDs

OVDs should be removed completely at the end of cataract surgery, because retained viscoelastic will clog the trabecular meshwork and can cause marked elevation in IOP for 24–48 hours after surgery. Such pressure spikes can cause pain and corneal edema. Some surgeons prefer to leave a small amount of viscoelastic in the eye at the end of trabeculectomy surgery to reduce the risk of chamber shallowing in the first 24–48 hours postoperatively. Cohesive OVDs can be removed more quickly than dispersive OVDs, since the former tend to coalesce into a large bolus during aspiration. To remove the material

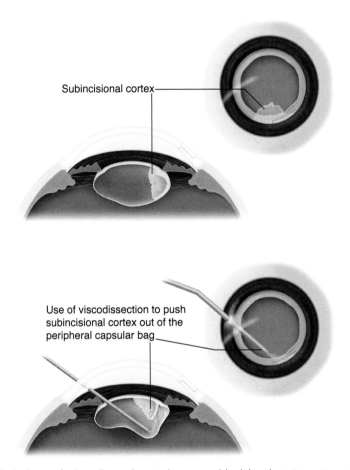

Subincisional cortex

Use of viscodissection to push
subincisional cortex out of the
peripheral capsular bag

Figure 16-4 Technique of viscodissection to loosen subincisional cortex. *(Illustration by Mark M. Miller.)*

completely, the surgeon may need to place the irrigation/aspiration tip behind the lens implant, or to rock the lens from side to side while aspirating.

Retained viscoelastic may also cause capsular distension syndrome. In this condition, retained viscoelastic between the IOL and capsular bag cannot escape anteriorly when the capsulorrhexis edge overlaps the anterior IOL surface for 360°. Osmotic flow of aqueous into the viscoelastic behind the intraocular lens over time eventually pushes the lens forward and causes a myopic shift. The trapped material appears distinctly gray between the posterior IOL surface and the posterior capsule and can make it difficult to focus the helium-neon aiming beam if YAG laser capsulotomy becomes necessary.

Irrigating Fluids

Irrigating fluid is necessary in phacoemulsification to cool the phaco tip and prevent wound burn. The basic intraoperative irrigating fluid is balanced salt solution (BSS). The addition of 0.5 mL of epinephrine 1:1000 to the 500 mL of BSS (final dilution of 1:1,000,000) helps enhance pupillary dilation and reduce bleeding when lysis of posterior synechiae is required. The addition of glutathione (BSS Plus, Alcon, Fort Worth, Texas) may provide better endothelial cell protection than BSS alone. Some clinicians recommend using chilled irrigating solution in eyes with compromised endothelial function. In all circumstances, the surgeon should strive to minimize the volume of irrigating solution used during surgery, since the turbulence of flow within the eye may damage endothelial cells. The irrigating ports of the phaco and irrigation/aspiration handpieces should be directed away from the endothelium during surgery.

Finally, antibiotics such as vancomycin 20 mcg/mL added to the irrigating solution have been shown to reduce bacterial load in the anterior chamber at the end of surgery. However, controlled clinical trials have not demonstrated a reduction in postoperative endophthalmitis with the use of irrigative antibiotics (as opposed to intracameral injections), and any potential benefit must be weighed against possible toxicity, including cystoid macular edema and endothelial damage (especially if a dilutional error is made in adding the antibiotic).

Mydriatics and Miotics

The use of epinephrine in the irrigating fluid to enhance dilation and reduce bleeding is discussed in the previous section. Intracameral mydriatics can be used to supplement or replace dilating drops. Before injection of viscoelastic, 0.5 mL of preservative-free epinephrine 1:1000 diluted 1:10 with BSS may also be injected directly into the anterior chamber for the same purposes. Some surgeons advocate the use of a high-concentration epinephrine/lidocaine solution to provide anesthesia and to keep intraoperative dilation more consistent and prolonged during cataract surgery, particularly in eyes of patients who have taken tamsulosin (Flomax) and are at risk for intraoperative floppy iris syndrome (IFIS). In order to provide adequate buffering of the solution (nonpreserved, bisulfate-free epinephrine 1:1000 is acidic enough to damage the corneal endothelium), the proper mixture is 3 parts BSS Plus to 1 part preservative-free 4% lidocaine, which is in turn mixed 3:1 with preservative-free 1:1000 epinephrine. For each anterior chamber injection 0.5–2.0 mL is used. Shortages of preservative-free epinephrine have occurred, in which case preservative-free phenylephrine 1.5% can be substituted.

Intracameral miotics are used in glaucoma surgery to constrict the pupil to facilitate creation of an iridectomy, in corneal transplant surgery to help protect the crystalline lens during trephination, and in cataract surgery to prevent iris capture of the intraocular lens. Miotics are also helpful in identifying vitreous strands that may be extending to the wound margin after capsular ruptures (Fig 16-5), and they may help reduce the risk of postoperative pressure spikes. Miotics are usually unnecessary in routine cataract surgery if the intraocular lens is completely covered by the anterior capsular rim. Furthermore, miotics are potentially pro-inflammatory, and for this reason are best avoided if possible following surgery for uveitic cataracts.

The miotics commercially available are acetylcholine 1% (Miochol) and carbachol 0.01% (Miostat). Both are direct-acting parasympathomimetics. About 0.5 mL is an adequate volume for injection. Acetylcholine causes pupillary constriction within seconds

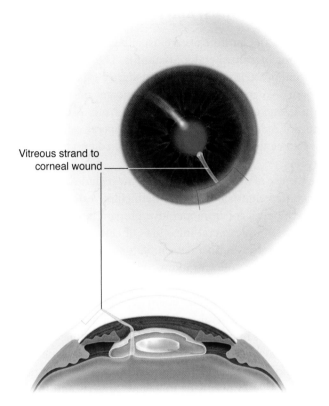

Vitreous strand to
corneal wound

Figure 16-5 Use of intracameral miotics to help identify vitreous incarceration into the wound. *(Illustration by Mark M. Miller.)*

but lasts only several hours, while carbachol may take 2–5 minutes to induce miosis but may last up to 24 hours. Both miotics will also reduce IOP. Carbachol will therefore provide more sustained IOP control, but it will also result in a small pupil on the first postoperative day, making visualization of the retina more difficult. Some surgeons use diluted carbachol to reduce this postoperative miosis.

Anesthetics

Intracameral anesthetics are sometimes used to supplement topical anesthetics in cataract surgery, providing a small but statistically significant reduction in pain compared to topical anesthesia alone. Their use may reduce the discomfort patients can feel when there is stretching of the ciliary body, as occurs when going to foot position 1 in phacoemulsification. Preservative-free lidocaine 1% must be used because the preservatives may cause severe corneal endothelial damage (the use of preservative-free tetracaine has been reported). The injection (no more than 0.5 mL) is usually given prior to injection of the viscoelastic. Intracameral lidocaine also enhances mydriasis, even without concurrent epinephrine.

Corticosteroids, Antibiotics, and Antifungals

Intravitreous antibiotics and antifungals are usually given only following open globe repair or as treatment for presumed endophthalmitis. The drug is injected through a pars plana incision 3–4 mm posterior to the limbus, using a 30-gauge needle. Typical regimens include amphotericin 5–10 mcg in 0.05–0.1 mL, vancomycin 1.0 mg in 0.1 mL, clindamycin 1.0 mg in 0.1 mL, and ceftazidime 2.25 mg in 0.1 mL. A large European study demonstrated a significant reduction in the risk of postoperative endophthalmitis following cataract surgery when cefuroxime 1 mg/mL was injected into the anterior chamber at the conclusion of surgery.

Drawbacks to the use of intracameral cefuroxime include limited effectiveness against gram-negative bacteria, enterococci, and methicillin-resistant *Staphylococcus aureus* (MRSA), as well as the need for intraoperative preparation of the drug and therefore a risk of dilutional errors. Intracameral injections of cefuroxime have been rarely associated with postoperative serous retinal detachment and macular edema, especially when given at inadvertently higher concentrations. Intracameral vancomycin 0.1 mg/mL has been recommended because it is effective against MRSA, but it, too, has been associated with the development of cystoid macular edema as a result of dilutional errors. Whether the potential benefits of intracameral antibiotic injections outweigh these risks remains unproven. Aminoglycosides in particular are toxic to the retina and should not be used.

Intravitreous injections of corticosteroids in the form of dexamethasone sodium phosphate or triamcinolone acetonide have been used recently to help treat or prevent cystoid macular edema due to uveitis or following surgery, and to treat choroidal neovascularization. While limited publications have shown considerable benefit, controlled studies are lacking, and caution is recommended. Triamcinolone acetonide preparations contain various preservatives and inactive ingredients that can cause a sterile endophthalmitis. True infectious endophthalmitis has also been reported, and sterilization of the conjunctiva with povidone-iodine solution prior to intraocular injection is mandatory. Intravitreous dexamethasone 400 mcg in 0.1 mL may also be useful in reducing inflammation in cases of gram-positive endophthalmitis.

Diluted and rinsed triamcinolone acetonide has been shown to be safe and effective in identifying vitreous prolapse as part of anterior vitrectomy in eyes with capsular rupture at the time of cataract surgery. Better identification of vitreous prolapse with this technique may reduce the risk of vitreous wick syndrome and retinal detachment after complicated cataract surgery.

Capsular Staining Agents

In cases of dense white cataracts, staining the anterior capsule greatly enhances visualization of the capsulorrhexis. The dye can either be injected underneath an air bubble and allowed to stay in place for 20–30 seconds, and then exchanged for BSS or viscoelastic, or injected without air and irrigated out immediately. It often helps to inject a small amount of viscoelastic just inside the paracentesis before injecting the air bubble; the viscoelastic helps keep the air bubble inside the eye as the dye is injected. Small pupils must be dilated prior to injection of the dye, as only the exposed anterior lens capsule will take up the stain. Indocyanine green 0.5% was first used by surgeons for this purpose, although such usage is not FDA-approved. Trypan blue is more effective than indocyanine green.

Although trypan blue is commercially available as an FDA-approved 0.06% solution (Vision Blue, Dutch Ophthalmic USA, Kingston, New Hampshire), concentrations of up to 1% have been used. Potential complications of trypan blue injections include inadvertent staining of the vitreous and posterior capsule in eyes with compromised zonules, resulting in loss of the intraoperative red reflex that may take up to 10 days to clear as well as possible retinal toxicity. Toxic anterior segment syndrome has been attributed to the use of compounded trypan blue. Using only the FDA-approved formulation and injecting a dispersive viscoelastic to prevent migration of the dye posterior to the lens equator, or staining the capsule underneath a large amount of viscoelastic using a "windshield wiper" technique (Video 16-1), may reduce potential toxicity. Testing of trypan blue–stained human lens capsule *in vitro* has shown increased capsular stiffness compared to unstained capsules, especially in eyes from diabetic patients, but the clinical significance of this finding is unclear.

An Ophthalmic Technology Assessment report from the American Academy of Ophthalmology found good evidence to support the use of capsular dye staining in pediatric and white cataracts, but emphasized that its benefit in less severe adult cataracts remains unproven. Nonetheless, many surgeons find it extremely useful for beginning resident surgeons who are first learning to perform capsulorrhexis.

 VIDEO 16-1 Anterior Capsular Staining (00:48)
Courtesy of Bryn Burkholder, MD

Vascular Endothelial Growth Factor Antagonists

Intravitreal injections of anti-VEGF agents such as aflibercept, bevacizumab, and ranibizumab are often used in the treatment of exudative macular degeneration, macular edema following retinal vein occlusion, diabetic macular edema, and neovascular glaucoma. The systemic safety profile appears excellent. However, rare local adverse events include acute glaucoma, vitreous hemorrhage, retinal detachment, and endophthalmitis (0.02%–0.2% per injection). The injections should always be done under sterile conditions, using a lid speculum (or manual retraction of the lids by an assistant) to keep the lashes away from the injection site, and the eye should be treated immediately beforehand with topical povidone-iodine 5%. Routine use of fluoroquinolone drops prior to injection may actually increase the risk of endophthalmitis through selection of resistant organisms after multiple injections.

Compounding Intraocular Drugs

Compounding errors (dilutional or contamination) become an increasing concern as cost control efforts compete with drug availability and patient safety issues. Prior to any intraocular injection, confirmation of the drug, dosage, expiration date, and volume between the injecting physician and the nurse or technician should be done. While the legal issues regarding compounding pharmacies is changing rapidly, the guiding principle is that the ophthalmologist should always have the highest assurance that any compounded drug is free of contamination or impurities before it is used.

Key Points

- Intraocular fluids can be classified into 7 categories: ophthalmic viscosurgical devices; irrigating fluids; mydriatics and miotics; anesthetics; corticosteroids, antibiotics, and antifungals; capsular staining agents; and biologic agents, including vascular endothelial growth factor (VEGF) antagonists.
- OVDs are primarily composed of hyaluronic acid and are commonly classified as either cohesive or dispersive. Cohesive OVDs fragment less, are better for maintaining space in the eye, and are more easily removed. Dispersive OVDs fragment more and provide better coating of the corneal endothelium, but are more difficult to remove from the eye.
- Injection of any intraocular fluid carries a small risk of endophthalmitis, and clinicians should obtain such solutions from a reputable source when compounding is necessary.
- Intracameral miotics acetylcholine and carbachol may be used to identify vitreous strands, protect the lens in penetrating keratoplasty, facilitate iridectomy, and prevent iris capture of the intraocular lens.
- Corneal endothelial damage may be reduced by using preservative-free intracameral solutions and by the addition of glutathione to irrigating solution.
- Anterior chamber irrigation with antibiotics such as cefuroxime may reduce the risk of endophthalmitis, but extreme care is necessary to prevent dilutional errors.

AAO Quality of Care Secretariat, Hoskins Center for Quality Eye Care. "Drug Shortage: Non-preserved, Bisulfate-Free Epinephrine" [Clinical Statement]. San Francisco: American Academy of Ophthalmology; 2012.

Bar-Sela SM, Fleissig E, Yatziv Y, et al. Long-term outcomes of triamcinolone acetonide-assisted anterior vitrectomy during complicated cataract surgery with vitreous loss. *J Cataract Refract Surg.* 2014;40(5):722–727.

Bissen-Miyajami H. Ophthalmic viscosurgical devices. *Curr Opin Ophthalmol.* 2008;19(1): 50–54.

Ezra DG, Allan BD. Topical anesthesia alone versus topical anesthesia with intracameral lidocaine for phacoemulsification. *Cochrane Database Syst Rev.* 2007;18(3):CD005276.

Jacobs DS, Cox TA, Wagoner MD, Ariyasu RG, Karp CL. Capsule staining as an adjunct to cataract surgery: a report from the American Academy of Ophthalmology. *Ophthalmology.* 2006;113(4):707–713.

Jonas JB, Akkoyun I, Budde WM, Kreissig I, Degenring RF. Intravitreal reinjection of triamcinolone for exudative age-related macular degeneration. *Arch Ophthalmol.* 2004;122(2): 218–222.

Kim SJ, Chomsky AS, Sternberg P Jr. Reducing the risk of endophthalmitis after intravitreous injection. *JAMA Ophthalmol.* 2013;131(5):674–675.

Liesegang TJ. Intracameral antibiotics: questions for the United States based on prospective studies. *J Cataract Refract Surg.* 2008;34(3):505–509.

Lorente R, de Rojas V, Vásquez de Parga P, et al. Intracameral phenylephrine 1.5% for prophylaxis against intraoperative floppy iris syndrome: prospective, randomized fellow eye study. *Ophthalmology.* 2012;119(10):2053–2058.

Nicholson BP, Schachat AP. A review of clinical trials of anti-VEGF agents for diabetic retinopathy. *Graefes Arch Clin Exp Ophthalmol.* 2010;248(7):915–930.

Parke DW. "Opthalmology and Compounding Pharmacies." Available at www.aao.org /publications/eyenet/201301/current_perspective.cfm. Accessed September 14, 2014.

Parikh CH, Edelhauser HF. Ocular surgical pharmacology: corneal endothelial safety and toxicity. *Curr Opin Ophthalmol.* 2003;14(4):178–185.

Regillo CD, Brown DM, Abraham P, et al. Randomized, double-masked, sham-controlled trial of ranibizumab for neovascular age-related macular degeneration: PIER Study year 1. *Am J Ophthalmol.* 2008;145(2):239–248.

Rodrigues EB, Costa EF, Penha FM, et al. The use of vital dyes in ocular surgery. *Surv Ophthalmol.* 2009;54(5):576–617.

Tognetto D, Cecchini P, Ravalico G. Survey of ophthalmic viscosurgical devices. *Curr Opin Ophthalmol.* 2004;15(1):29–32.

Self-Assessment Test

1. Name the primary component of most ophthalmic viscosurgical devices (OVDs).
2. Advantages of cohesive OVDs include which of the following? (Choose all that apply.)
   a. ease of removal
   b. better coating of corneal endothelium
   c. more effective space maintenance
   d. less likely to "drag" iris or vitreous out of incision
3. Why should OVDs be completely removed at the close of surgery? (Choose all that apply.)
   a. to avoid postoperative IOP elevation
   b. to prevent endothelial toxicity
   c. to prevent macular edema
   d. to prevent vitreous hemorrhage
4. Corneal endothelium injury during intraocular irrigation may be reduced by which of the following? (Choose all that apply.)
   a. directing irrigation port away from endothelium
   b. limiting use of intraocular antibiotics
   c. addition of intraocular glutathione
   d. use of chilled irrigating fluid
5. Name 3 uses for intraoperative miotics.

For preferred responses to these questions, see Appendix A.

CHAPTER 17

Patient Safety Issues

Andrew G. Lee, MD

The ophthalmologist in training should be cognizant of the specific issues and precautions that are necessary to ensure the safety of the patient during ophthalmic surgery. This chapter discusses 5 major areas of patient safety in the ophthalmic operating room: infection prophylaxis, surgery on the incorrect eye, improper intraocular lens insertion, medication errors, and iatrogenic fires in the operating room. Systematic practices can prevent these and other errors from occurring. The recommendations in this chapter are guidelines for patient safety and should not be construed as a "standard of care." Surgeons, hospitals, or operating rooms may differ in individual approaches, documentation, detail, or scope of their safety protocols and procedures. The content of this chapter is in no way intended to substitute for or replace local institutional policies. (See the references at the end of this chapter for further reading.)

Infection Prophylaxis

Prophylaxis against infectious endophthalmitis after cataract and other intraocular surgery is an important patient safety issue (AAO Preferred Practice Pattern, "Cataract in the Adult Eye"). Some potential risk factors include older age, a leaky incision, and a communication between the anterior and posterior chambers (eg, posterior capsular tear). Prophylaxis with 5% topical povidone-iodine in the conjunctival cul-de-sac is generally recommended. There is also supportive evidence for using a bolus of intracameral antibiotic at the conclusion of surgery, but there is only weak evidence supporting subconjunctival antibiotics. Alternatively, topical antibiotics given on the day of surgery rather than postoperatively may be a reasonable practice option. Unfortunately, due to the low incidence of endophthalmitis, there is insufficient evidence to support any specific type, route, or dose of antibiotic for infection prophylaxis for cataract surgery.

Surgery on the Incorrect Eye

Surgery on the incorrect eye is the most feared but fortunately preventable medical error in the ophthalmic operating room. Wrong-site surgery is not unique to ophthalmology; it is a significant medical, legal, and public relations problem affecting all surgical specialties. The wrong-site error is usually the result of a system or process failure in patient identification, confirmation, or verification of the site of surgery. These types of errors are preventable if the appropriate precautions are taken routinely. From 1985 to 1986, the Physician Insurers Association of America reported 331 closed claims for wrong-site surgery. The Joint Commission on Accreditation of Healthcare Organizations reported that wrong-site surgery (1995–2001) was one of the top 10 reported medical errors ($n=152$). Ambulatory care centers were a common location (58%) for this error. JCAHO continues to collect reports of wrong-site, wrong-patient, wrong-procedure events (www.jcaho.org). Surgery on the wrong eye (eg, enucleation) can be particularly devastating if the fellow unoperated eye still requires surgery despite having had the normal eye removed.

Common causes for wrong-site surgery include poor communication between the surgeon and the patient; inadequate communication among members of the surgical team; reliance upon memory only for the site identification; inadequate preoperative assessment of the patient; or insufficient or inaccurate verification procedures of the operative site. Patients might not identify the surgical site accurately during the informed consent process (eg, patients with language barriers, cognitive impairment, or anxiety over the procedure), in the preoperative area, or during the surgical marking of the site. Surgical team members and ancillary personnel might not properly verify the site of surgery or might over-rely upon the surgeon to make the correct decision. It has been documented that members of the surgical team in some wrong-site cases feared pointing out the error to the operating surgeon.

Additional contributory factors in wrong-site surgery include involvement of more than one surgeon; performance of multiple procedures on the same patient; time pressure to complete the preoperative procedures more quickly; physical deformity or morbid obesity that might alter the usual setup of equipment or positioning of the patient; distractions during the identification process; and failure to confirm the site.

In order to prevent wrong-site surgery, the verification process for the operative site should be performed consistently and routinely, including:

- formal written procedures and protocols for surgical team members to identify and confirm the operative eye (Surgeons should review their individual hospital or operating room protocols periodically.)
- informed consent form that clearly and explicitly states the operative procedure and the operative eye without the use of potentially confounding abbreviations (eg, OD, OS, IOL)
- review of the chart, the preoperative orders for pupil dilation, the regional anesthesia orders, and the surgical prep site by the nurse, anesthetist, resident, fellow, and other surgical team members. (All team members should be in agreement.)
- verification with the patient (or patient's family if the patient is unable to respond or is a minor) prior to pupillary dilation, anesthesia, surgical prep and drape, or the incision
- oral verification of the correct operative site by multiple members of the surgical team
- availability of the medical record in the room with explicit written documentation of the operative site
- availability and review of the pertinent imaging studies in the operating room

- marking of the operative eye (eg, using a marking pen and writing the surgeon's initials at the site)
- review of the written verification checklist of all documents referencing the intended operative procedure and site (eg, the medical record, preoperative dilation and surgical preparation orders, the imaging studies and their reports, the informed consent document, the operating room record, the anesthesia record, and direct observation of the marked operative site on the patient)
- on the case of enucleation, evisceration, or exenteration, the surgeon should perform a final additional verification of the preoperative pathology (eg, intraocular tumor) in the operative eye by direct examination (eg, dilated fundus exam in the operating room)
- signature confirmation of completion of the checklist to ensure that all of the above intraoperative steps have been performed
- a final confirmatory check by the surgeon in the operating room before the incision is made (without relying on memory alone)

In 2003, the AAO and 50 other professional health care organizations endorsed the Joint Commission's "Universal Protocol for Preventing Wrong Site, Wrong Procedure, and Wrong Person Surgery." Key points included

- completing a preoperative verification process
- marking the operative site
- taking a time-out immediately before starting the procedure
- adapting these requirements to non-operating room setting

Simon et al performed a retrospective series of 106 cases, including 42 from the Ophthalmic Mutual Insurance Company (OMIC) and 64 from the New York State Health Department. The most common error was wrong IOL in 67 cases (63%). Wrong-eye operations occurred in 15 cases, wrong-eye block in 14, wrong patient or procedure in 8, and wrong corneal transplant in 2. The authors concluded that the Universal Protocol would have prevented 85% of the wrong incidents analyzed had it been implemented.

Incorrect Intraocular Lens Placement

In addition to wrong-eye surgery, ophthalmic surgeons must prevent errors related to intraocular lens (IOL) placement after cataract extraction. IOL errors may relate to power, size, or type of lens. These errors may lead to a suboptimal postoperative corrected acuity, may require additional optical correction, or may require additional surgery (eg, IOL exchange). In one series of 700 medico-legal cases in ophthalmology, 154 (22%) cases were related to cataract extraction. Of these, IOL errors were the primary cause in one-third of claims. Between 1987 and 2008, about 220 cases of cataract surgery mistakes were filed with OMIC, and about 80% of those involved wrong power, wrong measurement or wrong IOL implantation, Numerous errors may contribute to an incorrect IOL insertion:

- use of an outdated or inaccurate IOL power calculation formula
- use of the incorrect A-constant in IOL power calculation formula

- incorrect axial length (biometry) or keratometry measurements for IOL power calculations
- transcription or data entry errors into the IOL power calculation program
- inappropriate surgeon selection of postoperative refractive target or IOL style
- calculation of IOL insertion for the incorrect patient or incorrect eye
- insertion by the surgeon of an incorrect IOL for the particular patient (eg, wrong patient, patients with the same or similar name operated on the same day, wrong eye, wrong procedure)
- incorrect labeling or packaging of the IOL by the manufacturer or defective IOL

In one study ($n=154$) of cataract surgery IOL-related errors, 54% were due to erroneous axial length measurement, 38% were anterior chamber depth estimation errors, and 8% were corneal power measurement errors. Errors in IOL manufacturing, packaging, or labeling represented less than 1% of the total errors. In order to prevent IOL-related errors, the surgeon or appropriate team member should consider the precautions shown in Table 17-1.

Minimizing Medication Errors: Communication About Drug Orders

Medication errors are preventable events that may threaten patient safety in the operating room. In 1999, the Institute of Medicine of the National Academies reported that 44,000 to 98,000 deaths occur each year in the United States from medical errors; medication errors constitute a significant proportion of these cases. Common medication errors include

Table 17-1 Precautions for IOL Procedures

In order to prevent IOL-related errors, the surgeon or appropriate team member should consider the following precautions:

1. Ensure that technicians are adequately trained in the techniques for biometry and keratometry measurements and perform periodic technician quality control checks.
2. Perform periodic calibrations of the ultrasound A-scan unit and keratometer.
3. Perform measurements (eg, axial lengths, keratometry) in both eyes for comparison (internal control) and to identify outlying values.
4. Repeat measurements in difficult or complex cases (eg, high myopia, asymmetric refraction) to document the reproducibility of the results.
5. Confirm by repeat measurements results that appear unexpectedly high or low.
6. Review preoperative biometry and keratometry results. (surgeon)
7. Maintain a written IOL calculation checklist that contains patient information, keratometry, axial length, and primary and alternate IOL power, style, and size. (surgeon)
8. In the operating room, check actual IOL information directly against the IOL calculation checklist information. (surgeon)
9. Show the IOL label and verbally confirm the IOL model number and power as the lens is passed to the surgeon for implantation. (circulating nurse, scrub nurse, surgical assistant, with confirmation by the surgeon)
10. Perform a final visual inspection of the IOL under the microscope for any lens defects or deposits. (surgeon)

incorrect administration (type, dose, or route); inaccurate product labeling, packaging, and nomenclature; and inaccurate compounding, dispensing, or distribution.

Like wrong-site surgery, medication errors are a common cause of malpractice claims; in the Physician Insurers Association of America database (n=117,000 claims), medication errors were the second most common cause for a claim. In a review of 700 medicolegal cases in ophthalmology, medication errors were the third most frequent complaint. In data from OMIC, claims for medication errors are more costly than the average claim and more likely to result in indemnity payments.

Factors that might contribute to medication errors include:

- incomplete, inaccurate, or unreviewed patient information (eg, known allergies, complete list of medications, complete medical history, complete surgical history, laboratory or radiographic results)
- incomplete or unavailable drug information (eg, lack of up-to-date warnings, product information, or drug interactions)
- use of standing preoperative or postoperative orders without physician review of patient allergies, potential drug interactions, or duplication of medications
- use of standing orders to "continue preoperative medications" without physician review of existing medication list for allergies, indications, contraindications, drug interactions, or adverse effects
- miscommunication between surgeon and other members of the surgical team (eg, nurse, technician, or pharmacist) regarding drug orders (eg, not hearing the complete order, deleting or inserting a word like "with" or "without" epinephrine from the verbal order)
- illegible handwriting, confusing letters (eg, lowercase letter "l" and the number "1", letter "o" for number "0", or letter "z" for number "2"), or incomprehensible verbal order
- confusion between drugs with similar sounding or similar written names or packaging. These medications should be identified as "high risk," labeled with trade and generic names, and should not be stored in close proximity. Examples of ophthalmic and systemic medications that might be confused and have been reported to the United States Pharmacopeia include the following (brand names are capitalized):
  - atropine and Akarpine
  - Betagan and Betoptic
  - Betoptic and Betoptic S
  - erythromycin and azithromycin
  - Murocel and Murocoll-2
  - Ocufen and Ocuflox
  - Ocufen and Ocupress
  - Refresh (lubricant eye drops) and ReFresh (breath drops)
  - TobraDex and Tobrex
  - Voltaren and tramadol
  - Voltaren and Ultram
- misuse or misinterpretation of zeroes and decimal points in drug dosing

- confusion of metric and English system units in dose
- use of illegible, inaccurate, or inappropriate abbreviations
- inaccurate or inappropriate labeling as a drug is prepared and repackaged into smaller units or into different delivery instruments (eg, syringes mislabeled)
- environmental factors (eg, poor lighting, heat, noise and interruptions) that can distract health professionals from their medical tasks
- failure to follow institution/facility policies and procedure
- presence of medications that may be safe in one route (eg, topical or subconjunctival) but devastating if administered via a different route (eg, intraocular gentamicin causing macular infarction)
- lack of confirmation of medication order and verification of dose, route, and medicine prior to administration of drug

Table 17-2 lists procedures that help minimize the possibility of medication errors.

Preventing Surgeon-Related Fire in the Operating Room

Most hospitals and operating rooms have internal policy and procedure manuals regarding fire prevention and safety. Hart et al described common misconceptions about OR fires including "(1) OR fires do not happen in today's hospitals; (2) if fires do occur, they were not preventable; (3) fires only occur at inferior facilities; and (4) all staff in the OR know what to do if a fire occurs." The Anesthesia Patient Safety Foundation (APSF) and

---

Table 17-2 Procedures That Help Minimize Medication Error

1. Complete and accurate medication list in the chart
2. Careful review of all relevant patient information by the surgeon (eg, known allergies, complete list of medications, complete medical history, complete surgical history, and laboratory or radiographic results)
3. Avoidance of the use of "standing orders" to "continue preoperative medications" without review of medication list, indications, allergies, and doses
4. Explicit communication between surgeon and other members of the surgical team (eg, nurse, technician, pharmacist) regarding drug orders including "digit by digit" repetition of dose (ie, two-three rather than twenty-three)
5. Legible handwriting with block handwriting; avoidance of abbreviations and Latin; complete spelling of drug names, route, and dosage; and avoidance of inappropriate or illegible decimal points in dosage orders
6. Use of leading zero before decimal points (eg, 0.1) and avoidance of use of trailing zero after decimal point (eg, 5. rather than 5.0)
7. Complete adherence to institutional, hospital, and facility policies and procedures regarding labeling of all medications, containers (eg, syringes), and solutions
8. Discarding unlabeled solutions or medications in the operating room
9. "Forcing functions" that eliminate the presence of medications from the surgery table that may be safe in one route but unsafe via a different route (eg, gentamicin, cytotoxic agents, and hypertonic saline)
10. Review of patient allergies prior to administration of drug
11. Individual verbal and written confirmation of medication orders and verification of dose, route, and medicine prior to administration

ECRI released in 2011 *New Clinical Guide to Surgical Fire Prevention* with specific fire reduction strategies including:

- recommendations for open oxygen delivery during procedures on the head, face, neck, and upper chest
- recommendations for the use of supplemental oxygen during procedures on the head, face, neck, and upper chest
- recommendations for implementing a preoperative time-out to assess fire risk potential for every patient for every procedure

The surgeon in training should be familiar with these rules and regulations. The Massachusetts Department of Public Health reviewed incidents of fire in the operating room. It identified 3 key elements necessary for combustion: an oxidizer, a fuel source, and an ignition source. Although a patient may require oxygen in the operating room, an oxygen-enriched environment is a major factor in many surgical fires. In an oxygen-enriched or nitrous oxide–enriched environment, surface fibers (eg, fabric, body hair, vellus hair) can flash (propagate flames) and then ignite more-combustible fuels at the edge of the initial surface.

The patient's health status should be reviewed carefully and the requirement for oxygen should be documented and confirmed as necessary. Oxygen and nitrous oxide levels can build up under the surgical drapes, and tenting of the operative drape (eg, with a Mayo stand) may allow the oxygen to dissipate and gravitate toward the floor. Oxygen can also build up from leakage around endotracheal tube cuffs.

Ophthalmic surgeons should avoid, if possible, creating an "oxygen tent" that could allow unnecessary buildup of oxygen. A spark or other ignition source can precipitate a fire in this highly oxygen-enriched environment. The risk for these fires can be reduced by prepping and exposing the patient's full face, with nasal cannula oxygen allowing the oxygen to dissipate more rapidly.

Cautery units and lasers may act as an ignition source and are more hazardous with oxygen in use because of the lowered temperature threshold for ignition. These units should be activated only when the tip is in view and should not be allowed to contact drapes or other combustible material. Hot-wire cautery devices (Fig 17-1) should not be set down on or near flammable material (eg, gauze or drapes) while still hot. A safety holster should be employed for all devices with active electrodes and set with the tip away

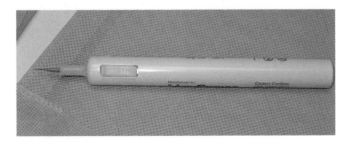

Figure 17-1 Cautery unit. *(Courtesy of Andrew G. Lee, MD.)*

from flammable items. If oxygen must be employed, then the lowest temperature setting for the cautery unit to achieve therapeutic effect should be employed. If possible, the oxygen should be held for at least 1 minute prior to use of the cautery and then restarted after the cautery is completed. Other potential ignition sources in the operating room include electrosurgical units, surgical lasers, fiber-optic light sources, and incandescent or static discharge sparks. Electrosurgical or cautery units should only be activated when the tip is visible and should be deactivated before the tip is removed from the surgeon's view.

Combustible substances that may ignite or act as fuel after a fire in the operating room (Fig 17-2) include surgical drapes and material (eg, gauze, sponges, adhesive tape, drape, hoods, and gown); surgical equipment (eg, plastic or rubber products, anesthesia masks, and tubes); operating room ointments, solvents, and solutions (eg, degreasers, petrolatum, aerosols, paraffin, wax, alcohol, adhesives, and tincture solutions); and the patient's hair (eg, head hair, eyebrows, mustache, or beard).

Consider taking these precautions:

- In ophthalmic surgery, the drapes may cover the eyebrows but in other cases the brow is exposed in the surgical field, and coating the eyebrows might be of benefit if oxygen will be in use.
- The hair can be made less flammable by coating with water-soluble lubricating jelly preoperatively.

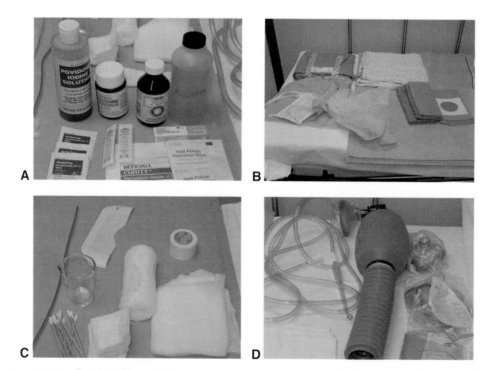

Figure 17-2 Combustible substances that may ignite or act as fuel in an operating room fire. **A,** Solvents and solutions (eg, alcohol, adhesives, tincture solutions). **B,** Surgical drapes, patient's cap and gown. **C,** Dressings (gauze, sponges, adhesive tape). **D,** Surgical tubing. *(Courtesy of Andrew G. Lee, MD.)*

- Volatile solutions (eg, liquid alcohol) should not be allowed to pool in the field, on the patient, or in open containers. Sufficient time should be allowed for drying of any topically applied solutions (eg, adhesives, tinctures, surgical prep solutions, and ointments).
- Alcohol-based surgical preps may contribute to fires if the vapors are trapped by the drapes and come into contact with a heat source.
- Patients should be advised preoperatively against the use on the day of surgery of skin, facial, and hair care products or medications that may contain potential combustible substances (eg, alcohol-based solutions). This includes skin care creams, moisturizers, hair tonics, conditioners, and topical ointments.

Key Points

- Steps to avoiding wrong eye surgery include formal written protocols for preoperative confirmation of correct eye, avoidance of abbreviations for proposed operated eye in the consent form, surgeon use of marking pen to identify correct eye in the operating room, and final verification of correct eye pathology by direct surgeon's examination.
- Incorrect IOL insertion may be caused by faulty power calculations, data transcription errors, surgeon judgment errors, and manufacturer labeling errors.
- Steps to avoid medication errors include ensuring presence and review of complete and accurate medication list in the chart, avoidance of standing orders and abbreviations, reconfirmation of dosage digit by digit between surgeon and medical team members, and eliminating potentially unsafe medications from the surgical suite.
- Causes of operating room fires include oxygen-enriched environment (under surgical drape), contact of cautery unit with flammables, excess flammable solutions such as cosmetics, and volatile operating room solutions.

AAO Cataract and Anterior Segment PPP Panel, Hoskins Center for Quality Eye Care. "Cataract in the Adult Eye—2011" [Preferred Practice Pattern]. Available at aao.org/ppp. Accessed September 12, 2014.

AAO Wrong-Site Task Force, Hoskins Center for Quality Eye Care. "Recommendations of American Academy of Ophthalmology Wrong-Site Task Force—2014." Available at http://one.aao.org/patient-safety-statement/recommendations-of-american-academy -ophthalmology. Accessed September 12, 2014.

American Academy of Ophthalmology, the American Society of Ophthalmic Registered Nurses, and the American Association of Eye and Ear Hospitals. *Minimizing Medication Errors: Communication about Drug Orders* [Patient Safety Bulletin]. 2005. Available at http://one.aao.org/patient-safety-statement/minimizing-medication-errors -communication-about-d. Accessed September 12, 2014.

American Academy of Orthopaedic Surgeons and American Association of Orthopaedic Surgeons. *Wrong-Site Surgery* [Information Statement]. 2010. Available at www.aaos.org /about/papers/advistmt/1015.asp. Accessed September 12, 2014.

American Academy of Orthopaedic Surgeons. *Report of the Task Force on Wrong-Site Surgery.* Rosemont, IL: American Academy of Orthopaedic Surgeons; 1998.

American Board of Ophthlamology. "Patient Safety Education." Available at http://abop .org/maintain-certification/part-2-lifelong-learning-self-assessment/cme/patient-safety/. Accessed October 10, 2014.

Brandt RW. Daily safety for you and your patient. *AORN J.* 1972;16(5):64–67.

Brick DC. Risk management lessons from a review of 168 cataract surgery claims. *Surv Ophthalmol.* 1999;43(4):356–360.

Courtright P, Paton K, McCarthy JM, Sibley LM, Holland SPl. An epidemiologic investigation of unexpected refractive errors following cataract surgery. *Can J Ophthalmol.* 1998;33(3): 210–215.

ECRI Institute. Fire hazard created by the misuse of Duraprep solution. *Health Devices.* 1998; 28(2):400–402.

ECRI Institute. Fires during surgery of the head and neck area (Update). *Health Devices.* 1980;9(3):82.

ECRI Institute. Fires from oxygen use during head and neck surgery. *Health Devices.* 1995; 24(4):155–156.

ECRI Institute. New clinical guide to surgical fire prevention. *Health Devices.* 2009;38(10): 314–332.

ECRI Institute. The patient is on fire! A surgical fires primer. *Guidance.* 1992;21(1):19–34.

Ellis JH. Faulty A-scan readings present potential liability. *ARGUS.* 1994. From OMIC Publication Archives. Available at www.omic.com/faulty-a-scan-readings-present -potential-liability-2/. Accessed September 12, 2014.

Hart SR, Yajnik A, Ashford J, Spring R, Harvey S. Operating room fire safety. *Ochsner J.* 2011;11(1): 37–42.

Institute of Medicine. *To Err Is Human: Building a Safer Health System.* Washington, DC: National Academies Press; 2000.

Joint Commission on Accreditation of Healthcare Organizations. *Lessons Learned: Wrong Site Surgery.* Sentinel Event Alert [serial online]. August 28, 1998;6. Follow-up alert December 5, 2001. Available at www.jointcommission.org/sentinel_event_alert_issue_6 _lessons_learned_wrong_site_surgery/. Accessed September 12, 2014.

Kirkner RM. How to manage your malpractice risks. *Rev Ophthalmol.* 2009;Jan 14: 45–48.

Kohnen S. Postoperative refractive error resulting from incorrectly labeled intraocular lens power. *J Cataract Refract Surg.* 2000;26:777–778.

Massachusetts Department of Public Health. 2002. "Health Care Quality Safety Alert: Preventing Operating Room Fires During Surgery." Available at www.mtpinnacle.com /pdfs/hospital_alerts_or_fires.pdf. Accessed September 12, 2014.

Morris R. Wrong power IOL inserted during cataract surgery [serial online]. *OMIC Digest.* 2000:11. Available at http://www.omic.com/wrong-power-iol-inserted-during-cataract -surgery/. Accessed September 17, 2014.

Murphy EK. Liability for incorrect intraoperative medications. *AORN J.* 1989(5);50:1106–1108.

National Patient Safety Foundation. *Agenda for Research and Development in Patient Safety.* 2000. Available at www.npsf.org/wp-content/uploads/2011/10/Agenda_for_RD_in_Patient _Safety.pdf. Accessed September 12, 2014.

Norrby N, Grossman L, Geraghty E, et al. Accuracy in determining intraocular lens dioptric power assessed by interlaboratory tests. *J Cataract Refract Surg.* 1996;22(7):983–993.

Olsen T, Olesen H. IOL power mislabeling. *Acta Ophthalmol (Copenh).* 1993;71(1):99–102.

Olsen T. Sources of error in intraocular lens power calculation. *J Cataract Refract Surg.* 1992; 18(2):125–129.

Simon JW, Ngo Y, Khan S, Strogatz D. Surgical confusions in ophthalmology. *Arch Ophthalmol.* 2007;125(11):1515–1522.

Smith HE. The incidence of liability claims in ophthalmology as compared with other specialties. *Ophthalmology.* 1990;97(10):1376–1378.

Weber P. "Wrong Eye, Wrong IOL, Wrong Patient" [serial online]. *OMIC Digest.* Summer 2008. Available at www.omic.com/wrong-eye-wrong-iol-wrong-patient. Accessed September 12, 2014.

Self-Assessment Test

1. Procedures to prevent wrong-eye surgery include which of the following? (Choose all that apply.)
   a. formal written procedures and protocols for surgical team members to identify and confirm the operative eye
   b. informed consent form that clearly and explicitly states the operative procedure and the operative eye without the use of potentially confounding abbreviations
   c. availability of the medical record in the room with explicit written documentation of the operative site
   d. marking of the operative eye (eg, using a marking pen and writing the surgeon's initials at the site)

2. Factors in incorrect IOL insertion include which of the following? (Choose all that apply.)
   a. incorrect perimetry data
   b. incorrect axial length (biometry) or keratometry measurements for IOL power calculations
   c. calculation of IOL insertion for incorrect patient or incorrect eye
   d. incorrect optical coherence tomography measurement of macular thickness

3. Common sources of medication error include which of the following? (Choose all that apply.)
   a. use of standing preoperative or postoperative orders without physician review of patient allergies, potential drug interactions, or duplication of medications
   b. miscommunication between surgeon and other members of the surgical team (eg, nurse, technician, and pharmacist) regarding drug orders
   c. patient self-medication in the operating room
   d. illegible handwriting, confusing letters, or incomprehensible verbal order
   e. confusion between drugs with similar sounding or similar written names or packaging

4. Combustible substances that may ignite in the operating room include which of the following? (Choose all that apply.)
   a. surgical drapes and material
   b. anesthesia masks and tubes
   c. operating room ointments, solvents, and solutions
   d. the patient's hair

For preferred responses to these questions, see Appendix A.

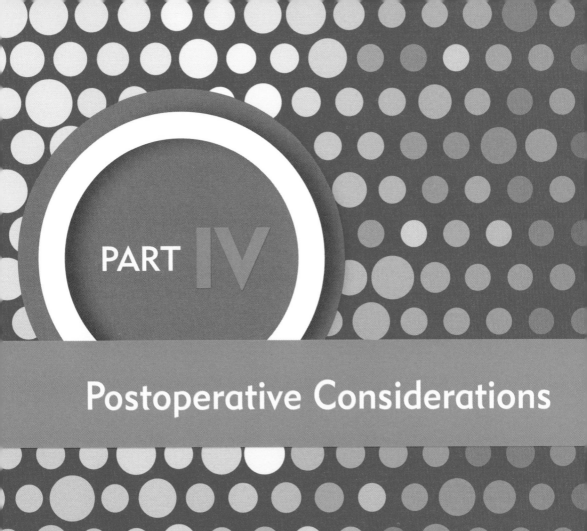

PART **IV**

Postoperative Considerations

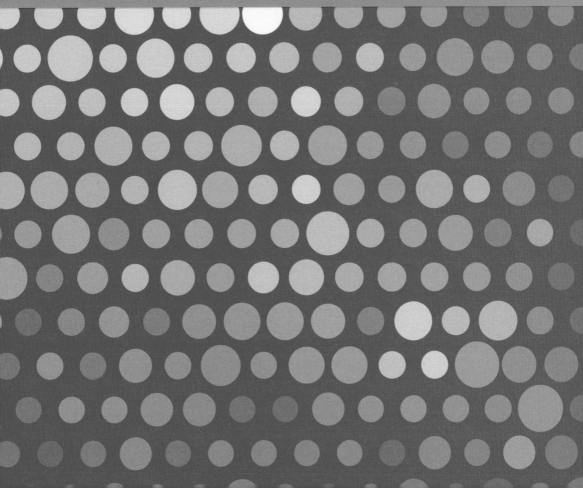

CHAPTER 18

Postoperative Management

Nicholas J. Volpe, MD
Dmitry Pyatetsky, MD

The care of patients undergoing ophthalmic surgery does not end in the operating room. Provision of appropriate postoperative care and prompt, effective management of complications are critical to successful surgery. Postoperative care is the surgeon's responsibility to the patient and should not be relegated to another physician or assistant.

This chapter describes components of successful postoperative management, including

- communicating postoperative instructions to nursing staff and your patient
- scheduling timely postoperative examinations
- ensuring properly focused postoperative examinations
- recognizing and treating common complications
- knowing when to get assistance from others

Most patients with complications can be managed successfully with an excellent outcome if complications are recognized early and treated appropriately. These patients will require you to focus the most, because they need your expertise much more than the patient with uncomplicated surgery. Certainly these patients and the conversations you have with them must not be avoided. You must acknowledge the "bump in the road" to your patient, be calm, and outline a careful treatment plan.

Postoperative Instructions

At the conclusion of any procedure the surgeon must write appropriate orders in the patient medical record and communicate postoperative care issues and instructions to the patient and the patient's family, both verbally and in writing (Fig 18-1). Postoperative orders vary from procedure to procedure and from surgeon to surgeon. However, certain issues should be addressed in most patients:

- name of the procedure
- orders to follow the usual discharge or admission procedure of the short procedure unit
- instructions for body positioning and wound care
- antiemetic medications
- pain medications

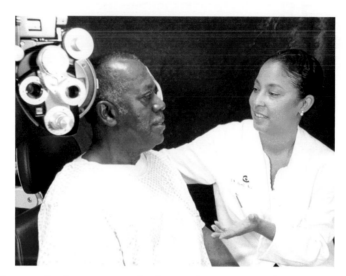

Figure 18-1 Communicating postoperative instructions to your patient—and the patient's family, if appropriate—is important to successful postoperative management. Other components are timely, focused postoperative examinations and effective management of complications. *(Image courtesy of National Eye Institute, National Institutes of Health.)*

- instructions to advance diet and discontinue intravenous fluids
- specific nursing instructions (eg, vision checks, use of ice, use of intravenous antibiotics)
- postoperative ocular medications (eg, antibiotic drops)

Patients (and family when appropriate) should hear the surgeon's initial impression as to the success of the surgery and the plan for postoperative care. This is of paramount importance to assure a good outcome. Patients must be instructed as to

- the appropriate care of surgical wounds or dressings
- the timing of postoperative evaluations and the application of medication
- the type and amount of pain to be expected and how to manage it
- activity restrictions
- warning signs or symptoms requiring contact with physician and immediate attention
- methods and phone numbers to contact the operating surgeon

Additional issues related to postoperative care and complications vary depending on the type of procedure that was performed. Detailed discussion of specific procedures and their complications is beyond the scope of this book. However, a general discussion here focuses on the timing of postoperative care and possible complications of 6 broad categories of ophthalmic procedures:

- anterior segment surgery
- strabismus surgery
- eyelid and orbital surgery

- retinovitreous surgery
- laser surgery
- intravitreal injection

Timing of Postoperative Care

The timing of appropriate postoperative care varies from procedure to procedure. Most patients are not examined on the same day of the surgery after they leave the operating room. A dressing such as an eye patch and shield are applied and then removed by the surgeon at the first follow-up visit. However, there are certain circumstances in which a brief examination should be performed the same day shortly after performing the procedure. These include

- after any type of surgery to check for recovery of motility and eyelid function following local anesthetic injection
- after orbital or optic nerve surgery to perform vision check and rule out bleeding
- after strabismus surgery to perform adjustment of adjustable suture
- after vitreoretinal surgery with gas injection to check intraocular pressure (IOP)

After intravitreal injection, it is important to check IOP, ascertain perfusion of the retina, and rule out inadvertent perforation of the retina with the needle. Specific schedules for postoperative care are determined on an individual basis determined by the surgeon and each patient's needs. The following are approximate guidelines for the 6 broad categories of patients.

Anterior Segment Surgery

Patients who undergo cataract surgery, glaucoma surgery, or corneal transplantation are examined for the first time within 24 hours of the surgical procedure. This initial examination is the most critical for ruling out unexpected intraoperative complications, measuring the initial level of visual acuity, determining the anatomic success of the procedure (eg, position of the iris or intraocular lens, depth of anterior chamber, appearance of filtration bleb, position of corneal transplant button), testing the security and watertight nature of all surgical wounds, measuring IOP, and looking for early signs of infection. For uncomplicated cataract surgery, the subsequent examinations are generally done 1 week later (optional) and 1 month after that.

Endophthalmitis generally presents between the first and seventh day postoperatively; therefore, if infection is suspected based on initial examination findings or symptoms of decreased vision, pain, or redness, sooner follow-up than 1 week would be needed.

Examinations of patients undergoing filtration surgery for glaucoma are often more frequent in the first week. These patients may initially have overfiltration or leaking wounds that need to be monitored or treated (patching, bandage contact lens) or underfiltration that either needs to be watched or treated with laser suture lysis. Antimetabolites may also be used during this time. If IOP is low, careful examination for choroidal detachments is necessary.

Corneal transplant patients need to be followed closely for evidence of graft failure and/or rejection that requires specific treatment.

Strabismus Surgery

Because strabismus surgery is extraocular, the risk of vision-threatening complications is lower than for intraocular procedures. Most strabismus surgeons schedule the first postoperative visit between the first day and 2 weeks after surgery. If the patient is not being seen on the first postoperative day, however, careful instructions are given to the patient or parents to call if excessive redness, discharge, pain or swelling develop that would suggest infection or if initial alignment of the eyes does not appear satisfactory. If adjustable sutures are used, then initial exam may be on the same day or first postoperative day for suture adjustment. For adults with multiple eye muscles operated, there is a small risk of anterior segment ischemia, and these patients are examined on the first day and in the following weeks for signs of this condition.

Eyelid and Orbital Surgery

Eyelid surgery patients are seen within a few days of the procedure provided there are no complaints of swelling or unexpected tenderness that would suggest infection. If adjustable suture technique is used or office modification of ptosis surgery is planned, the timing of follow-up is adjusted accordingly. Patients undergoing orbital surgery are often admitted to the hospital. Because of risk of bleeding and of injury to the optic nerve, ocular blood supply and adnexal structures they are examined on the first postoperative day and 2–3 times over the following month.

Retinovitreous Surgery

The widely varying types and complexities of retinovitreous surgeries require a flexible approach to timing of postoperative evaluations. These patients are always seen on the first postoperative day and followed closely in the weeks that follow. The frequency of postoperative visits is determined by the visual function as well as the status of detached retina and subretinal fluid, intraocular gas, IOP, and presence of intraocular bleeding.

Laser Surgery

Laser surgery procedures are generally performed on the anterior segment for glaucoma, the cornea for refractive surgery, the posterior lens capsule for capsulotomy, and the retina for various conditions including diabetic retinopathy, holes or tears, and choroidal neovascularization. Patients undergoing anterior segment laser procedures are often checked 1 or 2 hours after the procedure to measure IOP and 1 week later to determine success of the procedure. Refractive surgery patients are seen in the days after the surgery unless there are flap complications requiring more immediate attention. Patients undergoing laser surgery on the retina require follow-up at varying times in the days and weeks following the procedure, as some may require re-treatments (eg, choroidal neovascularization) and others need only be seen weeks later to determine whether treatments was successful (eg, macular treatment in diabetic retinopathy).

The use of femtosecond laser in cataract surgery for purposes of astigmatism-correcting corneal arcuate incisions, main and secondary corneal incisions, anterior capsulotomy, and/or nuclear fragmentation is becoming increasingly common. Postoperative care of these patients does not differ from those who have conventional phacoemulsification.

Intravitreal Injection

Intravitreal injections of therapeutic agents have become the standard of care for treatment of a number of ophthalmic diseases. The procedure offers the benefit of delivering a drug at a high concentration directly to the eye with minimal systemic absorption. (See "Intravitreal Injections" in *Basic Techniques of Ophthalmic Surgery* for procedural information.) Intravitreal injections are performed for a range of conditions, from treatment of macular degeneration with anti-VEGF agents, to delivery of antibiotics in the setting of endophthalmitis, to treatment of uveitis with antiviral, antifungal, and immunosuppressive agents. In addition, gas and implantable devices may be delivered intravitreally, but the discussion of these techniques is beyond the scope of this chapter.

Patients who undergo intravitreal injections should have a dilated funduscopic examination performed immediately after the procedure. The purpose of this examination is to ascertain that the retina and the optic nerve are perfused and not damaged by the needle and that the IOP is in an acceptable range. Subsequent examinations vary based on the indication for treatment, with daily examinations for patients with endophthalmitis and aggressive viral uveitis. Patients with noninfectious uveitis or cystoid macular edema should be re-examined 1–4 weeks after the procedure, and patients with neovascular macular degeneration should be examined 1 month after the procedure. For patients who are scheduled to be examined more than several days after the procedure, many practitioners employ a post-procedure telephone call, which may be performed by the surgeon or an assistant. The purpose of this phone call is to inquire about any evidence of endophthalmitis (severe pain, drastic drop in vision) and to reiterate to the patient the warning signs of problems and steps to take should such problems occur.

Focus of the Examination

Generally speaking, postoperative examinations are focused on determining whether the intended goal was accomplished, assessing the postoperative anatomy, looking for complications, and determining the timing of anticipated postoperative interventions such as medication changes and suture cutting. Once again the focus of the examination depends on the type of procedure performed.

Anterior Segment Surgery

The focus of this examination includes measurement of visual acuity, determining anterior segment anatomy (intraocular lens, corneal graft, or filtration bleb position), measurement of IOP, looking for intraocular inflammation (cells and flare in anterior chamber), looking for signs of infection (excessive injection, hypopyon), determination of the security of the surgical wound to be sure it is not leaking, and examination of the retina for perforations from anesthetic injection or retinal detachment. If visual acuity is decreased, an explanation must be found.

Strabismus Surgery

The focus of the postoperative strabismus examination is to ensure successful reattachment of muscles with normal function; to rule out scleral perforations, anterior segment ischemia, or infection; and to determine the success of the procedure. Successful strabismus surgery is characterized by maintenance of good visual acuity, successful motor alignment, and restoration of or facilitation of binocular single vision and fusion.

Eyelid and Orbital Surgery

Postoperative examination of eyelid surgery focuses on the security of skin wounds, resolution of swelling, absence of infection, and achievement of the surgical goal (eg, eyelid position in ptosis and ectropion surgery, and anatomic restoration and absence of tumor in cases of tumor excision). Postoperative evaluation after surgery for eyelid and orbital tumors must also include review of histopathology and specific diagnosis. This will help define further treatments as well as determine the adequacy of surgical margins. In patients undergoing orbital surgery, extraocular muscle function and optic nerve function should be measured.

Retinovitreous Surgery

After retinovitreous surgery, the focused examination includes a determination of whether the retina is attached, holes or breaks are adequately treated, and subretinal fluid is diminished. Many procedures involve the injection of intraocular gases and the level of fill and position of the gas bubble are important considerations. Examination of the anterior segment is required to assess corneal and lens clarity and should include an assessment of the IOP.

Laser Surgery

Laser surgery usually alters anatomy only minimally, so the postoperative examination centers on identifying secondary effects such as IOP spikes, corneal edema, and macular edema, as well as determining whether the goal of the procedure was accomplished. This involves assessment of uncorrected visual acuity in the refractive surgery patient, measurement of pressure in a patient undergoing trabeculoplasty, determination of anterior chamber depth and angle status in peripheral iridotomy patients, or adequacy of capsule opening in capsulotomy patients. The examination also assesses adequacy and extent of treatment in patients undergoing retinal laser treatment for diabetic macular edema, diabetic neovascularization (panretinal photocoagulation), and laser treatment for choroidal neovascularization.

Some retinal procedures (eg, photodynamic therapy) require repeated laser applications, and in this setting the examiner must determine if re-treatment is required for continued leakage from persistent neovascularization. For patients who underwent femtosecond laser-assisted cataract surgery, to rule out leakage, it is important to perform the Seidel test not only on the primary and secondary corneal incisions, but also the arcuate incisions.

Intravitreal Injection

A check of IOP and dilated funduscopic examination for the optic disc and the retina should be performed immediately after the procedure to ascertain perfusion and rule out inadvertent perforation of the retina. IOP is frequently elevated briefly immediately after the injection, but comes down spontaneously within minutes after the procedure. If the postoperative IOP is found to be very high (generally above 40 mmHg), the surgeon should consider performing an anterior chamber paracentesis to remove a small amount of aqueous. Look for a retinal tear, intraretinal or vitreous bleeding, or a retinal detachment. In cases where the injected substance is a particulate suspension or in cases of dense vitritis or small pupil, this examination may be difficult; if difficulty with the procedure is experienced, the surgeon may employ ultrasonography to rule out damage to the retina.

Subsequent examinations should focus on whether or not the goal of the treatment has been achieved, while also double-checking that there is no damage to the retina related to the injection and that the IOP is in an acceptable range, especially if a corticosteroid has been injected due to the risk of steroid-induced glaucoma.

Pain Management

Fortunately, most patients who undergo eye surgery will experience only mild to moderate pain. In fact, severe pain is often an important clue to a postoperative complication such as IOP spike, hemorrhage, or infection. Typical postoperative pain is generally managed with systemic medications and local maneuvers. Acetaminophen is often used as a first-line analgesic, as it is effective for mild to moderate pain and does not increase risk of hemorrhage. For more severe pain, after complications have been assessed and managed, narcotics such as codeine or oxycodone may be added. Helpful local maneuvers include the use of ice and elevation to modify pain and swelling in patients undergoing strabismus, eyelid, or orbital surgery.

Management of Complications

The term *complication* refers to an undesired outcome of surgery, related to an intraoperative event or a postoperative process that results in a suboptimal result. Postoperative management includes assessment for such processes and institution of measures to control the problems. It is beyond the scope of this text to detail management of specific complications; however, certain complications are more common, and assessment should include evaluation for them in each case. Full disclosure with careful discussion of the complication and the suggested course of action should always occur in your discussions with patients.

Retrobulbar or Peribulbar Anesthetic Injections

Complications related to these injections include

- retrobulbar hemorrhage
- puncture of the globe
- injection of anesthetic into the eye
- injection of anesthetic into the optic nerve or subarachnoid space
- injection into or trauma to an extraocular muscle

Retrobulbar hemorrhage is an ophthalmic emergency. An orbital compartment syndrome can develop, and elevation of the pressure in the orbit can be severe enough to compromise ocular blood flow or raise IOP to unsafe levels. If a retrobulbar hemorrhage is encountered, the ophthalmologist must decompress the orbit by performing a lateral canthotomy and cantholysis. Puncture of the globe and/or injection of anesthetic into the eye may result in a hypotonus eye; the red reflex may appear abnormal and the anterior chamber may be deeper than normal. The puncture can lead to retinal or vitreous hemorrhage, or retinal tear or detachment.

Unusual intraocular inflammation may result from the injection of anesthetic. Prompt treatment and retinovitreous surgery may be required. If the needle inadvertently is placed within the optic nerve sheath, it can cause a vision-threatening hemorrhage (sheath hematoma) requiring optic nerve sheath decompression surgery. The anesthetic can travel back to the brain and lead to seizures, respiratory depression, or cranial nerve palsies; neurologic consultation may be required for seizure control, and respiratory support may be necessary. Trauma and hemorrhage to an extraocular muscle during injection can lead to eye movement abnormality and double vision; typically, no acute intervention is required, but later correction may be necessary if muscle dysfunction persists.

General Principles of Management for Common Entities

A complete list of surgical complications requiring postoperative therapy is beyond the scope of this text, but some of the more common entities, along with general principles for management, are briefly described next by category.

Anterior segment surgery

Complications (and management) of cataract surgery include

- endophthalmitis, characterized by profound visual loss, severe pain, conjunctival injection, hypopyon, and vitreous opacity (vitrectomy or vitreous tap and culture, and intraocular antibiotic injection)
- uveitis (corticosteroid, topical and/or systemic)
- wound leaks (pressure patch, surgical closure)
- intraocular tissue prolapse through wounds (surgical replacement and closure)
- lost lens or lens fragments (corticosteroids, retinovitreous surgical removal)

- intraocular lens dislocation (surgical repositioning)
- elevation of IOP (pressure-lowering agents, paracentesis)
- corneal edema (manage IOP and inflammation)
- cystoid macular edema (topical anti-inflammatory agents)

Complications (and management) of corneal transplant surgery include

- graft rejection or primary graft failure (corticosteroid therapy)
- wound leak (surgical closure)
- suture abscess (suture removal if safe)
- persistent epithelial defects (patch, therapeutic contact lens)
- elevated IOP (pressure-lowering agents)

Complications (and management) of glaucoma surgery include

- persistence of high pressure (reinstitute medications, suture lysis, reoperation)
- flat or severely shallow anterior chamber secondary to overfiltration or bleb leaks (pressure patch, partial surgical closure)
- hyphema (pressure management; rarely, surgical evacuation)

Strabismus surgery

Complications (and management) of strabismus surgery include

- overcorrections and undercorrections (documentation, observation for stability, prisms, possible reoperation)
- scleral perforations (evaluation for retinal tear or detachment, laser or retinovitreous surgery if necessary)
- lost or torn muscles (surgical exploration and repair)
- anterior segment ischemia (anti-inflammatory therapy)

Eyelid and orbital surgery

Complications (and management) of eyelid and orbital surgery include

- orbital hemorrhage (emergent canthotomy and cantholysis, possible orbital exploration to control persistent bleeding)
- optic nerve damage after orbital surgery (neuroimaging to assess for bone fragments, intrasheath hemorrhage, possible reoperation for optic nerve sheath decompression)
- orbital cellulitis (neuroimaging to assess for abscess, systemic antibiotics, possible surgical drainage)
- eyelid hematoma (ice) or infection (systemic antibiotics)
- lagophthalmos and exposure keratitis (intensive lubricants, possible surgical repositioning)

Retinovitreous surgery

Complications (and management) of retinovitreous surgery include

- failure to achieve retinal reattachment or closure of holes or tears (observe, possible reoperation)

- intraocular hemorrhage (observe, possible reoperation)
- new retinal tears (re-treatment)
- IOP elevation, particularly when long-acting gases are used (pressure-lowering agents)

Laser surgery

Complications (and management) of laser surgery include

- glaucoma laser surgery: intraocular hemorrhage, elevated IOP (pressure-lowering agents)
- YAG capsulotomy: intraocular lens damage, IOP elevation, uveitis (pressure-lowering agents, topical corticosteroids), and retinal detachment
- keratorefractive surgery: corneal flap complications (possible surgical correction), corneal infections (antibiotics)
- retinal laser surgery: choroidal effusions (management of IOP)

Intravitreal Injection

Complications (and management) of intravitreal injection include

- significant post-procedure IOP elevation (topical IOP-lowering agents, anterior chamber paracentesis with removal of small amount of aqueous)
- long-term steroid-induced glaucoma (topical IOP-lowering agents, glaucoma surgery)
- infectious endophthalmitis (intravitreal injection of antibiotics with or without pars plana vitrectomy)
- sterile endophthalmitis (may be difficult to differentiate from infectious endophthalmitis; treat with topical steroids and monitor every few hours, being ready to switch to infectious endophthalmitis treatment strategy should the process worsen)
- retinal tear/perforation, inadvertent injection of therapeutic agent into the subretinal space (barrier laser photocoagulation)
- retinal detachment (surgical repair by pars plana vitrectomy or scleral buckle placement)
- development or progression of cataract, damage to the lens capsule by the needle (cataract extraction, may require advanced techniques and need for vitrectomy at time of cataract surgery in cases where lens capsule is damaged)

Key Points

- Postoperative counseling of the patient includes care of surgical wounds, dressings, and the application of medication, type and amount of pain to be expected, activity restrictions, and warning signs or symptoms requiring contact with physician and immediate attention.
- At the first postoperative visit after anterior segment surgery, the examination should include determining the anatomic success of the procedure, testing the

security and watertight nature of the surgical wound, measuring IOP, and looking for early signs of infection.

- Complications of cataract surgery include endophthalmitis, uveitis, wound leaks, intraocular tissue prolapse, lost lens or lens fragments, intraocular lens dislocation, elevation of IOP, corneal edema, and cystoid macular edema.
- Complications of strabismus surgery include overcorrections and undercorrections, scleral perforations, lost or torn muscles, and anterior segment ischemia.
- Complications of intravitreal injection include endophthalmitis, postoperative elevation of IOP, and damage to the retina or the lens with the needle.

American Academy of Ophthalmology. *An Ophthalmologist's Duties Concerning Postoperative Care.* Policy Statement. Available at http://bit.ly/1vC9Wwh. Accessed October 10, 2014.

Self-Assessment Test

1. Postoperative counseling of the patient should include which of the following? (Choose all that apply.)
   a. expected level of pain
   b. activity restrictions
   c. warning signs or symptoms requiring contact with physician and immediate attention
   d. the appropriate care of surgical wounds or dressings
   e. the timing of postoperative evaluations and the application of medication

2. For the first postoperative visit after anterior segment surgery, what are the key features of the examination? (Choose all that apply.)
   a. correcting residual astigmatic error
   b. determining the anatomic success of the procedure
   c. testing the security and watertight nature of the surgical wound
   d. measuring IOP
   e. looking for early signs of infection
   f. cleaning the posterior capsule of opacities

3. What should be the focus of the postoperative strabismus examination? (Choose all that apply.)
   a. Prescribe the appropriate prism spectacle correction.
   b. Remove muscle sutures.
   c. Ensure successful reattachment of muscles with normal function.
   d. Rule out scleral perforations, anterior segment ischemia, or infection.

4. Which of the following are possible complications of retrobulbar or peribulbar anesthetic injections? (Choose all that apply.)
   a. retrobulbar hemorrhage
   b. puncture of the globe
   c. injection of anesthetic into the eye
   d. injection of anesthetic into the optic nerve or subarachnoid space
   e. injection into or trauma to an extraocular muscle

5. Which of the following are possible early complications of cataract surgery? (Choose all that apply.)
    a. endophthalmitis
    b. strabismus
    c. wound leak
    d. intraocular tissue prolapse
    e. peripheral iridectomy
    f. intraocular lens dislocation
    g. elevation of IOP

6. Severe eye pain several days after intravitreal injection of bevacizumab for neovascular age-related macular degeneration may be a sign of which significant complication? How soon should the patient with this complaint be evaluated?
    a. endophthalmitis—examine in 1 week.
    b. retinal detachment—examine immediately.
    c. endophthalmitis—examine immediately.
    d. retinal detachment—examine in 1 week.
    e. keratitis—examine immediately.

For preferred responses to these questions, see Appendix A.

CHAPTER 19

The Healing Process

Frank Moya, MD
Peter A. Quiros, MD
Casey Mickler, MD

Healing in ophthalmic surgery involves several tissues with differing characteristics. Although many features are common to all tissue types, the processes involved in healing vary accordingly. This chapter addresses the stages and factors involved in healing and the ways in which they impact ocular surgery. An introduction to the basic science of wound modulation will place the surgeon in good stead to improve surgical outcomes in the coming years. In the future, modulation of wound healing is likely to become more sophisticated as manipulation of growth factors, cytokines, and cellular messengers that were once thought to be only basic science research likely will be indispensable in the operating room and outpatient settings.

Healing by Intention

Traditionally, 3 types of wound healing are described: healing by first intention, second intention, or third intention.

Healing by first intention involves approximation of the wound edges with sutures or adhesive strips, usually after surgical incision (Fig 19-1A). Wounds healed by primary intention are associated with minimal basement membrane interruption, tissue loss, and cellular damage.

Healing by second intention is associated with more extensive loss of tissue and unapposed wound edges (Fig 19-1B). Granulation tissue is formed and subsequently connective tissue deposited. A prominent feature of healing by second intention is wound contracture, the process whereby the surrounding normal tissue is pulled toward the area of the initial wound by the scarring process.

Healing by third intention (also called *delayed primary intention*) entails septic wounds (Fig 19-1C). Typically such a wound is debrided, treated, and left open until such time it is deemed suitable to be closed. It is important to remember that the sequence of healing events is the same regardless of the type of wound.

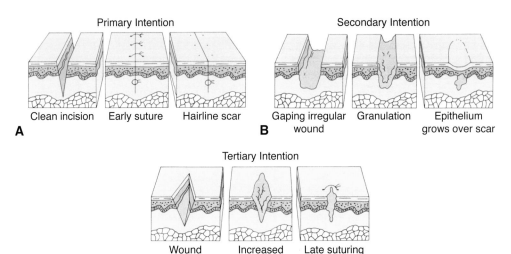

Figure 19-1 Healing by intention. **A,** Primary intention. **B,** Secondary intention. **C,** Tertiary intention. *(Reproduced with permission from Raymond-Seniuk C. Postoperative nursing management. In: Smeltzer SC et al, eds.* Brunner & Suddarth's Textbook of Medical Surgical Nursing. *11th ed. Philadelphia: Lippincott Williams & Wilkins; 2:538.)*

The Process of Healing

The process of wound healing has classically been divided into 3 phases: inflammation, proliferation, and tissue maturation. These stages are not mutually exclusive. They are a continuum of events, and all 3 stages may occur simultaneously. Vascular tissue injury causes bleeding that initiates a hemostatic response. In the inflammatory phase, neutrophils infiltrate and protect the site from microbes and begin the process of cleaning up necrotic tissue and cells. Macrophages continue the role of debridement and secrete factors that initiate the proliferative phase. In this phase, fibroblasts begin secreting connective tissue proteins. Vascular endothelial cells initiate the process of angiogenesis. Epithelial cells migrate over the wound surface and myofibroblasts, through cell–matrix interactions, contract the wound, and facilitate wound closure. In the maturational stage, fibroblasts continue to secrete the structural proteins and proteases necessary for the reorganization of collagen fibrils; both aid in increasing wound strength and tissue flexibility. The process of wound healing varies in different ocular tissues. Fig 19-2 illustrates a summary of the wound healing process.

The time needed for wound healing depends on many factors, including tissue vascularity, availability of chemoattractant factors, and cellular proliferation rates. In general, the more vascular the tissue, the quicker it tends to heal, as increased vascularity allows for a more robust cellular response and can support greater cellular proliferation. Because regulating the vascularity of a tissue without causing injury is more complex, modulation of wound healing is often accomplished by diminishing and slowing cellular response and proliferation mechanisms. For example, facial skin is usually sutured with nylon or polypropylene (Prolene) monofilaments. These minimize localized cellular response at the wound site, helping to prevent scarring. Similarly, medications such as

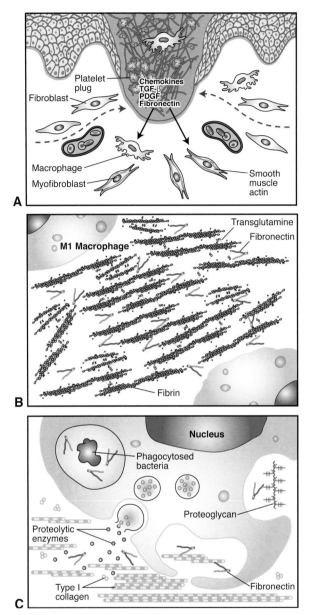

Figure 19-2 Summary of the healing process. **A,** Inflammatory cell migration. A low-power view of the wound site depicts the migration of macrophages, fibroblasts, and smooth muscle actin–containing myofibroblasts as they migrate to the wound from the surrounding tissue into the provisional matrix. Fibronectin, growth factors, chemokines, cell debris, and bacterial products are chemoattractants for a variety of cells that are recruited to the wound site (2–4 days). The initial phase of the repair reaction typically begins with hemorrhage into the tissue. **B,** A fibrin clot forms from plasma and platelets, and it fills the gap created by the wound. Fibronectin in the extravasated plasma binds fibrin, collagen, and other extracellular matrix components within fibrin strands that are cross-linked by the action of transglutaminase (factor XIII). This cross-linking provides a provisional mechanical stabilization of the wound (0–4 hours). Neutrophils rapidly infiltrate in the presence of bacteria or damaged tissue. **C,** Macrophages recruited to the wound area further process cell remnants and damaged extracellular matrix. The binding of fibronectin to cell membranes, collagens, proteoglycans, DNA, and bacteria (opsonization) facilitates phagocytosis by these macrophages and contributes to the removal of debris (1–3 days).

(Continued)

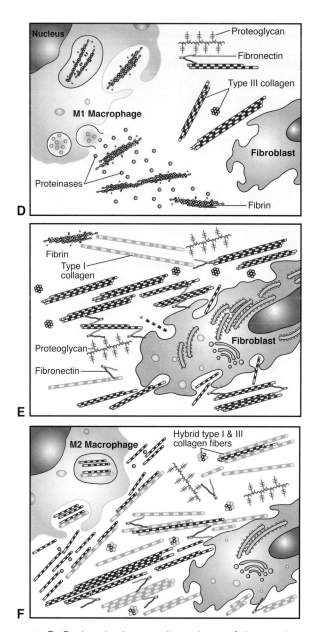

Figure 19-2 *(continued)* **D,** During the intermediate phase of the repair reaction, recruited fibroblasts deposit a new extracellular matrix of primarily smaller collagen type III fibers at the wound site, while the initial fibrin clot is lysed by a combination of a temporary matrix, including proteoglycans, glycoproteins such as polymerized cellular fibronectin, and fibers enriched in type III collagen (2–5 days). **E,** Concurrent with fibrin removal by macrophages, there is a continued fibroblast production of a temporary matrix, including proteoglycans, glycoproteins such as polymerized cellular fibronectin and fibers enriched in type III collagen (2–5 days). Integrin receptors act to form polymers of fibronectin, and integrins and fibronectin help form collagen fibrils. **F,** Final phase of the repair reaction. Gradually, the fibroblasts convert to production of thicker collagen fibers rich in type I collagen, and the temporary, thinner collagen III–enriched fibers are turned over, leading to the stronger definitive matrix (5 days to weeks). Summary of the wound healing process. *(Reproduced, with permission, from Sephel CG, Davidson JM. Repair, regeneration, and fibrosis. In: Rubin E, Reisner HM, eds.* Essentials of Rubin's Pathology. *6th ed. Baltimore: Lippincott Williams & Wilkins; 2014:59.)*

steroids can be used to slow the cellular response or the proliferation of certain cells in deference to others. As you will see, these techniques are applied to tissues differentially depending on the demands of the wound healing process, and techniques vary from tissue to tissue.

Wound Healing in Dermal/Conjunctival Tissue

Conjunctiva and dermis both are highly vascular tissues with like cellular and stromal structure and similarity in wound healing issues.

Inflammatory Phase

When tissue injury occurs, the inflammatory stage of wound repair begins. The injury often involves vascular damage, leading to the extravasation of blood into soft tissues. Tissue hemostasis involves an orchestration of many cellular components including vascular endothelial cells, platelets, and the coagulation cascade. The initial clot structure that fills the wound space has functions in addition to simple hemostasis. The newly formed structure is rich in fibrin and glycoproteins that facilitate binding of cellular adhesion molecules necessary for cellular migration. The clot also serves as a storage site for various growth factors that further aid in directing cellular migration and wound repair.

Many of the protein factors involved in the coagulation cascade also play a role in stimulating inflammation. The kinin enzymatic cascade triggers the complement system producing strong mediators of inflammation, including bradykinin, which increases vascular permeability and vasodilatation. The endothelium secretes enzymes that degrade the fibrin clot into *fibrin split products* or *fibrin degradation products,* which are chemotactic for neutrophils. Early in the process, neutrophils are recruited to the site of damage and provide important functions including debridement and microbe control at the wound site by ingesting foreign bacteria, antigens, necrotic tissue, and nonviable cells.

Macrophages arrive hours after the inflammatory response begins. As well as being proinflammatory, macrophages are crucial to tissue debridement by clearing any residual bacteria, necrotic tissue, and senescent neutrophils. Macrophages synthesize proteases capable of degrading a wide range of extracellular matrix constituents. Several of the zinc-dependent matrix metalloproteinases (MMPs) are synthesized as well. MMPs are important for many biologic functions, including cell migration, angiogenesis, extracellular matrix (ECM) breakdown, and in tissue remodeling.

Proliferative Phase

The formation of granulation tissue is a hallmark of the proliferative stage. It is marked histologically by the presence of invading fibroblasts and vascular endothelial cells. Key to wound healing, fibroblast activation results in secretion of growth factors, synthesis of connective tissue proteins, and expression of receptors for growth factors. The fibroblasts begin to secrete ECM proteins and ground substance components. The ECM is composed mainly of collagen, reticular, and elastin fibers. Wound healing relies upon proper synthesis and deposition of collagen, and wound mechanical strength corresponds with the amount of collagen in the wound.

Released from platelet granules and inflammatory cells, platelet-derived growth factor (PDGF) is an important regulator of fibroblast function. Synthesis of PDGF is induced in response to factors commonly present in the wound environment such as low tissue partial pressures of oxygen, thrombin, or by other cytokines and growth factors. PDGF functions as a potent chemoattractant and mitogen for fibroblasts and has been shown to stimulate protein synthesis of many matrix proteins such as collagen, fibronectin, and hyaluronic acid. It also induces synthesis of MMPs. During times of inflammation, fibroblasts and other connective tissue cells up-regulate expression of the PDGF receptor.

Angiogenesis

Angiogenesis is essential in normal wound healing and occurs through a series of orderly events. The first step is activation of the endothelial cell, which entails the secretion of proteolytic enzymes. Two important proteolytic enzyme groups are the tissue plasminogen activator (t-PA)/plasmin system and the MMPs. Endothelial cells behind the leading edge of migration begin to proliferate.

All of the processes necessary for formation of new vessels are mediated by a wide range of angiogenic agonists, including growth factors, chemokines, angiogenic enzymes, endothelial specific receptors, and adhesion molecules. While many factors have been documented to be angiogenic, evidence points to the potent role of vascular epithelial growth factor (VEGF). It is involved in angiogenesis, as a chemoattractant and mitogen to vascular endothelium, and guiding new vessel formation.

Epithelialization

The most basic function of the epithelial layer is to protect the organism from environmental insults. Between adjacent epithelial cell membranes are specialized adhesion proteins that form occluding or tight junctions. Additionally, epithelial cells are anchored to a basement membrane; this layer contains many of the same components as the extracellular matrix but has a predominance of type IV collagen, laminin, and heparan sulfate. In wound healing, basement membrane provides adhesion sites and migratory signals to proliferating cells.

After injury, it is imperative for the epithelium to seal off the wound from the external environment. Epithelial cells must disassociate from anchoring fibers and migrate over the matrix of the initial clot in the wound. In wound healing, basement membrane provides adhesion sites and migratory signals to proliferating cells, and must be replaced if disrupted as epithelial cell anchor to the basement membrane. Growth factors have also been implicated in inducing the migratory and proliferative responses of epithelial cells after injury. The tear film component epithelial growth factor (EGF) is a key regulator of migration and proliferation of epithelial cells of all types.

Wound contraction

In conjunction with re-epithelialization, contraction of the wound helps close it and decrease its size. Substantial evidence points to a differentiated form of fibroblast, the myofibroblast, as the cause of contraction. Within granulation tissue, these altered cells acquire features typical of smooth muscle.

Tissue Maturation Phase

The tissue maturation phase of healing is characterized by the modification of the granulation tissue into a scar combined with a decrease in cellularity of the scar. Components of the granulation tissue begin to transform from the initial fibrin- and fibronectin-rich network deposited in the wound site at the initial stages to a collagen-rich scar tissue. Remodeling of the wound tissue is a net result of a degradative versus synthetic process. As reflected earlier, the synthetic processes are carried out chiefly through the actions of the fibroblast. The degradative processes are influenced heavily by the enzymatic actions of MMPs and their endogenous inhibitors (tissue inhibitors of metalloproteinases, sometimes called TIMPs). Remodeling can begin early at the wound edges and can continue for months. While the fibrin clot is being degraded, collagen and other proteins are being synthesized and deposited in the wound site.

Practical Considerations

In general, primary closure of conjunctiva and dermis allows for more controlled healing and is used on the skin of the face and exposed conjunctiva. This type of wound closure is preferable as it minimizes scarring, while healing by secondary intention takes much longer and often leaves more prominent scars. Healing by secondary intention may be useful in cases of anterior segment reconstruction or reconstructive oculoplastic surgery. For example, healing by secondary intention is often applied after the removal of conjunctival and/or dermal tumors in which a large graft is needed, and the wound cannot be closed by primary intention.

The average time to re-epithelialization of conjunctiva and facial skin is quite short, on the order of several days. By postoperative day 5, the edges of most skin incisions will have re-epithelialized. However, wounds of the facial skin may require attention for longer periods in order to prevent scar formation. For example, sutures in facial skin are usually removed in 5–7 days in order to avoid an inflammatory reaction to the suture material. The wound only has 10% of its tensile strength at this time and usually requires at least an additional week of suppression of the cellular response in order to avoid scar formation. Supplemental support (eg, Steri-Strips) may be required to maintain tissue apposition.

Wounds of the facial skin achieve greater than 50% tensile strength within about 2 weeks, 70%–80% by 3 months. Conjunctival wounds achieve similar strengths in nearly half the time. The choice of suture material, as well as the type of suture placed, alters the way in which the tissue heals. Generally, nonorganic nylon or polypropylene monofilaments are used on the skin of the face in order to minimize scar formation. Fig 19-3 shows an example of primary closure of a wound and healing by first intention.

Topical steroids are then often used to further slow the cellular response. Whereas these measures also slow cellular proliferation to a certain extent, causing the wound to heal slower, the decreased cellular response produces a more favorable outcome. Conjunctival closures, in which a more robust cellular response is generally desired, usually utilize polyglactin (Vicryl) sutures. These result in a greater cellular response at the wound site, allowing for faster healing and increased tensile strength in a shorter time, as well as increased scar formation.

The short period to re-epithelialization can be problematic in cases where the wound was improperly constructed or where the wound margins were unapposed. The

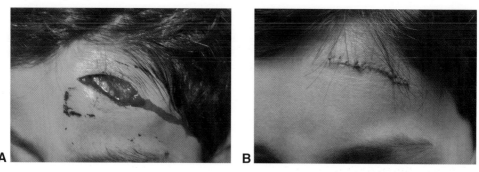

Figure 19-3 Example of primary closure of wound and healing by first intention. **A,** The muscle layer was closed with 4-0 polyglactin sutures. **B,** The skin was closed using a 6-0 running polypropylene suture that was removed after 7 days to decrease scar formation. *(Courtesy of Frank Moya, MD.)*

intervening gap will now heal by secondary intention, causing a visible scar. In these cases, wounds must be revised by creating "fresh" margins and reapposing them. Removal of any granulation tissue must also be accomplished as this will speed healing and avoid cyst formation. If this removal is not possible, there must be minimal disturbance of the granulation tissue in order to prevent scarring. This can be achieved using topical steroid/antibiotic combinations, but at the cost of very prolonged healing time.

During a glaucoma filtration surgery, special care to achieve hemostasis is required. We have learned that residual bleeding and clots can spur early bleb failure by acting as a source and reservoir for many inflammatory components. It is a delicate balance when aiming to achieve a watertight incision while adjacent tissue inflammation is suppressed. This is done by using a dissolvable suture like polyglactin to close the incision, while utilizing antifibrotic agents like mitomycin C and 5-fluorouracil to impair scar formation that would lead to bleb failure (Fig 19-4).

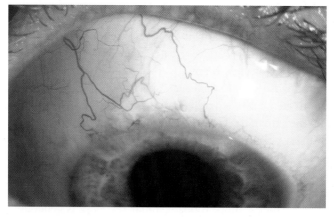

Figure 19-4 A broad diffuse bleb in a trabeculectomy performed with a subconjunctival injection of mitomycin C at the end of the case. The mitomycin C was then diffusely spread over a broad area using forceps as a squeegee. Note the 9-0 polyglactin closure of the fornix-based incision, with epithelial migration over the suture. There is minimal inflammation on topical steroids. Intraocular pressure is in single digits. *(Courtesy of Frank Moya, MD.)*

Corneal Wound Healing

The healthy cornea is devoid of vessels; therefore, corneal stromal wound healing is characterized by the absence of a vascular stage. Instead of granulation tissue, there is formation of fibroblastic tissue, a similar tissue without blood vessels. The corneal stroma has 3 major components: proteoglycans, keratocytes, and collagen, predominantly type I. When corneal tissue is damaged, fibrin and fibronectin aggregate at the wound. Fibrin derives from anterior chamber exudates in penetrating wounds, limbal vessels, and conjunctival vessels; keratocytes produce fibronectin. These elements are essential for cellular migration, proliferation, and collagen remodeling. Keratocytes are essential cells in the healing process and perform multiple functions depending on the chemical messengers in the stroma, including actions as fibroblasts, myofibroblasts, and phagocytic cells. Fibroblasts, keratocytes, and monocytes may show fibroblastic behaviors as well as phagocytic activity. Neutrophils are involved in phagocytosis of dead cells and damaged stromal constituents, and they defend against infection. Cells with fibroblastic activity deposit proteoglycans and collagen fibrils, forming a scar. The stromal scar is remodeled, with constituency becoming more like healthy tissue with time. However, the scar may never have the same tensile strength as surrounding healthy tissue.

Epithelial cell wound healing involves multiple phases, including sliding of superficial cells, cell mitosis, and stratification for normal epithelial anatomy. Should the wound involve Bowman layer and superficial stroma, the epithelium will fill in the extra space, forming an epithelial facet; Bowman layer and superficial stroma are not regenerated. Epithelial anchoring to the underlying stroma is rapid when a basement membrane is present; anchoring is significantly delayed if the basement membrane was ablated. Cell migration begins at approximately 5 hours after injury at 60 to 80 μm per hour. Intact epithelium increases the tensile strength of the underlying stroma, but an epithelial plug may prevent healing of a stromal wound.

Ablation of corneal tissue using an excimer laser induces a healing response as well. Initially epithelial cells migrate and proliferate over the wound bed using collagen, fibronectin, and various glycoproteins as described earlier in this chapter. Re-epithelialization of the wound bed usually is complete within a few days. Stromal reaction to ablation follows that of connective tissue in general. There is a migration, proliferation, and activation of stromal keratocytes that begin to secrete collagen, glycoproteins, and various components of the ECM. In time, the anterior stromal surface achieves a relatively normal lamellar appearance.

Following refractive keratotomy procedures, the corneal epithelium migrates and proliferates into the wound, forming an unpredictably persistent epithelial plug that initially retards normal wound healing. This plug has been shown to persist for up to 70 months in incision sites, but the corneal basement membrane with all of its attachments ultimately regenerates. After the initial stromal inflammatory response with edema, the keratocytes ultimately fill the plug with connective tissue, forming 2 distinct morphologically variable scars. These scars have been described as thin with feathery edges extending from the incision site, or as rougher and broad with an increased width containing epithelial inclusions. Fig 19-5 shows a post-LASIK cornea with an interface stromal scar.

Figure 19-5 Five-year post-Lasik cornea with an easily identifiable interface stromal scar *(arrows)* *(Modified from Dawson DG, Holley GP, Geroski DH, Waring GO, Grossniklaus HE, Edelhauser HF. Ex vivo confocal microscopy of human LASIK corneas with histologic and ultrastructural correlation. Ophthalmology. 2005;112:640.)*

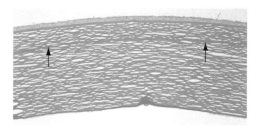

Following full-thickness incisions or lacerations, collagen and Descemet membrane retract due to their inherent elasticity. Fibrin and fibronectin fill the wound space providing a scaffold for migrating cells. As migrating epithelium fills the wound site, proper care should be given to appose the wound edges to prevent epithelial downgrowth. A stromal reaction ensues with production of ECM by fibroblasts. The endothelium heals in a similar manner to that described for all epithelial tissue. Initially, there is a migration of cells over the wound site. If there is compromise of the basement membrane, in this case Descemet membrane, there is synthesis of a new one.

Due to the avascular nature of the cornea, incisional wounds tend to heal slowly. Animal models show that central corneal wounds with respect to time have less than 5% tensile strength compared to that of intact tissue at 1 week and 45% at 2 months. Also of importance is the fact that a denuded cornea significantly slowed underlying stromal healing, demonstrated by a delay in gain of tensile strength as compared to wounded, non-denuded corneas. Highlighting the importance of vascular supply with respect to speed of healing is the fact that corneoscleral wounds showed 14%–24% tensile strength compared to that of intact tissue at 1 week and by 6 weeks the wound strength was recorded at 50% that of intact tissue.

Practical Considerations

Due to the nature of the tissue and its anatomic function, healing by primary intention (suture or glue closure) is required in full- and partial-thickness corneal wounds. Epithelial injury, however, is usually left to heal by secondary intention since the epithelial cells migrate over denuded areas in a very short period. In fact, most epithelial injury is fully healed in 72 hours.

As previously mentioned, the avascular nature of the cornea is the single greatest obstacle to wound healing in this tissue. Accordingly, the surgeon must account for this fact in the choice of suture and technique. For example, central corneal wounds can take months to achieve even 50% tensile strength; therefore, semipermanent sutures are placed in order to maintain wound integrity during this prolonged period. Once again, in order to minimize scar formation (the cornea must remain clear), nylon monofilaments are used because they will minimize any cellular response. Topical steroids or immunosuppressants such as cyclosporine and tacrolimus are again used to further retard cellular response. This process will take several months. Interestingly enough, corneal epithelial healing seems to be only minimally retarded by steroid use in an otherwise healthy cornea. The same is not true of anesthetic corneas, where lack of neurotropic factors retards epithelial healing. In these instances, steroid use must be modulated to avoid complications. Autologous serum drops are often used in corneas to replace the trophic factors that are absent in neurotrophic corneas. The technique with which the sutures are applied is also important in wound contracture modulation. Given the circular nature of most central corneal wounds as well as the anatomic curvature of the cornea, the use of interrupted sutures is necessary in order to be able to modify the wound contracture to avoid astigmatism.

Scleral Wound Healing

Scleral tissue heals by the formation of granulation tissue despite its relatively few native vessels. Depending on the anatomic site of injury, the sclera derives the cellular constituents needed for healing from nearby vascular components. Superficial scleral injury engages the overlying episcleral vessels. If the inner sclera is compromised, the underlying choroidal vessels contribute. A perforating injury results in granulation tissue derived from both vascular sources.

Pertinent to the issue of scleral wound healing is the topic of strabismus surgery. Animal studies have shown that after muscle surgery there is an initial lag phase for approximately 4–5 days, followed by a linear increase in tensile strength of the musculoscleral junction. By day 8, a tensile strength of 300 grams (well over the tension produced by the muscle in extreme lateral gaze of 100 grams) was found in both recession and resection surgeries.

Practical Considerations

Due to the nature and function of the sclera, healing by primary intention is necessary. Scleral wounds, similar to corneal wounds, require longer healing time due to the relative avascularity of the tissue. Prevention of scleral scar formation is less important, as clarity of the tissue is not primary. Nonetheless, wound contracture and cellular response must be mitigated as they can affect visual outcome.

The relatively avascular nature of the tissue mandates choice of suture material, but only in part; the size and anatomic location of the scleral wound determines which material to use. For example, the scleral wounds created in the pars plana during some larger gauge vitrectomy surgeries are usually closed with polyglactin sutures. The absorbable material increases cellular response at the wound site and speeds the repair process. In this case, there is no underlying retina, and the danger of neovascularization is minimal. In contrast, more posterior scleral wounds, such as those seen in ruptured globe cases, must be closed with nonabsorbable nylon monofilaments. In these cases, tensile strength is paramount. It may take sclera several months to achieve 50% tensile strength, and the tissue may never achieve the same tensile strength as the surrounding uninjured tissue. Therefore, there is an increased risk of rupture at this site. In addition, the choroid underlies these wounds and the nylon monofilaments minimize the risk of neovascularization.

Strabismus surgery presents a different aspect of scleral healing. The musculoscleral wounds in these surgeries heal at a much faster rate due to the highly vascularized muscle.

The vascularity of the muscle provides a desirable increased cellular response that speeds healing; the process also may be increased by the use of absorbable suture material (polyglactin). However, the fact that healing times are not significantly prolonged by use of the "hang back" technique (in which the suture is merely a placeholder) as compared to the "crossed swords" technique (in which the muscle is tightly reapposed to the scleral insertion) would seem to indicate that the presence of suture material minimally influences cellular response in these cases.

Uveal Wound Healing

While the ciliary body and choroid heal through deposition of granulation tissue and subsequent scar formation, the iris behaves differently. The anatomy of the iris lesion dictates whether healing takes place. A lesion oriented perpendicularly to the radial fibers allows the radial muscles to pull the wound edges apart, gaping the wound. Wound healing usually does not extend across the gap. A lesion oriented parallel to the radial fibers leaves the wound edges closely approximated. Subsequently, iris epithelium begins to migrate to cover the wound and stroma begins to secrete collagen fibrils and ground substance.

Fig 19-6 shows examples of pathology related to laser peripheral iridotomies.

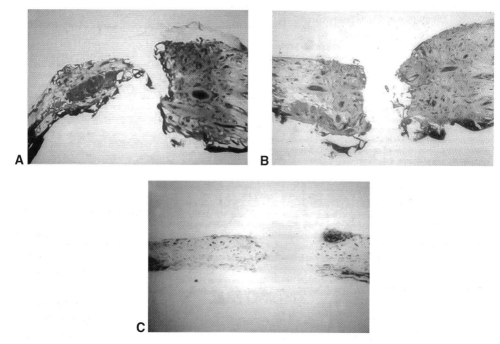

Figure 19-6 Argon **(A)**, diode **(B)**, and Nd:YAG **(C)** laser iridotomies. Note that iris pigment epithelium is intact up to the border of the argon and diode laser iridotomies, but is absent in the Nd:YAG laser iridotomy. This may account for the lower closure rate experienced with Nd:YAG laser iridotomy, as pigment migration and plugging accounts for most cases of closure. *(Reproduced, with permission, from Gamell LS, Saunders T, Schuman JS. Laser peripheral iridotomy. In: Kahook M and Schuman JS, eds.* Chandler and Grant's Glaucoma. *5th ed. Thorofare, NJ: Slack; 2013:503.)*

Modifying Wound Healing

Scarring of any ocular tissue can result in decreased vision and a subsequent increase in patient morbidity. Current research includes methods to modify the steps of wound healing to reduce poor visual outcomes.

Wound Closure Materials

A simple means of modifying wound healing is in the choice of suture materials. If more rapid healing is desired, then sutures capable of inducing an inflammatory reaction are used. These include gut, and silk. If inflammation is not desirable, monofilament sutures such as polypropylene and nylon may be used. In some surgeries it may be desirable to use both types of sutures. For example, in a limbal-based trabeculectomy, nylon sutures are used to close the scleral flap, as inflammation and scarring in this area are undesirable, inhibiting aqueous flow around the flap. However, when closing the conjunctiva, a polyglactin suture allows scarring and a watertight closure. Table 19-1 compares suture materials (also see Chapter 9).

Commercially available bioadhesives such as cyanoacrylate are used to aid in skin, conjunctiva, and cornea wound closures. Bioadhesives may even be able to replace sutures in some cases, possibly providing faster surgical times, lower risks, and improved healing times. Fibrin glue consists of fibrinogen and thrombin that when mixed form a fibrin clot. It has reported uses in many various ocular surgeries including pterygium repair, strabismus, glaucoma drainage devices, wound leaks, amniotic membrane transplant, vitreoretinal surgery, corneal surgery, eyelid and adnexal surgery, lens-fixation surgery, among others. ReSure (Fig 19-7) is a polyethylene glycol liquid that is placed on clear corneal incisions at the end of cataract surgery and then polymerizes into a hydrogel. It may be used in place of a suture in appropriate cases.

Table 19-1 Comparison of Suture Materials and Properties

Example	Material	Filament Type	Cellular Response	Absorbable?	Time to Resorption
Gut (plain)	Bovine intestine	Monofilament	Marked	Yes	5–7 days
Gut (chromic)	Bovine intestine	Monofilament	Marked	Yes	2–3 weeks
Mersilene	Polyethylene terephthalate	Braided	Mild	No	N/A
Nylon	Nylon	Mono- or multifilament	None to mild	No	N/A
Prolene	Polypropylene	Monofilament	None to mild	No	N/A
Silk	Silk	Braided	Mild to moderate	No	N/A
Vicryl	Polyglactin	Braided (monofilament available)	Moderate	Yes	6–8 weeks

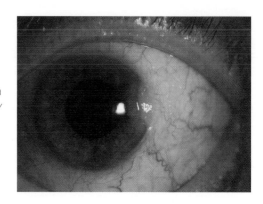

Figure 19-7 Hydrogel sealant (ReSure) on a clear cornea cataract incision. *(Courtesy of Terry Kim, MD.)*

Wound Healing Enhancers

Some wound healing enhancers may aid in both the speed and the strength of surgical and wound recovery. Amniotic membrane (AM) possesses many important properties that make it very useful in aiding wound healing or reconstruction of ocular surface tissues. It can be utilized as a basement membrane substitute or graft material. It encourages epithelial healing with its protein structure and growth factors, coupled with anti-inflammatory and anti-scarring modulators. Uses include reconstruction of the conjunctiva and corneal epithelium (Fig 19-8). ProKera (Bio-Tissue, Doral, FL) is amniotic membrane on a thermoplastic ring that can be placed in the clinic to treat ocular surface pathology.

Autologous serum drops have been shown to aid in corneal epithelial healing, due to its concentration of growth factors, nutrients, and antibodies. Uses include treatment for dry eye, persistent epithelial defects, and reconstruction of corneal or conjunctival surface.

Anti-Inflammatories

The administration of corticosteroids reduces postoperative inflammation, affecting all stages of wound healing. In the acute stages, they interfere with neutrophil adherence to vessel walls and migration. Later in the process, they inhibit the formation of plasmin through action on plasminogen activators, thereby preventing degradation of fibrin, whose products aid in recruitment of neutrophils, and preventing activation of MMPs. They further impair inflammation by lymphocytolysis.

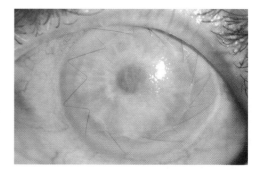

Figure 19-8 Slit-lamp photograph of an amniotic membrane disc sutured to the cornea with a 10-0 nylon running stitch, used to treat painful bullous keratopathy. Note the scalloped retraction between suture passes along the lower edge of the membrane. *(Modified from Said, DG et al. Histologic features of transplanted amniotic membrane: implication for corneal wound healing. Ophthalmology. 2009;116:1289.)*

Nonsteroidal anti-inflammatory drugs (NSAIDs) have been shown to inhibit some cell adhesion interactions in the early stages of inflammation. NSAIDs nonspecifically inhibit the isoforms of cyclooxygenase, the enzyme necessary for the transformation of arachidonic acid into prostaglandins, vasoactive substances that indirectly facilitate leukocyte migration. Later studies have shown that topical NSAIDs may have a negative effect on normal corneal wound healing, by destroying newly deposited ECM, through the induction of early synthesis of MMPs by corneal epithelium.

Antiproliferative Agents

The use of antiproliferative agents is the current gold standard in glaucoma filtration surgery to delay postsurgical scarring. The 2 most common agents are 5-fluorouracil (5-FU) and mitomycin C. 5-FU, a pyrimidine analog, inhibits RNA synthesis through its conversion to 5′-uridine monophosphate (5-UMP) and its subsequent incorporation into the mRNA. DNA synthesis is inhibited through its conversion to deoxyuridine 5′ phosphate, which inhibits thymidylate synthesis. Mitomycin C, an antibiotic, inhibits DNA synthesis through its ability to cross link DNA molecules and induce single-strand breaks.

While these therapies have improved the success of glaucoma surgeries (Fig 19-9), limitations remain. While single exposure to antiproliferatives impairs fibroblast replication, it does not stop them from secreting growth factors, expressing growth factor receptors, and producing ECM matrix molecules.

Administration of cyclosporine A, an immunosuppressive agent, may lead to a decrease in wound healing parameters. Anti-VEGF has been used in glaucoma filtering procedures with varying success. Caution is needed when using these treatments due to possible systemic health risks, as well as localized complications.

Possible future therapies include modification of gene expression, antisense oligonucleotides, gene transfers, neutralizing monoclonal antibodies, and ribozymes. It is likely

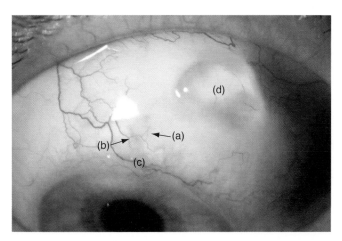

Figure 19-9 Two months after a trabeculectomy with mitomycin C and subsequent 5-fluorouracil injections given superotemporally. Note **(a)** the nylon sutures that had been lysed with laser and **(b)** gaping around sclera flap. The limbal polyglactin suture has dissolved **(c)**. Note **(d)** the avascular tissue and severe thinning of conjunctiva superotemporally as an effect of the antifibrotic agents. The lack of injection is due to aggressive topical steroid therapy. *(Courtesy of Frank Moya, MD.)*

that a "cocktail" of therapeutic agents, targeting different components of the wound healing process to optimize surgical outcomes, will be the standard of care.

The Ultimate Goal

In summary, this chapter has sought to provide a solid base of knowledge on the healing process. Young ophthalmologists who are the future of the field are challenged to spur novel ideas on how to modulate wound healing on the molecular level. The short- and long-term goals of improving surgical outcomes coincide well with the ultimate goal of optimal patient care.

Key Points

- Wound healing by first intention involves approximation of wound edges with sutures, resulting in less scarring, while healing by secondary intention involves unapposed wound edges and granulation tissue formation, with more scarring.
- Corneal wound healing is prolonged due to avascularity and requires permanent sutures to maintain wound approximation and prevent scarring.
- Wound healing may be modulated by the suture choice and closure type, as well as anti-inflammatory and other immunomodulatory agents that may either suppresses or encourage the healing process.

Apt L, Gaffney WL, Dora AF. Experimental suture studies in strabismus surgery. I. Reattachment rate of extraocular muscles after recession and resection operations. *Albrecht Von Graefes Arch Klin Exp Ophthalmol.* 1976;201(1):11–17.

Azar DT, Hahn TW, Khoury JM. Corneal wound healing following laser surgery. In: Azar DT, ed. *Refractive Surgery.* Stamford, CT: Appleton & Lange; 1997:41–62.

Bowman PH, Fosko SW, Hartstein ME. Periocular reconstruction. *Semin Cutan Med Surg.* 2003; 22(4):263–272.

Chabner BA, Ryan DP, Paz-Ares L, et al. Antineoplastic agents. In: Hardman JG, Limbird LE, Gilman AG, eds. *Goodman and Gilman's The Pharmacological Basis of Therapeutics.* 10th ed. New York: McGraw-Hill Professional; 2001:1389–1460.

Chang L, Crowston JG, Cordeiro MF, Akbar AN, Khaw PT. The role of the immune system in conjunctival wound healing after glaucoma surgery. *Surv Ophthalmol.* 2000;45(1):49–68.

Cordeiro MF. Beyond Mitomycin: TGF-beta and wound healing. *Prog Ret Eye Res.* 2002; 21(1):75–89.

Cordeiro MF, Schultz GS, Ali RR, Bhattacharya SS, Khaw PT. Molecular therapy in ocular wound healing. *Br J Ophthalmol.* 1999;83(11):1219–1224.

Daneshvar R. Anti-VEGF agents and glaucoma filtering surgery. *J Ophthalmic Vis Res.* 2013; 8(2):182–186.

Furie B, Furie BC. The molecular basis of blood coagulation. In Hoffman R, ed. *Hematology: Basic Principles and Practice.* 3rd ed. New York: Churchill Livingstone; 2000:1783–1804.

Gasset AR, Dohlman CH. The tensile strength of corneal wounds. *Arch Ophthalmol.* 1968; 79(5):595–602.

Geerling G, MacLennan S, Hartwig D. Autologous serum eye drops for ocular surface disorders. *Br J Ophthalmol.* 2004:88(11):1467–1474.

Hanna C, Roy FH. Iris wound healing. *Arch Ophthalmol.* 1972;88(3):296–304.

Hertle RW, James M, Farber MG. Insertion site dynamics and histology in a rabbit model after conventional or suspension rectus recession combined with ipsilateral antagonist resection. *J Pediatr Ophthalmol Strabismus.* 1993;30(3):184–191.

Hoffman GT, Soller EC, Bloom JN, Duffy MT, Heintzelman DL, McNally-Heintzelman KM. A new technique of tissue repair in ophthalmic surgery. *Biomed Sci Instrum.* 2004;40: 57–63.

Johnston WT, Filatov V, and Talamo JH. Corneal wound healing following refractive keratotomy. In: Azar DT, ed. *Refractive Surgery.* Stamford, CT: Appleton & Lange; 1997: 29–40.

Kim T, Levenson J, Tyson F. "Randomized Controlled Study of an Ocular Sealant to Prevent wound Leak After Cataract Surgery." Poster presented at American Academy of Ophthalmology Annual Meeting, Nov 16–19, 2013, New Orleans, LA.

Kinoshita S, Adachi W, Sotozono C, et al. Characteristics of the human ocular surface epithelium. *Prog Retin Eye Res.* 2001;20(5):639–673.

Kumar V, Abbass AK, Fausto N, Aster J. *Robbins and Cotran Pathologic Basis of Disease.* 8th ed. Philadelphia: Saunders; 2009.

McDermott M. Stromal wound healing. In: Brightbill FS, ed. *Corneal Surgery: Theory, Technique & Tissue.* St Louis: Mosby; 1999:40–48.

Meller D, Pauklin M, Thomasen H, Westekemper H, Steuhl K. Amniotic membrane transplantation in the human eye. *Dtsch Arztebl Int.* 2011;108(14):243–248.

Panda A, Kumar S, Kumar A, Bansal R, Bhartiya S. Fibrin glue in ophthalmology. *Indian J Ophthal.* 2009;57(5):371–379.

Phillips LG. Wound healing. In: Sabiston CM, ed. *Textbook of Surgery.* 16th ed. Philadelphia: Saunders; 2001:131–144.

Ribatti D, Vacca A, Presta M. The discovery of angiogenic factors: a historical review. *Gen Pharmacol.* 2000;35(5):233–239.

Sephel G, Davidson J . Repair, regeneration, and fibrosis. In: Rubin E, Reisner H, eds. *Essentials of Rubins Pathology.* 6th ed. Baltimore: Lippincott, William, and Wilkins; 2014: 49–70.

Stenn KS, Malhotra R. Epithelialization. In: Cohen KI, Diegelmann RF, Linblad WJ, eds. *Wound Healing: Biochemical & Clinical Aspects.* Philadelphia: Saunders; 1992:115–127.

Ware AJ. Cellular mechanisms of angiogenesis. Ware AJ, Simons M, eds. *Angiogenesis and Cardiovascular Disease.* New York: Oxford University Press; 1999:30–59.

Yanoff M, Fine BS. *Ocular Pathology: A Text and Atlas.* 3rd ed. Philadelphia: JB Lippincott; 1989:103–162.

Self-Assessment Test

1. Conjunctival and skin wound healing is characterized by which of the following? (Choose all that apply.)
   a. inflammation and coagulation
   b. invading fibroblasts and endothelial cells
   c. angiogenesis, modulated by VEGF
   d. epithelialization, modulated by EGF
   e. all of the above

2. Corneal wound healing differs from conjunctival and scleral wound healing in which of the following ways? (Choose all that apply.)
   a. lack of vascular stage
   b. neutrophils are not involved
   c. slower healing
   d. epithelial plugs may facilitate wound healing
3. Time to regain approximately 50% tensile strength after wound creation in cornea versus corneoscleral tissue is?
   a. 6 weeks versus >2 months
   b. >2 months versus 6 weeks
   c. 1 week versus 3 weeks
   d. 3 weeks versus 1 week
4. Which of the following may delay wound healing? (Choose all that apply.)
   a. corticosteroids
   b. 5-FU
   c. cyclosporine
   d. absorbable suture material

For preferred responses to these questions, see Appendix A.

CHAPTER 20

Dressings

David K. Wallace, MD, MPH

Dressings are placed at the conclusion of many ophthalmic procedures, although some surgeries do not require them, and they are used less frequently than in previous years. Each surgeon has his or her own preferences for the use and selection of dressings; for the same ophthalmic procedure, some surgeons will choose to use a dressing and others will not. This chapter reviews the major advantages and disadvantages of ophthalmic postoperative dressings, the major surgical procedures for which these dressings are typically used, the materials commonly used, and techniques for placement of pressure and nonpressure dressings.

Advantages and Disadvantages of Postoperative Dressings

The advantages of postoperative dressings include

- absorption of blood and ocular secretions
- reduction of postoperative edema, especially if applied with pressure
- reduction of injury risk to the operated site, especially in children
- in some cases, increased patient comfort (eg, in the presence of a large epithelial defect)
- prevention of exposure keratopathy after procedures involving an eyelid block and/or retrobulbar or peribulbar anesthesia
- in major orbital surgeries, prevention of the accumulation of fluid and blood in empty spaces (pressure dressing)

The disadvantages of postoperative dressings include

- patient discomfort, due to tightness, itching, and/or excessive warmth
- possible delay of the diagnosis of complications such as infection or excessive bleeding
- prevention of the administration of topical medications until removal of the dressing
- in some cases, delay of the healing process
- production of exposure keratopathy (if improperly applied)
- rare complications such as central retinal artery occlusion (with pressure dressings)
- damage to delicate eyelid tissues (if not carefully removed)
- skin irritation or allergic reactions from adhesive tapes

In selected cases, it may thus be preferable to defer the use of a dressing.

Indications

A dressing is typically applied after the following ophthalmic procedures:

- major ophthalmic plastic procedures, including surgery of anophthalmic sockets and orbital decompression
- vitreoretinal surgery, including posterior vitrectomy or scleral buckle
- penetrating keratoplasty
- trabeculectomy
- extracapsular cataract extraction
- adjustable suture strabismus surgery, in order to provide comfort and to protect the sutures from dislodgment
- any intraocular procedure in a child
- any procedure for which an eyelid block and/or retrobulbar or peribulbar anesthesia is used, to prevent exposure keratopathy from lagophthalmos
- any procedure in which a large epithelial defect is created, either intentionally or unintentionally
- any procedure in which considerable postoperative conjunctival edema is anticipated (eg, some strabismus reoperations)

A dressing is typically not applied after the following ophthalmic procedures:

- most minor ophthalmic plastic procedures, including ptosis surgery or minor eyelid procedures
- uncomplicated phacoemulsification with topical anesthesia (shield only)
- strabismus surgery

Supplies

Table 20-1 lists the soft dressing materials, eye shields, tape, and other supplies used in applying dressings. Key points about these items include

- Telfa (3M, St Paul, MN) nonadherent dressing is indicated as the first layer if removal of the patch could damage delicate tissues beneath it, such as skin grafts. One piece of Telfa is cut slightly larger than the wound or graft and is placed gently on the incision site (Fig 20-1).
- Oval eye pads are used for most dressings. The standard technique for nonpressure or pressure dressings is outlined in the next section.
- Gauze can be used as part of a large pressure dressing or in place of a dressing altogether. After some minor oculoplastics procedures, ice-soaked gauze is applied directly on the incision site immediately at the conclusion of surgery.
- Eye shields can be used with or without soft dressings beneath them. They are often used without a soft dressing after uncomplicated phacoemulsification with topical anesthetic. They are sometimes used at night only to prevent unintentional injury to the operative site from unconscious rubbing of it. A clear plastic eye shield without an underlying eye pad is particularly useful for monocular patients or those whose better-seeing eye is being shielded.

Table 20-1 Supplies for Dressings

	Category	Type
	Soft dressing materials	Telfa
		Oval eye pads
		Gauze
		Tegaderm
	Eye shields	Adult versus child size
		Right versus left
		Plastic versus metal
	Tape	Paper
		Silk
		Plastic
	Other	Steri-Strips
		Skin adhesive (eg, Mastisol)

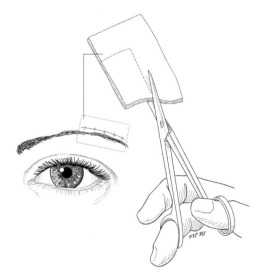

Figure 20-1 Telfa is cut to proper size to cover a surgical incision. *(Illustration by Mark M. Miller.)*

- Tape is available in many materials, including paper, silk, plastic, and Elastoplast (a stretchable dressing from Beiersdorf, Hamburg, Germany). Paper tape is extremely lightweight and generally causes less skin irritation than other types. Silk and plastic tapes are stronger than paper tape and are more easily torn into pieces with square edges. Elastoplast can be used when a large amount of pressure is required to the surgical site.
- Steri-Strips (3M) are thin, adhesive paper-based strips. They are sometimes used with a skin adhesive and without a dressing for minor oculoplastics procedures to reduce wound tension.
- Tegaderm (3M) is a transparent waterproof dressing with high adherence. It can be used as a postoperative eye dressing in children. Because children often attempt to remove dressings prematurely, Tegaderm can in some cases be more secure than using dressings or tape with loose ends that can be pulled.

Technique for Dressing Placement

If the decision is made to use a dressing, it should be placed neatly; it is the first impression of the results of surgery for both patient and family. The tape should be clean, its pieces should be approximately the same length, and its ends should be square. Dressings are almost never placed on both eyes because of the psychological impact of bilateral occlusion. Exceptions include bilateral enucleations and bilateral intraocular surgery, sometimes performed in infants with cataracts or glaucoma.

Nonpressure Dressing With a Shield

1. An eye drop or ointment is usually administered just before a dressing is placed.
2. Several (usually 4 or 5) pieces of tape of approximately the same length are prepared ahead of time and placed in a convenient location (eg, the edge of a table) near the patient's head.
3. An oval eye pad is oriented horizontally and placed directly above the *closed* upper eyelid.
4. The superior end of the first piece of tape is placed on the patient's forehead, and the tape is directed inferiorly and slightly temporally through the center of the eye pad to the patient's cheek (Fig 20-2). Great care is taken not to apply downward pressure on the eye during this maneuver. The inferior edge of the tape should be placed in the middle of the cheek and not too close to the corner of the patient's mouth. The tape should not be placed over the patient's hairline, or removal postoperatively will be difficult and painful, especially in children.
5. Other pieces of tape are applied in a similar manner, progressively nasal and temporal to the center piece until the entire eye pad is covered (Fig 20-3).

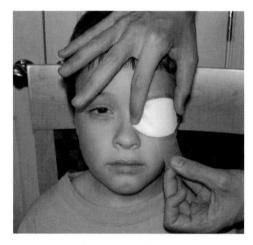

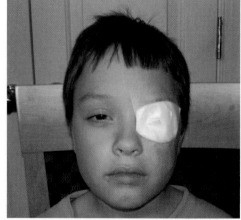

Figure 20-2 First piece of tape applied over center of eye pad. *(Courtesy of David K. Wallace, MD, MPH.)*

Figure 20-3 Appearance after all pieces of tape applied to soft dressing. *(Courtesy of David K. Wallace, MD, MPH.)*

6. A shield that is appropriate for the patient's eye (left or right) and age (child versus adult) is then applied over the patch.
7. A single piece of tape placed in the same orientation as the first piece placed over the eye pad is usually sufficient to secure the shield (Fig 20-4).
8. The edges of the shield should be in contact with the bones surrounding the orbital rim (Fig 20-5A). If the edges are not in contact with these bones, then any force exerted on the exterior of the shield is transmitted posteriorly to the eye instead of to the facial bones (Fig 20-5B).

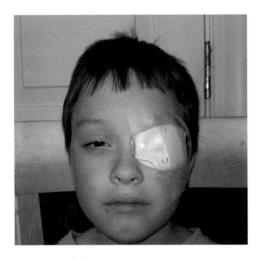

Figure 20-4 Final appearance of dressing after shield placement. *(Courtesy of David K. Wallace, MD, MPH.)*

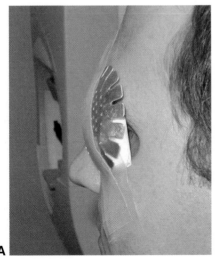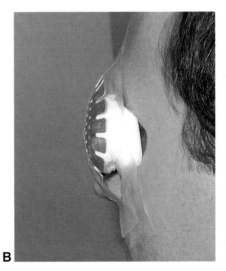

A   **B**

Figure 20-5 Shield placement. **A,** Proper placement of a shield in contact with facial bones (side view). **B,** Improper placement of a shield with edges not in contact with facial bones (side view). *(Courtesy of David K. Wallace, MD, MPH.)*

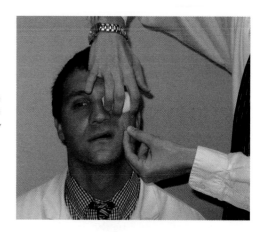

Figure 20-6 Technique for creating a pressure dressing by lifting the cheek superiorly before placing the inferior portion of the tape. *(Courtesy of David K. Wallace, MD, MPH.)*

Pressure Dressing

The technique is similar to that for a nonpressure dressing, except that with a pressure dressing, the goal is to exert significant downward pressure on the wound to prevent postoperative edema and/or hemorrhage. Two oval eye pads or an eye pad with gauze is used. It may be useful to have an assistant place gentle downward pressure on the dressing while the tape is placed. The maximum amount of pressure from the dressing is obtained by lifting the cheek superiorly before attaching the inferior end of each piece of tape (Fig 20-6). A skin adhesive such as Mastisol (Eloquest Healthcare, Ferndale, MI) can help to seal the tape in the proper position. An eye shield is generally not needed.

Postoperative Instructions

Patients should be instructed regarding the normal postoperative course and any signs or symptoms that should prompt a call to the surgeon. When a dressing has been applied, some tightness and/or itching may be anticipated. The dressing may normally become wet with tears or blood-tinged. Patients should be instructed to call if they experience excessive bleeding, pain, an unusual amount of swelling or bruising, or a fever. In some cases, the patient may be instructed to remove the dressing on the same day as surgery. In other cases, it is left in place as long as 2 days postoperatively. If the patient is examined on the first postoperative day, the dressing will usually be removed by the surgeon or by one of the office staff.

Dressing Removal

Dressings should be carefully removed by the surgeon, office staff, or, when appropriate, the patient or his or her caregiver at home. Care should be taken to avoid pressure on the eye during dressing removal. If the tape is stuck firmly to the skin or hair, then removal can be briefly painful, and reassurance is useful. If the eyelids are stuck together by dried secretions, then sterile irrigating solution can be used to cleanse the lashes and allow the eye to open.

Key Points

- Postoperative dressings protect the operative site from injury, reduce tissue fluid accumulation and absorb secretions, and may increase patient comfort.
- Disadvantages of dressings include patient discomfort, possible delay of the diagnosis of complications such as infection or excessive bleeding, prevention of the administration of topical medications prior to removal, and potential complications such as keratopathy, tissue damage, and allergic reactions.
- Dressings are typically applied after pediatric intraocular procedures, major intraocular procedures, procedures involving an eyelid and/or retrobulbar block, vitreoretinal surgery, and major oculoplastic procedures.
- Precautions for placing postoperative dressings include confirmation of eyelid closure before placing the dressing, placement of the shield so that its edges rest on the facial bones, and avoidance of excess pressure on the globe.

Lewis C, Traboulsi EI. Use of Tegaderm for postoperative eye dressing in children. *AAPOS*. 2008;12(4):420.

Self-Assessment Test

1. What are the benefits of postoperative dressings? (Choose all that apply.)
   a. reduction of tissue fluid accumulation
   b. prevention of infection
   c. protection of the operative site from injury
   d. prevention of central retinal artery occlusion
2. What are disadvantages of postoperative dressings? (Choose all that apply.)
   a. delayed diagnosis of complications
   b. prevention of application of topical medications
   c. identification of the surgical site
   d. possible tissue damage
3. What precautions should be taken when placing an ophthalmic postoperative dressing? (Choose all that apply.)
   a. Ensure that no antibiotic ointment touches the cheek.
   b. Confirm the lids are closed before placing the dressing.
   c. Make sure the edges of the shield rest on the facial bones.
   d. Avoid excess pressure to the globe while applying the dressing.
4. After which of the following surgical procedures are postoperative dressings commonly applied? (Choose all that apply.)
   a. trabeculectomy
   b. procedures involving an eyelid and/or retrobulbar block
   c. bilateral strabismus surgery
   d. vitreoretinal surgery

For preferred responses to these questions, see Appendix A.

CHAPTER 21

Handling of Ocular Tissues for Pathology

Mahendra K. Rupani, MD
Anvesh C. Reddy, MD

Ocular tissue is often removed for therapeutic or diagnostic reasons. Intraocular fluids such as vitreous may be removed as well. Most ophthalmic surgical specimens are small, and delicate. Consequently, it is important to handle specimens with proper care and planning, in order to facilitate accurate and timely diagnosis. This chapter is a brief introduction to the proper handling of ocular surgical specimens. Many books and institutional manuals are devoted to this subject. For further reading, refer to the selection of resources at this end of this chapter.

Preoperative Planning, Frozen and Routine Specimens

In the collection of frozen and routine specimens, the surgeon and the operating room staff must be familiar with the proper handling of ocular tissues. Specimens are sent for frozen sectioning in order to guide intraoperative patient management. These specimens are processed and read while the patient is still in the operating theater. Remaining or additional tissue is sent for permanent sections that are used to arrive at a final diagnosis. Preoperative planning with pathology is necessary to ensure that staff is available at the time of the procedure. Routine specimens are sent for processing fresh or in a fixative and are read after the patient has left the operating theater.

In preoperative preparations for working with specimens, consider the following steps:

1. *Become familiar with standard operating procedures.* Most institutions have standard operating procedures for specimen collection, handling, billing, and reporting. These have been developed in consultation with the laboratory that will handle and process the tissues as well as the pathologist who will examine the gross specimens and microscopic slides.
2. *Check supplies.* Specimen containers and preservatives, labels for the containers, requisitions, and packaging for transportation should all be immediately available.

3. *Check posted information.* Contact information for the laboratory and the pathologist should be posted. Procedures for billing and reporting on the specimen should
be outlined.

4. *Consult the pathologist and the laboratory in advance.* Consultation with the pathologist and the laboratory prior to starting a surgical procedure is paramount
if there is uncertainty about how to handle a particular specimen; if an urgent
diagnosis is required; if fresh material is to be sent; if specialized procedures (eg,
electron-microscopy, immunohistochemistry, flow cytometry) are anticipated; or
if a frozen section is planned or anticipated during surgery.

Supplies and Equipment, Requisitions

Table 21-1 lists common fixatives used in ophthalmic pathology. The most commonly
used fixative is 10% neutral buffered formalin. The general recommendation for the quantity of formalin is 10 times the volume of the tissue specimen. There are some important
exceptions to this general guideline for a fixative, depending on the type of tissue, the
clinical diagnosis and the reason for the biopsy. Saline is not a fixative. See guidelines later
in this chapter for individual tissue type and specialized procedures.

Table 21-2 lists common stains used in ophthalmic pathology; Figs 21-1, 21-2, and
21-3 show examples of various stains. Certain stains are useful only if they are on fresh or
properly fixed tissue. This should be coordinated with the laboratory prior to the day of
surgery. Often a specimen is divided with half submitted fresh and the other half in fixative. Formalin-fixed specimens should be submerged in sufficient quantity of formalin. It
is helpful to place membranous tissue such as the conjunctival biopsy, epithelial side up,
on a piece of paper and submerge it in the fixative.

Specimens that are to be sent fresh to the laboratory should not be allowed to be
dried. They should be placed on a piece of gauze moistened in saline in a labeled container, and refrigerated immediately. If microbiological culture will be obtained, the

Table 21-1 Common Fixatives Used in Ophthalmic Pathology

Fixative	Color	Examples of Use
Formalin	Clear	Routine fixation of all tissues
Bouin solution	Yellow	Small biopsies
B5	Clear	Lymphoproliferative tissue (eg, lymph node)
Glutaraldehyde	Clear	Electron microscopy
Ethanol/methanol	Clear	Crystals (eg, urate crystals of gout)
Michel fixative	Light pink	Immunofluorescence
Zenker acetic fixative	Orange	Muscle differentiation

Reprinted, with permission, from *Basic and Clinical Science Course, Section 4: Ophthalmic Pathology
and Intraocular Tumors.* American Academy of Ophthalmology, 2014.

Table 21-2 Common Stains Used in Ophthalmic Pathology

Stain	Material Stained: Color	Example
Hematoxylin and eosin (H&E)	Nucleus: blue Cytoplasm: red	General tissue stain
Periodic acid–Schiff (PAS)	Glycogen and proteoglycans: magenta	Descemet membrane
Alcian blue	Acid mucopolysaccharide: blue	Cavernous optic atrophy
Alizarin red	Calcium: red	Band keratopathy
Colloidal iron	Acid mucopolysaccharide: blue	Macular dystrophy
Congo red	Amyloid: orange, red-green dichroism	Lattice dystrophy
Ziehl-Neelsen	Acid-fast organisms: red	Atypical mycobacterium
Gomori methenamine silver (GMS)	Fungal elements: black	*Fusarium*
Crystal violet	Amyloid: purple, violet	Lattice dystrophy
Gram stain (tissue Brown & Brenn [B&B] or Brown & Hopps [B&H] stain)	Bacteria positive: blue Bacteria negative: red	Bacterial infection
Masson trichrome	Collagen: blue Muscle: red	Granular dystrophy Red deposits
Perls Prussian blue	Iron: blue	Fleischer ring
Thioflavin T (ThT)	Amyloid: fluorescent yellow	Lattice dystrophy
Verhoeff–van Gieson (elastic stain)	Elastic fibers: black	Temporal artery elastic layer (Fig 15-6B)
von Kossa	Calcium phosphate salts: black	Band keratopathy

Reprinted, with permission, from Basic and Clinical Science Course, Section 4: Ophthalmic Pathology and Intraocular Tumors. American Academy of Ophthalmology, 2014.

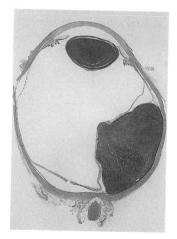

Figure 21-1 Hematoxylin and eosin–stained section of an intraocular tumor specimen. *(Courtesy of Hans E. Grossniklaus, MD.)*

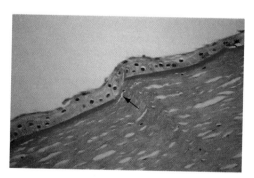

Figure 21-2 Keratoconus. Masson trichrome stain demonstrates focal disruption of the Bowman layer *(arrow). (Courtesy of Hans E. Grossniklaus, MD.)*

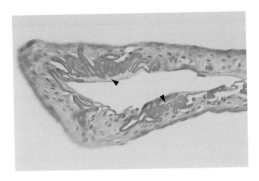

Figure 21-3 Epithelial basement membrane dystrophy (EBMD, map-dot-fingerprint dystrophy). Periodic acid–Schiff (PAS) stain highlights numerous folds *(arrowheads)* in the epithelial basement membrane. *(Courtesy of George J. Haracopos, MD.)*

microbiology laboratory should be alerted in advance for proper handling and transportation of the specimen.

Labeling of Specimen Containers

All specimens should be properly labeled with the patient's name and date of birth, patient location, type of specimen, surgical site (including laterality), surgeon's name, and the date and time of collection. When there are multiple specimens from the same patient, each specimen should be placed in a separate container with careful identification and labeling of each. If there are multiple fragments from the same specimen (such as a ruptured globe), these may be all placed in the same container.

Specimen Requisitions

There should be a separate requisition form for each specimen container, and the demographic information on the form and the container should match. For accurate interpretation of the findings, the pathologist needs adequate clinical information. The completed requisition form should include

- patient's name
- medical record number
- date of birth
- patient's sex
- name of surgeon
- date and time specimen obtained
- type and location of the specimen (a sketch would be helpful)
- laterality (right or left)
- relevant clinical information in adequate detail to guide the pathologist
- contact information of the clinician

Figure 21-4 shows an example of a pathology slip.

Wills Eye Hospital

WEH-262   STOCK # 1416130   REV. DATE 8-98

EYE PATHOLOGY LABORATORY   LAB (215) 928-3280

REQUEST FOR SERVICE

☐ BILL PATIENT ☐ BILL HOSPITAL ☐ INS. INFO ATTACHED

PATIENT NAME (LAST, FIRST, MI)

ADDRESSOGRAPH

DATE OF BIRTH	AGE	SEX	MEDICAL RECORD

PATIENT STREET ADDRESS

PATIENT CITY, STATE, ZIP

PHYSICIAN/HOSPITAL STREET ADDRESS

PHYS./HOSP. CITY, STATE, ZIP

SOURCE OF MATERIAL

☐ WILLS OPERATING ROOM   ☐ PRIVATE OUT-PATIENT
☐ EMERGENCY ROOM   ☐ OTHER

CONTRIBUTOR   DATE OF SURGERY

SERVICES

☐ RUSH   ☐ PHONE REPORT   ☐ ROUTINE

FOR LAB USE ONLY

PATHOLOGY NUMBER	DATE RECEIVED

PREVIOUS SURGERY (LIST) ☐ WILLS EYE ☐ OTHER

HISTORY, PHYSICAL EXAMINATION, PERTINENT LABORATORY DATA

OD

OS

OD

OS

OD   OS

OD   OS

PREOPERATIVE DIAGNOSIS

POSTOPERATIVE DIAGNOSIS

LIST SPECIMENS SUBMITTED

SURGICAL PROCEDURE

PROCEDURE	FOR OFFICE USE ONLY	PROCEDURE
GROSS ONLY (LEVEL I)	SPECIAL STAINS I (GROUP I)	FLOW CYTOMETRY
ROUTINE (LEVEL II)	NO. 1 2 3 4 5 6 7 8	NO. 1 2 3 4 5
ROUTINE (LEVEL III)	(each special stain)	CONSULTATION
ROUTINE MULTIPLE (IV)	SPECIAL STAINS II (GROUP II)	CONSULTATION BLOCK
ENUCLEATON (LEVEL V)	NO. 1 2 3 4 5 6 7 8	CONSULTATION COMPREHENSIVE
ORBITAL EXENTERATION (VI)	(each special stain)	VITRECTOMY (MILLIPORE)
FROZEN SECTION SINGLE	IMMUNOHISTOCHEMISTRY	VITRECTOMY (CELL BLOCK)
FROZEN SECTION NO. 1 2 3 4 5 6 7 8 (each additional)	NO. 1 2 3 4 5 6 7 8 (each antibody)	FNAB
	DECALCIFICATION	ELECTRON MICROSCOPY
NON-OCULAR BX	SMEAR	MISC$

Figure 21-4 Example of a pathology laboratory service request form. *(Courtesy of Wills Eye Hospital.)*

Transportation

The specimen containers, accompanied by the requisitions, should be transported as quickly as possible to the laboratory, taking care that the laboratory is aware of the plan.

A fresh specimen should be refrigerated then hand delivered by an operating room staff member or a courier as soon as possible. To assure proper preservation and handling of the fresh tissue, the laboratory should be alerted ahead of time, especially if the sample is to be delivered after regular hours. Sometimes the fresh specimen is placed in a transport media to prevent autolysis and stabilize crystals. Always consult the laboratory prior to surgically removing the tissue specimen to make certain that the proper preservative is readily available in the operating room. Surgical removal of the tissue specimen is beyond the scope of this chapter.

If the specimen is radioactive (eg, radioactive plaque used for melanoma), the institutional protocol should guide the handling of such specimens.

Frozen Sections

Indications for frozen sections include rapid diagnosis, evaluation of margins of resection, and determination of adequacy of tissue sample for permanent sections. The preparation of a frozen section sample requires close collaboration between the surgeon and the pathologist. It is desirable that both discuss the case prior to surgery.

The surgeon needs to be aware that there are limitations to the accuracy and type of information that can be obtained with a frozen section. Final diagnosis is always based on permanent sections. If only a small amount of tissue is available, the surgeon should opt for permanent rather than frozen section to improve diagnostic accuracy.

Pearls for Handling of Routine Specimens

Eyelids

Eyelid lesions are among the most common ophthalmic specimens sent for pathologic processing and analysis. Most eyelid specimens can be submitted in 10% neutral buffered formalin. If there is clinical suspicion for malignancy, proper orientation and marking of the specimen and margins is necessary to allow the pathologist to provide the surgeon with useful information on the adequacy of excision. If there is a suspicion for sebaceous cell carcinoma, consult with the pathology laboratory for the preferred method of handling as routine processing will leach the lipid from the specimen.

Commonly, in wedge resections, the surgeon uses suture to provide specimen orientation (ie, a short suture superior and a long suture lateral). Some surgeons elect to "ink" their specimen margins themselves to provide further orientation. It is also helpful to provide a diagram indicating specimen orientation, which may be of particular help if separate tissue margins from the primary resection are submitted.

Conjunctiva

Conjunctival specimens for routine pathology are typically submitted in 10% neutral buffered formalin. Conjunctiva tends to curl or roll up following removal; therefore, the specimen should be placed flat onto an absorbent surface such as filter paper or the cardboard tab used to turn a sterile gown and allowed sufficient time to adhere.

If possible, the specimen should be ink marked. Do not put ink on absorbent surface, as this will dissolve away in the formalin. Alternatively, the filter paper or cardboard can be notched to help orient the specimen (ie, 1 notch denoting superior and 2 notches denoting temporal, and so on.) This tissue filter paper complex can then be placed tissue face up in formalin and allowed to sink to the bottom as the fixative is absorbed.

If multiple biopsies are taken, for example to map intra-epithelial sebaceous cell carcinoma, a sketch should be provided to indicate from where the biopsies are taken. Each biopsy should be placed in a separate container and appropriately labeled to match its location on the sketch.

A clinical drawing aids the pathologist in orienting the specimen, especially in cases of neoplastic margins.

In suspected cases of lymphoma, consult with the pathology laboratory prior to resection, as special preparation may be required for flow cytometry evaluation.

Conjunctival biopsies for cystinosis should be placed in 100% ethanol, as opposed to formalin, as the cysteine crystals are water soluble.

Cornea

Routine corneal buttons may be placed in 10% neutral buffered formalin. If it is suspected that electron microscopy or assessment of lipid/crystalline deposits will be necessary, the pathology laboratory should be consulted prior to surgery. In either case, the corneal sample should not be allowed to desiccate in room air before placement in fixative.

Corneal biopsies and scrapings of corneal epithelium yield minute specimens that need to be handled appropriately if a diagnosis is to be obtained. If an infectious process is suspected, appropriate cultures should be sent to the microbiology laboratory. The quantity and the type of fixative used for the corneal biopsies/scrapings is critical in maintaining an adequate amount of viable tissue for cytology, as well as microbiological cultures.

Muscle

Routine muscle specimens may be placed in 10% neutral buffered formalin and submitted to pathology for light microscopy. This approach is useful for suspected inflammatory myopathies. If there is suspicion for a mitochondrial, congenital, or metabolic myopathy, fresh or frozen tissue may be required for enzyme histochemistry or immunohistochemical analysis. A section of fresh muscle may be wrapped in saline moistened gauze and then placed on ice for transport or may be directly frozen in liquid nitrogen in the operating room.

Although muscle biopsies are often taken from limb muscles, it is possible to use a section of orbicularis or levator, which can be taken at the time of ptosis repair or blepharoplasty. It is best to avoid cautery of the muscle to avoid tissue artifact. If there is interest in extent of an infiltrative or malignant lesion, a suture may be used to provide orientation to the pathologist.

Temporal Artery Biopsy

Temporal artery biopsies for cases of suspected giant cell arteritis should be 2 cm or greater in length due to the "skip" nature of these inflammatory lesions. The biopsy specimens should be placed on a piece of stiff paper or cardboard, stretched to the length of the resection, and pinned down before placing it in 10% neutral buffered formalin. Jars containing paraffin soaked in formalin and pins are commercially available as an alternative. If bilateral temporal artery biopsies are performed, they should be submitted separately in properly identified containers.

Lacrimal System

Most tissue from biopsy or excision of lacrimal gland and lacrimal sac can be placed in 10% neutral buffered formalin with the exception of suspected lymphoid lesions. Fresh tissue is often submitted for flow cytometry in addition to tissue for permanent sections in these cases.

Descemet Membrane

Tissue obtained after procedures such as DSEK, DSAEK, and DMEK is routinely submitted to pathology in 10% neutral buffered formalin. The specimen should be laid flat on a piece of paper prior to immersing in fixative.

Iris

Routine iridectomy specimens need not be sent to pathology. However, any iris tissue removed for treatment or diagnosis of a tumor and any unknown lesion should be submitted in 10% neutral buffered formalin for pathologic examination. A sketch of the clinical lesion should be included to provide proper orientation of the resection margins.

Ciliary Body or Iridocyclectomy

These specimens are usually removed due to suspicion of malignancy and are usually submitted in 10% neutral buffered formalin for confirmation of diagnosis and to study the surgical margins. The specimen should be accompanied by a detailed sketch to indicate the location of the tumor and to identify the resection margins. One of the margins, medial or lateral, should be identified by placement of a suture or surgical ink.

Evisceration

Eviscerated tissue is handled as any routine specimen and submitted in sufficient quantity of 10% neutral buffered formalin. The laboratory should be alerted if calcification or bone is suspected, and if there is any question about the presence of a tumor or a foreign body.

Exenteration

These specimens require special handling due to the size and variety of diagnosis. No incisions should be made in the globe. To help in proper orientation of the specimen, identify a horizontal and a vertical rectus muscle with a long and a short suture. The specimen should not be wrapped in paper or gauze. Entirely submerge the specimen in an appropriately sized container with 10% neutral buffered formalin, generally about 200 mL.

The pathologist should receive relevant clinical history that includes the diagnosis, previous surgical procedures, and presence of an intraocular lens or foreign body. Also include a sketch detailing the location of tumor, whether it is intraocular or external such as on the eyelid, or in the orbital space. If it is important to know the status of any resection margins, convey this information to the laboratory.

Enucleation

An enucleation specimen should be submitted in a container large enough to hold 10% neutral buffered formalin in a ratio of 10 times the volume of the globe. Do not make any incisions into the specimen. If placed in an appropriate volume of fixative, the globe will be properly fixed.

If the eye is enucleated for a tumor, submit a sketch indicating location of the tumor in the eye. If a foreign body, intraocular lens, calcification or bone is suspected, indicate this on the requisition. Also include a description of prior trauma or surgery involving the enucleated eye.

Choroidal and Retinal Tissue

Biopsies of choroidal and retinal tissue are rare. Since these specimens consist of sparse tissue that can not easily be identified, wrapping them in tissue paper or applying surgical ink aids in identification. If there is a need for cultures, the specimen should be placed in appropriate medium after consultation with the microbiology laboratory. If electron-microscopy or other special analysis is anticipated, the laboratory should be consulted in advance for instructions about preservatives and transportation.

Orbital Tissue

Orbital tissue is removed for diagnostic and/or therapeutic purposes. These specimens are usually submitted in a sufficient quantity of 10% neutral buffered formalin. Some orbital lesions such as orbital lymphoma or rhabdomyosarcoma require special handling and consultation with the laboratory, as discussed elsewhere in this section.

Orbital tissue removed during decompression and strabismus surgery does not need to be sent for histopathologic examination. However, if there is any doubt about the diagnosis, or to evaluate the degree of baseline inflammation and scarring, it would be appropriate to submit the tissue for evaluation.

Any foreign body or bone removed from the orbit should be submitted for gross description and documentation.

All lacrimal gland tissue should be sent to the laboratory for histopathologic diagnosis.

Vitreous

Vitreous samples are often obtained to assist in the diagnosis of tumors, intraocular infections, or lympho-proliferative disorders. Besides routine cytology and histology, special tests may be indicated, including cultures, polymerase chain reaction–based testing, cytokine analysis, flow cytometry, and immuno-histochemical tests. After appropriate specimens are taken for microbiology, an aliquot of the specimen should be fixed in an equal amount of preservation media or cytology fixative.

Some laboratories may require that the specimen be sent fresh, immediately, for lymphoma evaluation. Since the cellularity of vitreous is variable, it is best to send an undiluted aliquot taken before infusion is started, in addition to the entire vitrectomy fluid cassette at the end of the case. Contents of the vitrectomy fluid cassette can be spun down on a centrifuge to prepare a cell block or a cytospin prep, which is then processed like a block of tissue. Always consult the laboratory to determine which preservative and what quantity should be used. Refrigerate the specimen if there is any delay in transporting it to the laboratory.

Special Procedures

For the following special procedures, contact the laboratory and the ocular pathologist prior to obtaining the specimen to determine how it should be collected, preserved, and transported:

- immunohistochemistry
- immunofluorescence
- electron-microscopy (EM)
- special stains
- microbiological cultures
- genetic typing
- investigation of metabolic disorders such as gout, cystinosis, storage diseases, and so on

Special preservatives, such as the glutaraldehyde for electron-microscopy or 100% ethanol for storage disease such as cystinosis or gout, will have to be arranged with the laboratory.

Gross Specimens Only

Some specimens normally do not require microscopic evaluation. They should be submitted in 10% neutral buffered formalin for preservation and decontamination, and sent to the laboratory for gross description and documentation. Examples include lens, foreign bodies, and redundant eyelid skin.

Key Points

- The most common specimen preservative is formaldehyde (10% neutral buffered formalin).
- Always consult the laboratory for special instructions when requesting specialized tests such as tissue markers, electron microscopy, and immunofluorescence.
- The pathologist should receive the patient's detailed clinical history.
- All specimens should be properly labeled with the patient's name, date of birth, patient location, specimen type, site (including laterality), surgeon's name, date and time.
- The laboratory and the pathologist should be consulted ahead of surgery for complicated surgical excisions, for frozen sections, and when there is uncertainty about how to handle the specimens.

American Academy of Ophthalmology. *Basic and Clinical Science Course, Section 4: Ophthalmic Pathology and Intraocular Tumors.* San Francisco: American Academy of Ophthalmology; 2014.

Almousa R, Charlton A, Rajesh ST, Sundar G, Amrith S. Optimizing muscle biopsy for the diagnosis of mitochondrial myopathy. *Ophthal Plast Reconstr Surg.* 2009; 25(5):366–370.

Center for Cancer Research. "Laboratory of Pathology Online Policy Manual." Available at http://goo.gl/p9gUpr. Accessed November 15, 2014.

Department of Ophthalmology, University of Iowa Hospitals and Clinics, Ocular Pathology Laboratory. "Special Procedure Specimen Collection." Available at http:/goo.gl/U2RSgB. Accessed November 15, 2014.

Doan A. "Eight Pearls for Reducing Medical Errors in Eye Pathology." Available at http://goo.gl/MLUQKE. Accessed November 15, 2014.

Glasgow B. "Eye Pathology Specimen Processing Manual for Residents." Available at http://goo.gl/slVm3a. Accessed November 15, 2014.

Lott R, Tunnicliffe J, Sheppard E, et al; College of American Pathologists. "Pre-Microscopic Examination Specimen Handling Guidelines in the Surgical Pathology Laboratory." Available at http://goo.gl/vFYLIo. Accessed November 15, 2014.

National Cancer Institute. "Laboratory of Pathology Online Policy Manual." Available at http://goo.gl/dtiGjN. Accessed November 15, 2014.

The Children's Hospital of Philadelphia. "Muscle Biopsy—General Instructions." Available at http://goo.gl/OPUq9f. Accessed November 15, 2014.

"The David G. Cogan Ophthalmic Pathology Collecction." Available at http://cogancollection.nei.nih.gov. Accessed November 15, 2014.

University College London, Institute of Ophthalmology, Department of Eye Pathology. "Ophthalmic Pathology Diagnostic Service User Guide." Available at http://goo.gl/Z3KLHs. Accessed November 15, 2014.

Ypsilantis E, Courtney ED, Chopra N, Karthikesalingam A, et al. Importance of specimen length during temporal artery biopsy. *Br J Surg.* 2011; 98(11):1556–1560.

262 • Basic Principles of Ophthalmic Surgery

Self-Assessment Test

1. The ophthalmic surgeon takes several conjunctival biopsies for suspected sebaceous cell carcinoma. Which of the following is an appropriate way to handle the tissue?
   a. Put all specimens in one formalin-filled container.
   b. Submit each specimen in a separate formalin-filled container and properly label each container indicating the biopsy site.
   c. Submit all specimens fresh in one container.
   d. Wrap each specimen in moist gauze, submit in separate containers, and deliver to the laboratory expeditiously.
   e. b and d

2. What is the proper volume of fixative for an enucleation specimen?
   a. 5 times the tissue volume
   b. 10 times the tissue volume
   c. 15 times the tissue volume
   d. 20 times the tissue volume

3. Communication with the pathologist is recommended in situations below except which of the following?
   a. vitreous tap for evaluation of possible lymphoma
   b. planned conjunctival biopsy for cystinosis
   c. corneal biopsy for suspect *Acanthamoeba* ulcer
   d. extraction of a mature cataract
   e. assessment of resection margins by frozen section for an infiltrating malignant eyelid tumor

For preferred responses, see Appendix A.

CHAPTER 22

Complications and Their Consequences

Sarah W. DeParis, MD
M. Reza Vagefi, MD

Operative complications, while infrequent, are part of any surgical specialty. Accordingly, education about the implications of unanticipated outcomes as they apply to the patient, the physician, and the legal system is an important part of residency training in ophthalmology.

An adverse event can be defined as an unwelcome and unintended, though not necessarily unanticipated, result of a medical treatment. For example, an allergic reaction to an ophthalmic drop or an elevation of intraocular pressure after a glaucoma laser procedure is considered an adverse event associated with a particular treatment.

In contrast, the Institute of Medicine defines a medical error as an adverse event that could have been prevented given the current state of medical knowledge. In 2000, the Quality Interagency Coordination Task Force mandated by President Bill Clinton expanded the working definition of a medical error to cover as many types of errors as possible. As defined by the Task Force, a medical error is "the failure of a planned action to be completed as intended or the use of a wrong plan to achieve an aim. Errors can include problems in practice, products, procedures, and systems." A surgical complication is thus a specific type of medical error and may be defined as any undesirable, unintended, and direct result of surgery affecting the patient that would not have occurred had the surgery gone as well as could reasonably be hoped.

Care of the Patient

Foremost, care of the patient begins long before surgery with the preoperative visit when the patient-physician relationship is established and the informed consent process is initiated. All surgical procedures carry risk, and errors can occur despite appropriate and meticulous patient care. As such, a detailed discussion of the risks of surgery, including the possibility of the need for additional surgeries should an untoward event occur, can help prepare the patient for news of an unanticipated outcome.

When a surgical error does occur, immediate care of the patient takes first priority. This includes appropriate intraoperative management of the error, as well as subsequent postoperative care. After primary surgical management is complete and the patient is stable, consultation and referral to a subspecialist should promptly be initiated if indicated, preferably with direct communication between the physicians. In addition, the outcome and care plan should be communicated with the patient's primary care doctor and referring physician when applicable. Following the disclosure of the error to the patient as outlined below, contact information for the surgeon and care team should be provided. A clear plan should be outlined for close follow-up. If postoperative sequelae such as elevated intraocular pressure or inflammation occur, they should be treated promptly. If additional surgery is required, informed consent must be obtained for any new treatments.

It is a surgeon's ethical responsibility to promptly disclose an error that may affect a patient's well-being. Survey studies have indicated that patients want to be informed when a medical error occurs. Patients may experience a wide range of emotions after an error, such as feeling hurt, deceived, embarrassed, debased, and/or scared. Accordingly, when there is an unanticipated surgical outcome that will adversely affect the patient's visual or physical health, an initial disclosure discussion should be held once the patient is physically and psychologically able to receive this information. It is important to hold the discussion as soon as possible and as is appropriate at the physician's discretion, for example once the patient has adequately recovered from anesthesia. Responsibility of the error is shared with the attending physician supervising the case, and it thus may be appropriate for that person to be present for the discussion as well.

The objective of the disclosure discussion is to communicate sympathetically to the patient and family what occurred, to express regret of the event, and to explain how it will immediately affect the patient's health, vision, and prognosis. Part of the discussion should explain the patient's current needs and goals. This process helps ease patient confusion, anger, and distrust. Candid disclosure of the error also helps demonstrate a continued commitment to the care and well-being of the patient, thus ensuring much needed follow-up and possible need for additional interventions. Furthermore, patients often feel that they have played a role in the error, and the discussion can help alleviate some of these sentiments.

When choosing a location for the discussion, the resident must consider the patient's privacy and healthcare needs. One should use receptive body language with good eye contact and avoid creating physical barriers by crossing arms or legs. The surgeon should state that an error was made and convey a continued duty to the patient's care. Sympathy should be expressed for the patient and family, as this can help strengthen the patient-physician relationship. Examples of statements that can be used include

- "I am sorry that this has happened to you."
- "This should not have happened."
- "I understand how you must be feeling."

The physician should, however, avoid statements that assign blame or assume responsibility. The physician should validate the patient's concerns and give ample time for the patient to express his or her emotions and ask questions. It is not unnatural for the patient and/or family to become distressed or angered by the news of an error, but it is paramount for the physician to refrain from becoming defensive.

During the disclosure discussion, it is important that the physician acknowledge the error by stating the facts and using nontechnical language. Subjective opinion, such as speculation about the fault of others or of instrumentation involved in the incident, should be excluded. Criticizing any prior care that the patient has received should also be avoided. The surgeon should then verify the patient's understanding of what was discussed and of the plan for follow-up care. During this time and in subsequent moments, the surgeon may tend to unintentionally distance himself or herself from the patient because of the complexity the error adds to the patient-physician relationship. Rather, the surgeon should be available to see the patient as frequently as necessary in the recovery period, because it is not only essential in their care but also in restoring and maintaining their trust. Finally, if the patient requests a second opinion, the surgeon should be supportive and help him or her find another provider. A detailed documentation of the discussion should be recorded, including the follow-up plan.

Medicolegal Implications of an Error

During training, a resident may feel somewhat insulated from the medicolegal outcomes of an error. However, a physician-in-training should be aware of the legal implications of a medical error, not just for a better understanding of medical malpractice, but also because these issues may directly affect them and will apply to their future careers.

The occurrence of an error in itself does not necessarily mean that medical malpractice has ensued. To establish medical negligence, the plaintiff must prove:

- the existence of a duty of care owed to the patient by an established patient-physician relationship
- negligence, or violation of this duty, caused by a negligent act or omission on behalf of the physician
- a causal connection between the negligent act and subsequent injury to the patient
- injury to the patient, as demonstrated by pain and suffering, disability or disfigurement, or wrongful death

In the event of an error, proper postoperative management and thorough documentation can help prevent future legal action.

Initial Management Strategies

The informed consent discussion and preoperative visit are not only the first steps in proper patient care, but also in mitigating medicolegal risk in the event of an unanticipated surgical outcome. For example, the 2 most commonly cited issues in oculoplastic surgery cases that ended in litigation were an alleged lack of informed consent and a need for additional surgeries. A detailed, well-documented consent process is crucial to providing appropriate patient care and avoiding legal consequences for the physician.

After an error has occurred and the patient's immediate physical needs have been met, the initial disclosure discussion with the patient and family should be held. Hospitals are required to develop policies on disclosure of unanticipated outcomes to patients by Joint Commission regulations and thus the surgeon should be certain to follow the recommendations of his or her institution. From a legal standpoint, some states have implemented laws requiring healthcare organizations to disclose adverse events or unanticipated outcomes to patients. In other states, there is a legal precedence that stems from case law where a surgeon has a duty to disclose an error because of the fiduciary nature of the patient-physician relationship. Failure to do so has been recognized by courts as fraud and/or fraudulent concealment even in the absence of false statements. Moreover, disclosure may decrease the risk of litigation, as the desire to discover what led to the error is a frequent cause of many lawsuits.

Many physicians incorrectly perceive that an apology will increase the risk of legal proceedings, when there is actually little evidence to support this. While an apology is admissible into evidence, such an admission does not correlate to evidence of guilt, as it does not automatically prove that the surgeon departed from the standard of medical care. Moreover, case law supports that judges and juries like apologies and treat them favorably. In reality, cases of malpractice litigation have demonstrated that patients are incensed when there is a failure to acknowledge a mistake and apologize. Such a failure is thought to lie at the root of the majority of suits.

Complete documentation includes the facts of what occurred, the healthcare team's subsequent management of the error, what was covered in the disclosure discussion, who was present at the discussion (including names of family members), and the treatment and follow-up plans. All of this documentation should all be included in the medical record. The physician should consider filing an incident report or contacting hospital risk management if these options are available and appropriate.

Later Management

The surgeon should be actively involved in the patient's postoperative care well beyond the initial disclosure discussion. All patient requests and questions should be responded to promptly. If the patient requests a waiver of fees, a consideration can be made as doing so is not considered an admission of liability; however, the surgeon should consult with hospital risk management and/or office of general counsel, as certain contracts with third-party payers may restrict refunds, and state law may require this to be disclosed or reported. In the event of litigation, a physician should seek legal help from the institution's office of general counsel and disclose all events fully to the legal advisors.

If applicable, a case review or root cause analysis should be conducted following a surgical error in order to find the cause of the incident and improve future outcomes. Hospitals have quality improvement committees that are responsible for conducting the event analyses, and the surgeon and healthcare team will often be actively involved in this process. The goal of the event analysis is to develop a corrective action plan that will help to prevent the same error from occurring again in the future. Finally, throughout this process it is important to acknowledge the effect of the error on all members of the healthcare team, as these events can be unsettling for everyone involved.

Medicolegal Implications of Cataract Surgery Complications

Although the incidence of retained or dropped lens fragments during cataract surgery is a relatively infrequent surgical error (0.1%–1.6%), it is associated with 12.5% of malpractice claims related to cataract surgery. However, as good visual outcomes can often be achieved when this error is managed appropriately, the preoperative, intraoperative, and postoperative care of the patient are vital in determining both the visual outcome for the patient and the likelihood of legal consequences for the physician. In one study of cataract surgery litigation, a larger difference between preoperative and postoperative visual acuity was the strongest predictor of worse legal outcomes. Delay in diagnosis or delay in referral were additionally cited in 11% of claims related to retained or dropped lens fragments. As such, close follow-up care, prompt control of postoperative inflammation and elevated intraocular pressure, as well as early referral to a specialist if appropriate are crucial in the management of surgical errors for both the patient's and physician's well-being.

Care of the Surgeon in the Event of an Error

It is normal for a surgeon at any level of training to feel self-doubt following a surgical error, regardless of whether litigation results. There is a significant amount of pressure for perfection in medicine. Consequently, resident physicians may experience a spectrum of emotions including shock, guilt, shame, vulnerability, fear, anxiety, anguish and isolation. Moreover, they may worry about the ramifications to their professional relationships and reputation. Besides fear of the patient outcome, physicians place significant weight on fear of disciplinary action or punishment. Studies have found that 95% of physicians experience significant distress during litigation.

Several unfavorable coping mechanisms are often employed after an unanticipated event including denial, minimization of the outcome, and distancing from the error. Residents who experience a surgical error should acknowledge that it is normal to feel emotional and physical distress. They should bear in mind that by mere disclosure of the error to the patient, they will begin to obtain forgiveness and decrease their feeling of guilt. It is important that they remain levelheaded during this time. Residents should be aware that these feelings might create an inadvertent desire to distance themselves from the patient. However, residents should see the patient as frequently as is possible and appropriate in the recovery period, because it is not only essential in the patient's care, but in the resident's own learning and recovery.

Surgeons-in-training should make use of the support system available at their institution. First and foremost, they should review the error with the attending physician who participated in the surgery. Then, a discussion of the case at the department's morbidity and mortality or quality improvement conference can help facilitate insight while receiving support and suggestions from their peers on how to better prevent the error. In addition, they may find it not only educational but also therapeutic to seek relevant information in the medical literature in order to better understand what occurred and why. Should there be a need for further conversation, the program director should be approached.

Symptoms of ongoing depression or anxiety merit a consultation with a primary care physician or mental health expert. In addition, universities may have mental health services available at no cost for resident physicians, which can provide relief in the form of a safe, confidential space to share feelings and mitigate stress. Residents should continue to participate in leisure activities and exercise for the maintenance of their mental well-being. However, in reflecting on the event and internally processing, residents should try not to assign blame or be excessively critical of themselves.

Sharing feelings with trusted coworkers, family, or friends who were not involved can also help. Although one should avoid disclosing patient protected health information or details about the case, conferring with family or trusted friends can be therapeutic for those who experience great emotional distress following an error or in the event of litigation. Lastly, other support resources may be found online, such as the Physician Litigation Stress Resource Center (www.physicianlitigationstress.org) or Cooperative of American Physicians (http://www.capphysicians.com).

Key Points

- In the event of a surgical error, immediate care of the patient takes first priority.
- It is a surgeon's ethical responsibility to promptly disclose an error to the patient that may affect their well-being.
- Statements of empathy and apology can help build the patient-physician relationship and reestablish trust, but blame or assumption of responsibility should be avoided.
- Consultation with risk management and event or root cause analysis should be sought, if available.
- In a medical malpractice case, the plaintiff must prove duty of care, negligence, a causative link between the negligent act and injury to the patient, and damages.
- A detailed informed consent process is crucial to building the patient relationship and mitigating potential future risk.
- Negative emotional reactions are common and normal following surgical errors.
- Residents should seek support from their colleagues, friends and family, and institutional network to mitigate stress.

Charles SC. Coping with a medical malpractice suit. *West J Med.* 2001;174(1):55–58.

Engel KG, Rosenthal M, Sutcliffe KM. Residents' responses to medical error: coping, learning, and change. *Acad Med.* 2006;81(1):86–93.

Kim JE, Weber P, Szabo A. Medical malpractice claims related to cataract surgery complicated by retained lens fragments (an American Ophthalmological Society thesis). *Trans Am Ophthalmol Soc.* 2012;110:94–116.

Mazor KM, Simon SR, Gurwitz JH. Communicating with patients about medical errors: a review of the literature. *Arch Intern Med.* 2004;164(15):1690–1697.

Menke AM. Responding to unanticipated outcomes. San Francisco: Ophthalmic Mutual Insurance Company Risk Management; 2014.

Pinto A, Faiz O, Bicknell C, Vincent C. Surgical complications and their implications for surgeons' well-being. *Br J Surg.* 2013;100(13):1748–1755.

Porto GG. Disclosure of medical error: facts and fallacies. *J Healthc Risk Manag.* 2001;21(4): 67–76.

Rehm PH, Beatty DR. Legal consequences of apologizing. *J Disp Resol.* 1996;1:1–165.

Report of the Quality Interagency Coordination Task Force to the President. "Doing What Counts for Patient Safety: Federal Actions to Reduce Medical Errors and Their Impact." Available at http://archive.ahrq.gov/quic/report/mederr2.htm. Accessed November 15, 2014.

Sokol DK, Wilson J. What is a surgical complication? *World J Surg.* 2008;32(6):942–924.

Svider PF, Blake DM, Husain Q, et al. In the eyes of the law: malpractice litigation in oculoplastic surgery. *Ophthal Plast Reconstr Surg.* 2014;30(2):119–123.

Self-Assessment Test

1. In the event of a surgical error, it is in the surgeon's best interest to do which of the following?
   a. Avoid disclosure of events in order to avoid future medicolegal consequences.
   b. Do not apologize, as doing so is an admission of guilt.
   c. Promptly and fully disclose to the patient what happened.
   d. Assign blame for the error to others.
2. It is normal for surgeons to experience negative emotions following a surgical error. Good strategies to cope with these feelings include all EXCEPT which of the following?
   a. talking with trusted friends and family
   b. presenting the error at a morbidity and mortality conference
   c. seeking the care of a mental health professional
   d. distancing oneself from further care of the patient
3. In a medical malpractice case, the plaintiff must prove that which of the following things have occurred? (Choose all that apply.)
   a. duty of care
   b. negligence
   c. a causative link between the negligence and injury to the patient
   d. damages
4. Following an error, all activities should be done EXCEPT which of the following?
   a. prompt referral to a specialist or for a second opinion as appropriate
   b. frequent follow-up visits
   c. use of an intermediary (other physician, office staff, etc.) to avoid further direct contact with the patient
   d. consultation with risk management if available

For preferred responses to these questions, see Appendix A.

Preferred Responses, Chapter Self-Assessment Tests

Chapter 1

1. d
2. cardiac disease, systemic hypertension, pulmonary disease, diabetes
   mellitus, altered mental status, postural limitations
3. a, b, c

Chapter 2

1. b
2. d
3. f

Chapter 3

1. b, c, d
2. exercise, sleep deprivation
3. true
4. a, b

Chapter 4

1. d
2. b
3. d

Chapter 5

1. a
2. d
3. c
4. d

Chapter 6

1. d
2. a
3. d

Chapter 7

1. d
2. a, d
3. a, c, e, f
4. a, d

Chapter 8

1. d
2. c
3. c
4. a
5. d

Chapter 9

1. a
2. d
3. a
4. c

Chapter 10

1. c
2. d
3. a, b, e
4. a, b, c, d
5. b

Chapter 11

1. b
2. a
3. e
4. d

Chapter 12

1. a, b
2. b, d
3. b
4. a, c
5. d
6. b

Chapter 13

1. true
2. a
3. false
4. d
5. d
6. true
7. true

Chapter 14

1. a, c, d
2. a
3. a, d
4. excessive postoperative inflammation, sterile hypopyon in diabetics, intravenous infusion may be lethal
5. increased infusion pressure, gas bubble infusion

Chapter 15

1. b, d
2. a, b, c
3. a
4. a, b, d

Chapter 16

1. hyaluronic acid
2. a, c
3. a

4. a, b, c, d
5. identify vitreous strands, protect lens in penetrating keratoplasty, facilitate iridectomy, prevent iris capture of intraocular lens

Chapter 17

1. a, b, c, d
2. b, c
3. a, b, d, e
4. a, b, c, d

Chapter 18

1. a, b, c, d, e
2. b, c, d, e
3. c, d
4. a, b, c, d, e
5. a, b, c, d, f, g
6. c

Chapter 19

1. e
2. a, c
3. b
4. a, b, c

Chapter 20

1. a, c
2. a, b, d
3. b, c, d
4. a, b, d

Chapter 21

1. e
2. b
3. d

Chapter 22

1. c
2. d
3. a, b, c, d
4. c

Index

Page numbers followed by *f* denote figures; those followed by *t* denote tables.

A

Absorbable sutures, 112–114, 113*t*
Accommodation, 80
Accreditation Council for Graduate Medical Education
  case logs, 133–138
  definition of, 133
  informed consent core competencies, 25
  milestones, 137–138
  residency programs, 133, 134*t*, 137
  surgical logs, 133–138
  surgical training requirements, 133–138
Acetylcholine, 192
ACGME. *See* Accreditation Council for Graduate
  Medical Education
Adjuvant agents, 156–157
Adverse events, 263, 266
Advertising, 7–8
Aflibercept, 195
Akahoshi prechopper, 101*f*
Ak-Taine. *See* Proparacaine
Ak-T-Caine. *See* Tetracaine
Alcaine. *See* Proparacaine
Alcian blue stain, 253*t*
Alcohol, 144
Alizarin red stain, 253*t*
Allergic reactions, 263
α-1 blockers, 7
Altered mental status, 6
Alternatives to surgery, 11–12
American Heart Association, 12–13
Aminoglycosides, 194
Amphotericin, 194
Anesthesia
  brainstem, 166
  central nervous system spread of, 166
  complications of
    central nervous system spread of anesthesia, 166
    extraocular muscle trauma, 220
    injection into eye, 220
    injection into optic nerve, 220
    malignant hyperthermia, 167
    oculocardiac reflex, 166–167
    retrobulbar hemorrhage, 165–166
    scleral perforation, 166
    strabismus, 166
  general, 153, 163*t*, 163–164
  hypotensive, 171
  intracameral, 193
  local. *See* Local anesthesia
  overview of, 153
  patient's understanding of, 12
  regional. *See* Regional anesthesia
  safety during, 153–154
  special requirements or concerns, 13
  topical. *See* Topical anesthesia
Anesthetic blocks
  administration of, 14
  parabulbar, 162, 162*f*

  patient positioning and, 14
  peribulbar
    complications of, 220
    technique for, 161*f*, 161–162
  retrobulbar
    complications of, 220
    technique for, 159–161, 160*f*
Anethaine. *See* Tetracaine
Angiogenesis, 230
Animal eyes, as simulation models, 36, 36*f*–37*f*
Anterior chamber
  paracentesis, 219
  viscoelastic injection into, 189
Anterior chamber irrigating cannula, 100*f*
Anterior segment surgery. *See also* Cataract surgery
  advances in, 129
  complications of, 220–221
  examination after, 217–218
  postoperative care for, 215–216
Antibiotics, 194
Anticoagulants, 5
Antifungals, 194
Anti-inflammatories, 238–239
Antiproliferative agents, 239
Antiseptic agents
  application of, 144, 145*f*
  types of, 143–144
Anxiety, 268
Apology, 266
Armrests, 51*f*, 72, 73*f*
A-scan ultrasonography, 157
Aseptic techniques
  draping, 50*f*, 147, 149*f*
  gloving, 146–147, 148*f*
  gowning, 146–147
  hand scrubbing, 20, 144–145, 146*f*
  history of, 143
Atkinson needle, 159, 161

B

B5, 252*t*
Balanced salt solution, 191–192
Barraquer cilia forceps, 93*f*
Barraquer iris spatula, 99*f*
Barraquer needle holder, 99*f*
Barraquer wire, 87*f*
Barron radial vacuum trephine, 104*f*
Barron vacuum punch, 104*f*
Basement membrane, 230
Bechert nucleus rotator, 98*f*
Bed. *See* Surgical bed
Beer cilia forceps, 93*f*
Benzalkonium chloride, 155
Benzodiazepines, 153
Beta-blockers, 19
Betadine. *See* Povidone-iodine
Bevacizumab, 195
Bioadhesives, 237

Biosyn sutures, 112, 113*t*
Bishop-Harmon forceps, 93*f*
Blades. *See* Surgical blades
Bleb, 232*f*
Bleeding
    intraoperative, 171, 174
    prevention of, 171
    silicone oil control of, 174
Blocks. *See* Anesthetic blocks; Facial nerve blocks;
    specific block
Blunt-tip keratome, 107*f*
Body language, 264
Bouin solution, 252*t*
Bowman lacrimal probe, 89*f*
Bowman layer, 233
Bradykinin, 229
Braided sutures, 112
Brainstem anesthesia, 166
Brevital. *See* Methohexital
Bruch's membrane, 125
Bupivacaine, 155*t*, 156
Buried interrupted subcutaneous suture,
    184, 184*f*

C
Caffeine, 19
Calipers, 105*f*
Cannulas, 100, 100*f*–101*f*
Capsular staining agents, 194–195
Capsular tension rings, 96, 97*f*
Capsule polishers, 102, 102*f*
Capsule retractors, 96, 98*f*
Capsulorrhexis
    bent needle used for, 189
    forceps for, 95*f*
    simulation training tools for, 37, 38*f*
Capsulotomy, Nd:YAG laser, 124, 128
Carbachol, 192
Carbocaine. *See* Mepivacaine
Carbon dioxide laser, 173
Cardiac disease, 5
Cardiac valvular disease prophylaxis, 12–13
Case logs, 133–138
Case review, 266
Castroviejo caliper, 105*f*
Castroviejo needle holder, 100*f*
Castroviejo suturing forceps, 93*f*
Cataract surgery
    blades for, 107*f*
    capsulorrhexis step of, 75
    complications of, 220–221, 267
    concerns before, 4*t*
    examinations after, 215
    microscope light intensity for, 81
    patient evaluation before, 4*t*, 4–5
    postoperative care for, 215
    retained or dropped lens fragments during, 267
    simulation training tools for, 37, 38*f*
    virtual reality simulation tools for, 39, 40*f*
Cautery, 171
Cautery units, 205, 205*f*
Ceftazidime, 194

Chair
    ergonomic practices, 53–54, 54*f*
    office, 53–54
    surgical. *See* Surgical chair
Chalazion excision instruments, 88, 88*f*
Chang-Seibel chopper, 101*f*
Children, 6, 67–68
Chin-down position, 66, 66*f*
Chin-up position, 66, 66*f*
Chlorhexidine gluconate, 20, 144
Choroidal neovascular membrane, 125
Choroidal specimen, 259
Chromic gut sutures, 113*t*, 114, 237*t*
Chromophores, 121
Cilia forceps, 93*f*
Ciliary body specimen, 258
Clear cornea blades, 108*f*
Clindamycin, 194
Clinic ergonomics, 54–55, 55*t*, 56*f*–58*f*
Cocaine, 154, 154*t*
Coefficient of friction, 111
Cohesive viscoelastics
    advantages of, 187
    description of, 187–189
    indications for, 189, 190*f*
    removing of, 190–191
    viscodissection use of, 189, 191*f*
CO_2 lasers, 119
Colibri corneal forceps, 93*f*
Colloidal iron stain, 253*t*
Communication
    medication errors prevented by, 202–204
    operating room staff, 14
Complications
    anesthesia-related
        central nervous system spread of anesthesia, 166
        malignant hyperthermia, 167
        oculocardiac reflex, 166–167
        retrobulbar hemorrhage, 165–166, 220
        scleral perforation, 166
        strabismus, 166
    anterior segment surgery, 220–221
    cataract surgery, 220–221, 267
    corneal transplantation, 221
    definition of, 219
    eyelid surgery, 221
    glaucoma surgery, 221
    laser surgery, 222
    operative, 263–268
    orbital surgery, 221
    postoperative, 219–222
    retinovitreous surgery, 221–222
    strabismus surgery, 221
Compounding, of intraocular drugs, 195–196
Computer monitors, 53
Congenital heart failure, 5
Congo red stain, 253*t*
Conjunctival forceps, 95*f*
Conjunctival specimens, 257
Conjunctival wound, 231–232
Consent. *See* Informed consent
Continuous wave lasers, 120, 124

Cooperative of American Physicians, 268
Coping, with surgical error, 267
Cornea
  avascular nature of, 234
  diseases involving, 6
  edema of, 6
  epithelium of, 233
  specimens of, 257
  stroma of, 233
  suturing of, 180
  transplantation of, 216, 221
Corneal buttons, 257
Corneal endothelial guttata, 4
Corneal markers, 103
Corneal stromal flaps, 121
Corneal trephines, 104*f*
Corneal wounds
  central, 234
  healing of, 233–235
  tensile strength of, 234
Corticosteroids, 194
Counter touch with nondominant hand, for hand
    tremor, 75, 76*f*
Counterweight setting, 77, 77*f*
CPT codes, 134, 136
Crawford hook, 90*f*
Crawford stent, 90*f*
Crescent blade, 107*f*
"Crossed swords" technique, 236
Crystal violet stain, 253*t*
Cumulative trauma disorders. *See* Work-related
    musculoskeletal disorders
Curette, 88*f*
Cutting needles, 115, 117*f*
Cyclodialysis spatulas, 99*f*
Cyclosporine A, 239
Cystoid macular edema, 217
Cystotome, 106*f*

D
Depression, 268
Descemet membrane, 234
Descemet membrane punch, 105*f*
Desmarres lid retractor, 86*f*
Dexon sutures, 112, 113*t*
Diabetes mellitus, 6, 128
Diagonal chop, 101
Diathermy, 171–173, 172*f*
Dilating drops, 13
Dilators, 89*f*
Diopter setting, 78
Diprivan. *See* Propofol
Direct ophthalmoscopy, 55*t*, 58*f*
Dispersive viscoelastics
  advantages of, 187–188
  description of, 187
  indications for, 189–190
Douglas cilia forceps, 93*f*
Draping, 50*f*, 147, 149*f*
Dressing(s)
  advantages of, 243
  combustibility of, 206, 206*f*
  description of, 243
  disadvantages of, 243
  illustration of, 206*f*
  indications for, 244
  nonpressure, with shield, 246–247, 246*f*–247*f*
  placement of, 246–248
  postoperative instructions for, 248
  pressure, 248, 248*f*
  removal of, 248
  supplies for, 244–245, 245*t*
Dressing forceps, 92
Drysdale nucleus manipulator and polisher, 102*f*
Duranest. *See* Etidocaine

E
Elbows, raising of, 72
Electrons, 119
Embolization, 174–175
Endophthalmitis, 192, 194, 199, 215, 222
Endothelial cells, 229
Energy density, 124
Enucleation scissors, 92*f*
Enucleation specimen, 259
Epinephrine, 156*t*, 156–157
Epithelial basement membrane dystrophy, 254*f*
Epithelial cells
  description of, 226
  wound healing of, 233
Epithelial growth factor, 230
Epithelialization, 230
Ergonomic practices
  chair sitting, 54, 54*f*
  in clinic, 54–55, 55*t*, 56*f*–58*f*
  direct ophthalmoscopy, 55*t*, 58*f*
  indirect ophthalmoscopy, 55*t*, 57*f*
  microscope, 50*f*–51*f*
  in office, 53*f*, 53–54
  in operating room, 46, 48, 49*f*–52*f*
  during patient preparation, 49*f*–50*f*
  postoperative period, 52*f*
  slit lamp, 55*t*, 56*f*–57*f*
  surgical bed, 49*f*
Ergonomics
  definition of, 45
  office, 53–54
  risk factors, 47*t*–48*t*, 49*f*–52*f*, 54*f*, 55, 55*t*, 56*f*–58*f*
Errors
  medication, 202–204, 204*t*
  surgical. *See* Surgical errors
Ethanol/methanol, 252*t*
Ethical considerations, 7–8, 26
Etidocaine, 155*t*, 156
Evisceration specimen, 258–259
Excimer lasers, 119
Exenteration specimen, 259
Exercise, 18
Extracellular matrix, 229, 231
Extraocular muscle
  specimen of, 257–258
  trauma to, 220
Extraocular simulation, 38
Eyelid clamp, 88*f*

Eyelid specimens, 256
Eyelid surgery, 216, 221
"Eye parallel to floor" position, 64–65, 65f, 67
Eye shields
    description of, 244
    nonpressure dressing with, 246–247, 246f–247f
    placement of, 246f–247f
Eyesi surgical simulator, 39, 40f

F
Facial nerve blocks
    description of, 164
    Nadbath-Ellis block, 164f, 165
    O'Brien block, 164f, 165
    Van Lint block, 164f, 164–165
Family members, 12
Fechtner conjunctival forceps, 95f
Femtosecond laser, 121
Fibrin, 233–234
Fibrin degradation products, 229
Fibrinogen, 173
Fibroblast, 226, 228–229, 233
Fibroin, 114
Fibronectin, 233
Field of view, 82
Fine–Thornton fixation ring, 105f
Fire, in operating room
    cautery units, 205, 205f
    combustible substances for, 206f, 206–207
    oxygen-enriched environment and, 205
    precautions to prevent, 206–207
    prevention of, 204–207
First intention, wound healing by, 225, 226f
Fixatives, 252t
Flat-shaped hydrodissection cannula, 100f
Flieringa scleral fixation ring, 105f
Fluence equations, 124
Fluid–gas exchange, 175
5-Fluorouracil, 239
Forceps, 92, 93f–95f, 102, 102f
Forearm scrubbing, 144, 146f
Formalin, 252, 252t
Formalin-fixed specimens, 252
Freer periosteal elevator, 106f
Frozen sections, 256
Frozen specimens, 251–252, 256

G
Gass retinal detachment hook, 98f
Gauze, 244
General anesthesia, 153, 163t, 163–164
Glaucoma surgery, 215, 221
Global Rating Assessment of Skills in Intraocular
    Surgery, 137, 138f
Globe puncture, 220
Gloving, 146–147, 148f
Glutaraldehyde, 252t, 260
Glutathione, 192
Gomori methenamine silver stain, 253t
Gowning, 146–147
Graefe iris forceps, 93f
Gram stain, 253t

Granulation tissue, 226f, 230
GRASIS. See Global Rating Assessment of Skills in
    Intraocular Surgery
Gripping of instruments, 52f, 74–75, 75f
Gross specimens, 260–261
Growth factors, 230
Guideline for Prevention of Surgical Site Infection, 143
Gut suture, 113t, 114, 237t

H
Halstead mosquito clamp, 106f
Hand(s)
    poor positioning of, 75
    scrubbing of, 20, 144–145, 146f
    during slit lamp use, 56f
    stabilization process for
        large arm muscles, 72
        raised elbows and, 72
        relaxation of small hand muscles, 74–75
        shoulder muscles, 72
        steps involved in, 72
        at wrist, 74, 75f
Hand grip, 75f
Hand lifting, 75
Hand tremor
    caffeine and, 19
    counter touch with nondominant hand to reduce,
        76, 76f
    hand stabilization to minimize. See Hand(s),
        stabilization process for
"Hang back" technique, 236
Harmonic generation, 120
Headrest, 64, 65f
Healing of wound. See Wound healing
Heating, for hemostasis
    cautery, 171
    diathermy, 171–173, 172f
    laser photocoagulation, 173
Heat transfer, using laser, 124–125
Hematoxylin and eosin stain, 253t, 253f
Hemostasis
    biochemical enhancement of, 173–174
    description of, 229
    embolization for, 174–175
    heating for, 171–173
    mechanical tamponade for, 174
    vasoconstriction for, 173
Henderson capsular tension ring, 97f
Herbal supplements, 5, 12
Hibiclens. See Chlorhexidine gluconate
Hockey stick blade, 107f
Honan balloon, 13, 160
Hooks, 90f, 98, 98f
Horizontal mattress suture, 182f, 182–183
Human eyes, as simulation models, 36, 37f
Hyaluronic acid, 189
Hyaluronidase, 156t, 157
Hydrodissection, 81
Hydrogel sealant, 238f
Hydroxypropyl methylcellulose, 187–189
Hypertension, 5, 171
Hypotensive anesthesia, 171

I

Illness, 19–20
Incisions
  site marking of, 13
  surgical instrument centering in, 76
Incompetent individuals, 12
Indirect ophthalmoscopy, 55t, 57f
Infants, 67–68
Infection prophylaxis, 199
Inflammatory phase, of wound healing, 229
Informed consent
  Accreditation Council for Graduate Medical
    Education core competencies for, 25
  alternatives to surgery, 11–12
  in compromised patient, 28
  consent element of, 27
  in dementia patient, 26, 28–29
  description of, 7, 11
  discussions included in, 27
  elements of, 11–12, 26–28
  importance of, 25–26
  with incompetent individuals, 12
  information included in, 27
  malpractice claim prevention through, 26
  medicolegal considerations, 25–26, 265
  with minors, 12
  obtaining of, by resident, 26, 28–31
  preconditions, 26–27
  procedure-related, 12, 128
  questions asked by patients during, 29–30
  scenarios involving, 28–31
  summary of, 31
  surgical risks-related, 12
  voluntariness as condition of, 26–27
Injections
  complications associated with, 220
  ergonomic practices during, 50f
  intravitreal. See Intravitreal injections
  local anesthetic agents, 155
  viscoelastics, 189
Instruments. See also specific instrument
  calipers, 105f
  cannulas, 100, 100f–101f
  capsule polishers, 102, 102f
  centering of, in incision, 76
  chalazion excision, 88, 88f
  corneal markers, 103
  curette, 88f
  description of, 85
  forceps, 92, 93f–95f, 102f
  gripping of, 52f, 74–75, 75f
  hooks, 90f, 98, 98f
  lacrimal, 88–89, 89f–90f
  lens loop, 105f
  needle holders, 99, 99f–100f
  nucleus choppers, 101, 101f
  nucleus splitters, 101
  posterior capsule polishers, 102f
  punches, 104f
  retractors, 85, 86f, 95–96, 96f, 98f
  scissors, 90, 91f–92f
  spatulas, 99, 99f

speculums, 86, 87f
surgeon's familiarity with, 18
trephines, 104f
Interrupted sutures
  buried subcutaneous, 184, 184f
  simple, 181, 181f
Intracameral miotics, 192, 193f
Intraocular anesthesia, 155, 158
Intraocular drugs, compounding of, 195–196
Intraocular fluids
  anesthetics, 193
  antibiotics, 194
  antifungals, 194
  capsular staining agents, 194–195
  corticosteroids, 194
  description of, 187
  irrigating fluids, 191–192
  miotics, 192–193, 193f
  mydriatics, 192–193
  viscoelastics. See Viscoelastics
Intraocular lens placement
  errors in, 201–202
  precautions for, 202t
Intraocular pressure, 164, 174, 217, 219
Intraocular simulation, 36–38, 36f–38f
Intraoperative floppy iris syndrome, 5–6, 95, 192
Intravitreal injections
  advantages of, 217
  complications of, 222
  dilated funduscopic examination after,
    217, 219
  follow-up evaluations, 217, 219
  indications for, 217
  intraocular pressure measurement after, 217,
    219, 222
  speculums for, 86
  vascular endothelial growth factor antagonists,
    195
Iodophors, 143–144
Iridectomy, 120, 258
Iridocyclectomy, 258
Iridotomies, 236, 236f
Iris
  abnormalities of, 6–7
  specimen of, 258
Iris forceps, 93f
Iris hooks, 98f
Iris retractors, 96f
Iris spatula, 99f
Irradiance equation, 124
Irrigating fluids, 191–192

J

Jaeger lid plate, 86f
Jaffe scissors, 91f
Jaffe wire retractor, 86f
Jamison muscle hook, 98f
Jensen posterior capsule polisher, 102f
Jeweler forceps, 94f
Joint Commission on Accreditation of Healthcare
    Organizations, 21, 200–201
J-shaped hydrodissection cannula, 100f

K

Katzin corneal transplant scissors, 92f
Kelly Descemet membrane punch, 105f
Kelman-McPherson angled tying forceps, 94f
Keratocytes, 233
Keratome, 107f
Keyboard, 53
Kimura spatula, 99f
Kitaro simulation training systems, 37, 38f
Knots
    simple square, 177–179, 178f
    tying of, 178f
Koch phaco spatula, 99f
Kratz-Barraquer speculum, 87f
Kuglen iris hook, 98f
Kyphosis, 48, 48f, 51f

L

Laboratory testing, 12
Lacrimal cannula, 100f
Lacrimal instruments, 88–89, 89f–90f
Lacrimal specimen, 258
Laser(s)
    burn considerations, 124–125
    CO_2, 119
    continuous wave, 120, 124
    controllable variables of, 125–126
    definition of, 119
    energy control, 124–125
    excimer, 119
    expectations of patients regarding, 128
    eyewear protection for, 127
    femtosecond, 121
    filters on, 127
    fluence equations for, 124
    foot switch for activation of, 127
    future directions for, 129
    harmonic generation, 120
    heat transfer considerations, 124–125
    irradiance equation for, 124
    media opacity considerations, 126
    Nd:YAG, 120–121, 124, 128
    ocular-cardiac responses to noxious stimuli from, 128
    organic dye, 120
    patient issues regarding, 127–129
    photoablation use of, 121
    photochemical use of, 123
    photocoagulation uses of, 121, 122f, 124, 127, 173
    photodisruption use of, 120–121
    physics of, 119–120
    "pulsed," 120
    safety considerations, 127
    spot size considerations, 125–126
    surgeon protections while using, 127
    surgery using, 216–219, 222
    tissue and, interactions between, 120–123, 121f–122f
    wavelength of, 123f, 123–124
Laser safety officer, 127
LASIK surgery, 121
Legal guardian, 12
Lens, 7
Lens loop, 105f

Lester IOL manipulator, 98f
Lidocaine
    administration of, 158
    intracameral, 192
    regional anesthesia uses of, 155t
    topical uses of, 154t, 155
Lighting
    for microscope, 81
    for surgical loupes, 82
Lister, Joseph, 143
Local anesthesia
    agents
        administration of, 154
        cocaine, 154, 154t
        injection of, 155
        intraocular, 155
        lidocaine, 154t, 155
        proparacaine, 154t, 154–155
        tetracaine, 154t, 155
    intraocular, 158
    topical
        advantages of, 157–158, 158t
        agents for, 154t, 154–155
        delivery of, 158
        description of, 157
        disadvantages of, 158, 158t
        patient selection for, 157
Lordosis, 48, 48f
Loupes. See Surgical loupes
Low back pain, 46
Lumbar kyphosis, 51f

M

Mackool capsular retractor, 98f
Macrophages, 229
Magnification
    using microscope
        description of, 63–64
        level of, 81
    using surgical loupes, 82
Malignant hyperthermia, 6, 167
Malpractice, 25–26, 203
Malyugin ring, 96f
Mandell eye mount, 36
Marcaine. See Bupivacaine
Masson trichrome stain, 253f, 253t
Matrix metalloproteinases, 229, 231, 238–239
McNeill-Goldman scleral fixation ring and
    blepharostat, 88f
McPherson tying forceps, 94f
Mechanical tamponade, 174
Medical clearance, 12–13
Medical negligence, 265
Medications. See also specific medication
    errors in, 202–204, 204t
    preoperative administration of, 13
Medicolegal considerations
    informed consent, 25–26, 265
    surgical errors, 265–267
Mental status alterations, 6
Mepivacaine, 155t, 156
Mersilene sutures, 237t

Methohexital, 153
Michel fixative, 252*t*
Microscope
  accommodation through, 80
  advantages of, 63–64
  bumping of, 68
  ceiling-mounted, 77
  counterweight setting, 77, 77*f*
  disadvantages of, 63–64
  ergonomic practices in using, 50*f*–51*f*
  floor-mounted, 77
  focus-related problems with, 81
  gross maneuvering of, 77–78
  hand stabilization process for. *See* Hand(s),
      stabilization process for
  light intensity of, 81
  magnification using, 63–64
  maneuvering of, 79–81
  oculars positioning and setting, 78–79
  operating steps for, 79
  patient positioning for
    chin-down position, 66, 66*f*
    chin-up position, 66, 66*f*
    problems in, 66–68
    surgical eye parallel to floor, 64–65, 65*f*
  pedals. *See* Microscope pedals
  positioning of, 14
  surgeon positioning for
    ergonomic practices, 50*f*
    foot clearance, 70*f*, 71–72
    overview of, 68
  surgical loupes vs, 81
  temporal approach, 69, 69*f*, 77
  vibration concerns for, 64
Microscope head
  centering button for, 77, 78*f*
  positioning handles on, 77–78, 78*f*
  swinging positioning arm for, 77, 77*f*
Microscope pedals
  elements of, 79, 80*f*
  illumination switch on, 80*f*
  illustration of, 80*f*
  joystick on, 79–80, 80*f*
  surgeon positioning for, 68, 68*f*, 78
Microsurgical forceps and handles, 102, 102*f*
Midazolam, 153
Minors, 12
Miostat. *See* Carbachol
Miotics, 192–193, 193*f*
Mitomycin C, 239
Model eyes, 37–38, 38*f*
Monitors, 53
Mono-Crawford stent, 90*f*
Monofilament sutures, 111–112
Morcher capsular tension ring, 97*f*
Mouse, computer, 53
MST capsule retractor, 98*f*
MST system, 102*f*
Multifilament sutures, 111
Muscle specimens, 257–258
Music, in operating room, 21
Mydriatics, 192–193

N
Nadbath-Ellis block, 164*f*, 165
Nd:YAG laser
  capsulotomy using, 124, 128
  description of, 120–121
Near–far vertical mattress suture, 182, 182*f*
Neck pain, 46, 47*t*
Needle holders, 99, 99*f*–100*f*
Needle knife, 108*f*
Needle point scissors, 91*f*
Negligence, medical, 265
Neutrophils, 229
Nitrous oxide gas, 164
Nominal hazard zone, 127
Nonpressure dressings, 246–247, 246*f*–247*f*
Nonsteroidal anti-inflammatory drugs, 5, 239
Nuclear disassembly, simulation training tools for,
    37, 38*f*
Nucleus choppers, 101, 101*f*
Nucleus splitters, 101
Nylon sutures, 114*t*, 115, 237*t*

O
O'Brien block, 164*f*, 165
Oculars, 78–79
Oculocardiac reflex, 166–167
Office ergonomics, 53–54
Operating room
  environment of
    equipment in, 18
    ergonomic issues, 20
    music in, 21
    preparation of, 20–21
    surgeon's familiarity with, 18
    time-out checklist for, 20–21
  ergonomic practices by surgeon in, 46, 48, 49*f*–52*f*
  fire in
    cautery units, 205, 205*f*
    combustible substances for, 206*f*, 206–207
    oxygen-enriched environment and, 205
    precautions to prevent, 206–207
    prevention of, 204–207
  incision sites, 13
  patient preparations in, 13–14
  patient's comfort in, 14
  staff communication in, 14
Operative site
  cleaning of, 144
  skin preparation, 143–144
  wrong-site surgery, 20, 199–201
Ophthaine. *See* Proparacaine
Ophthalmic anesthesia. *See* Anesthesia
Ophthalmic pathology
  specimens. *See* Specimens
  stains, 252, 253*t*
  supplies and equipment used in, 252, 252*t*
Ophthalmoscopy
  direct, 55*t*, 58*f*
  indirect, 55*t*, 57*f*
Ophthetic. *See* Proparacaine
Orbital lymphoma, 259
Orbitals, 119

Orbital surgery, 216, 221
Orbital tissue specimen, 259–260
Organic dye laser, 120
Osher/Malyugin ring manipulator, 96f
Otto device, 36
Oval eye pads, 244
Overuse syndromes. See Work-related musculoskeletal disorders
"Oxygen tent," 205

P

Pain
    low back, 46
    management of, 219
    neck, 46, 47t
    upper extremity, 46, 47t
Panretinal photocoagulation, 129
Parabulbar block, 162, 162f
Patient(s)
    boosting of, onto bed/cart, 49f
    comfort of, 14
    disclosure of surgical error to, 264–265
    draping of, 50f, 147, 149f
    expectations of, 3
    laser discussions with, 127–129
    lifting of, 49f
    postoperative instructions, 213–215
    preparation of
        ergonomic considerations during, 49f–50f
        ergonomic risk factors, 47t
        informed consent. See Informed consent
        medical clearance, 12–13
        in office, 11–13
        in operating room, 13–14
    safety issues and concerns for. See Safety issues
    surgeon meeting with, 13, 17
    treatment-related decision making by, 7
Patient positioning
    children, 67–68
    chin-down position, 66, 66f
    chin-up position, 66, 66f
    description of, 14
    "eye parallel to floor" position, 64–65, 65f, 67
    on headrest, 64, 66f
    infants, 67–68
    local anesthetic blocks, 14
    for microscope, 14, 64–68
    problems in, 66–68
    Trendelenburg position, 67, 67f
Perfluorooctane, 174
Peribulbar block
    complications of, 220
    technique for, 161f, 161–162
Periodic acid-Schiff stain, 253t
Periosteal elevator, 106f
Peripheral iridectomy, 120
Peripheral iridotomies, 236, 236f
Perls Prussian blue stain, 253t
Phaco chopper, 101f
Phacoemulsification grooving, 37
Photoablation, 121
Photochemical, 123

Photocoagulation
    lasers for, 121, 122f, 124, 129, 173
    retinal, 121, 124, 126, 129
    safety during, 127
Photodisruption, 120–121
Photons, 119–120
Physician Litigation Stress Resource Center, 268
Pigtail probe, 89f
Platelet derived growth factor, 230
Polishers, 102, 102f
Polyester sutures, 114, 114t
Polyglactin sutures, 112, 113t, 237t
Polypropylene sutures, 112, 114t, 115, 237t
Polysorb sutures, 112, 113t
Pontocaine. See Tetracaine
Positioning
    of bed, 70f, 70–72
    of hands, 75
    of patient. See Patient positioning
    of surgeon, 68–70
Posterior capsule polishers, 102f
Postoperative care
    anterior segment surgery, 215, 217–218
    ergonomic practices, 48t, 52f
    examinations, 217–219
    eyelid surgery, 216
    laser surgery, 216–219
    orbital surgery, 216
    pain management, 219
    retinovitreous surgery, 216, 218
    strabismus surgery, 216
    timing of, 215–217
Postoperative instructions, 213–215
Postoperative management, 213–224
Posture
    ergonomic risk factors for, 47t–48t
    good, 48f
    importance of, 5
    seated, 53f
    surgical risks and, 5
Povidone-iodine, 143
Power density, 124
Preconditions, of informed consent, 26–27
Pressure dressings, 248, 248f
Probes, 89f
Procedure. See also specific procedure
    discussion about, 12
    ergonomic practices during, 50f
    informed consent about, 12
    surgeon's familiarization and understanding of, 18
Proparacaine, 154t, 154–155
Propofol, 153
Proteases, 229
Proteoglycans, 233
Pulmonary disease, 5–6
"Pulsed" lasers, 120
Pumping, 119
Punches, 104f
Punctate keratopathy, 154
Pupillary dilation, 6
Pupillary distance, 78

Q

Quickert lacrimal probe, 89*f*

R

Ranibizumab, 195
Red reflex, 66, 220
Re-epithelialization, 231–232
Refractive keratotomy, 233
Regional anesthesia
 adjuvant agents for, 156–157
 advantages of, 159, 159*t*
 agents for
  bupivacaine, 155*t*, 156
  description of, 155–157
  etidocaine, 155*t*, 156
  lidocaine, 156
  mepivacaine, 155*t*, 156
 central nervous system spread of, 166
 complications of, 166
 description of, 158–159
 disadvantages of, 159, 159*t*
 epinephrine for, 156*t*, 156–157
 hyaluronidase for, 156*t*, 157
 parabulbar block, 162, 162*f*
 peribulbar block, 161*f*, 161–162, 220
 retrobulbar block. *See* Retrobulbar block
 sodium bicarbonate for, 156*t*, 157
Rehabilitation, 12
Remodeling of wound, 231
Repetitive motion/strain disorders. *See* Work-related
  musculoskeletal disorders
Requisitions, for specimens, 254, 255*f*
Residency programs, 133, 134*t*, 137
Residents
 informed consent obtained by, 26, 28–31
 questions asked of, by patients, 29–30
 surgical errors by, 267–268
 training of, 8
Retina
 photocoagulation of, 121, 124, 126, 129
 specimen of, 259
 translucency of, 126
Retinal pigment epithelium cells, 121, 122*f*
Retinal proteins, 126
Retinovitreous surgery, 216, 218, 221–222
Retractors
 capsule, 96, 98*f*
 general types of, 85
 iris, 95, 96*f*
Retrobulbar block
 complications of, 220
 description of, 159, 160*f*
Retrobulbar hemorrhage, 165–166
Reverse cutting needles, 115, 117*f*
Reverse Trendelenburg position, 171
Rhabdomyosarcoma, 259
Root cause analysis, 266
Routine specimens, 251–252
Ruedeman lacrimal dilator, 89*f*
Running horizontal mattress suture, 183–184, 184*f*
Running subcuticular sutures, 184–185, 185*f*
Running suture, 183–184, 184*f*

S

Safety issues
 anesthesia, 153–154
 infection prophylaxis, 199
 intraocular lens placement errors, 201–202
 lasers, 127
 medication errors, 202–204, 204*t*
 operating room fires
  cautery units, 205, 205*f*
  combustible substances for, 206*f*, 206–207
  oxygen-enriched environment and, 205
  precautions to prevent, 206–207
  prevention of, 204–207
 wrong-site surgery, 20, 199–201
Schepens orbital retractor, 106*f*
Schepens scleral depressor, 106*f*
Schocket scleral depressor, 106*f*
Scissors, 90, 91*f*–92*f*
Sclera
 perforation of, 166
 wound healing of, 235–236
Scleral blades, 107*f*–108*f*
Scleral depressors, 106*f*
Scleral fixation ring, 88*f*, 105*f*
Screw-type speculums, 87*f*
Scrubbing of hands, 20, 144–145, 146*f*
Scrub technician, 146
Seated posture, 53*f*
Second intention, wound healing by, 225, 226*f*
Sedation, 153–154
Seeley flat-shaped hydrodissection cannula, 100*f*
Serrefine, 106*f*
Sheath hematoma, 220
Sheets irrigating vectus, 105*f*
Shoulder muscles
 hand stabilization and, 72
 "shrugging" of, 72, 73*f*
 sustained retraction of, 51*f*
 work-related disorders involving, 47*t*
Silicone oil, 174
Silk sutures, 112, 114*t*, 114–115, 237*t*
Simple continuous (running) suture, 183, 183*f*
Simple interrupted suture, 181, 181*f*
Simple square knot, 177–179, 178*f*
Simulation
 benefits of, 35
 extraocular, 38
 intraocular, 36–38, 36*f*–38*f*
 virtual reality, 39–40
 wet laboratory, 35, 35*t*
Simulation models
 animal eyes, 36, 36*f*–37*f*
 human eyes, 36, 37*f*
 model eyes, 37–38, 38*f*
 Styrofoam head, 36, 37*f*
 suturing, 38, 39*f*
Sinskey hook, 98*f*
Skin preparation, 143–144
Sleep deprivation, 18–19
Sleeve spreading forceps, 95*f*
Slit lamp, 55*t*, 56*f*–57*f*
Smooth forceps, 92

Sodium bicarbonate, 156t, 157
Sodium hyaluronate, 174
Soft shell technique, 188, 188f
Spatula, 99, 99f
Spatula needles, 117, 117f
Special procedures, 260
Specimens
  choroidal, 259
  ciliary body, 258
  conjunctival, 257
  corneal, 257
  enucleation, 259
  evisceration, 258–259
  exenteration, 259
  eyelid, 256
  formalin-fixed, 252
  frozen, 251–252, 256
  frozen sections, 256
  gross, 260–261
  handling of, 252, 254, 256–260
  iris, 258
  labeling of containers for, 254
  lacrimal, 258
  muscle, 257–258
  orbital tissue, 259–260
  preoperative preparations for, 251–252
  requisitions for, 254, 255f
  retinal tissue, 259
  routine, 251–252
  special procedures, 260
  temporal artery biopsy, 258
  transportation of, 256
  vitreous, 260
Speculums, 86, 87f
Spot size, for lasers, 125–126
Stab knife blades, 107f
Staff, 14
Stainless steel sutures, 114t, 115
Stains, 252, 253t
Sterile field, 150
Steri-strips, 245
Stevens hook, 98f
Stevens tenotomy scissors, 91f
Strabismus, after regional anesthesia, 166
Strabismus surgery
  complications of, 221
  examination after, 218
  postoperative care, 216
  scleral healing, 235
  success criteria for, 218
  suturing in, 180
Substance use/abuse, 19
Superior rectus forceps, 93f
Surgeon
  apology by, 266
  bed positioning for, 70f, 70–72
  beta-blocker use by, 19
  caffeine use by, 19
  communication by, in operating theater, 21
  disclosure of surgical error to patient, 264–265
  experience of, 8
  familiarization of, 17–20

feet clearance for, 70f, 71–72
  flaring of knee by, 71, 71f
  handwashing by, 20
  illness effects on, 19–20
  instrumentation familiarity of, 18
  magnification level preferences, 81
  operating room fires caused by. See Operating room,
    fires in
  patient's interaction with, 13, 17
  performance of, 18–20
  physical factors that affect, 18–20
  positioning of, for microscope use, 50f, 68–70
  preparation of, 17–21
  procedure understood by, 18
  sleep deprivation effects, 18–19
  surgical error effects on, 267–268
  training of, 8
  voice quality of, 21
Surgeon's knot, 179
Surgery
  anterior segment. See Anterior segment surgery
  cataract. See Cataract surgery
  concerns before, 4t
  criteria for, 3
  "dry run" before, 18
  eyelid, 216
  glaucoma, 215
  goals of, 12
  laboratory testing before, 12
  laser. See Laser(s)
  orbital, 216
  patient's expectations about, 3
  patient's questions about, 29–30
  preoperative medical evaluation, 4–5
  resident in training, 8
  side-to-side eye movement during, 76
  temporal approach to, 69, 69f
Surgical bed
  bumping of, 70–71
  ergonomic practices, 49f
  illustration of, 65f
  lifting/lowering of, 49f
  positioning of, 70f, 70–72
Surgical blades
  cataract surgery, 107f
  clear cornea, 108f
  scleral, 107f–108f
  stab knife, 107f
Surgical case logs, 133–138
Surgical chair
  armrests on, 51f, 72, 73f
  height of, 72, 72f
  illustration of, 73f
Surgical errors
  disclosure of, 264–265
  intraocular lens placement, 201–202
  medicolegal implications of, 265–267
  patient care after, 263–265
  by residents, 267–268
  root cause analysis for, 266
  surgeon's response to, 267–268
Surgical instruments. See Instruments

Surgical loupes
  advantages of, 63, 81
  description of, 63
  field of view for, 82
  lighting for, 82
  magnification using, 82
  microscope vs, 81
  working distance with, 82
Surgical microscope. See Microscope
Surgical risks
  factors that affect, 4–7
  patient's understanding of, 12
  types of, 12
Suture(s)
  absorbable, 112–114, 113t
  Biosyn, 112, 113t
  braided, 112
  buried interrupted subcutaneous, 184, 184f
  characteristics of, 111
  chromic gut, 113t, 114, 237t
  classification of, 111–115
  Dexon, 112, 113t
  extraocular surgery, 116t
  gut, 113t, 114, 237t
  horizontal mattress, 182f, 182–183
  internal structure of, 112
  intraocular surgery, 116t
  material of, 112
  Mersilene, 237t
  monofilament, 111–112
  multifilament, 111
  near–far vertical mattress, 182, 182f
  nomenclature for, 111
  nonabsorbable, 112, 114t, 114–115
  nylon, 114t, 115, 237t
  polyester, 114, 114t
  polyglactin, 112, 113t, 237t
  polypropylene, 112, 114t, 115
  Polysorb, 112, 113t
  running horizontal mattress, 183–184, 184f
  running subcuticular, 184–185, 185f
  silk, 112, 114t, 114–115, 237t
  simple continuous (running), 183, 183f
  simple interrupted, 181, 181f
  size of, 115, 116t
  stainless steel, 114t, 115
  tensile strength of, 111
  vertical mattress, 181f, 181–182
  Vicryl. See Polyglactin
  wound healing affected by, 237, 237t
Suture needles, 115, 117, 117f
Suture scissors, 91f
Suturing
  corneal, 180
  needle position for, 179f, 179–180
  principles of, 179–180
  simulation models for, 38, 39f
  in strabismus surgery, 180

T
Tamsulosin, 5
Tape, 245

Taper point needles, 115, 117f
Telfa, 244, 245f
Temporal approach
  bed positioning for, 70, 70f
  microscope positioning for, 77
  surgeon positioning for, 69, 69f
Temporal artery biopsy specimen, 258
Tennant tying forceps, 94f
Tenotomy scissors, 91f
Tensile strength, 111
Tetracaine, 154t, 155
Thioflavin stain, 253t
Third intention, wound healing by, 225
Thrombin, 173–174
Throw, 178
Tilt, 78–79
Time-out checklist, 20–21
Tissue forceps, 92
Tissue inhibitors of metalloproteinases, 231
Tissue plasminogen activator, 230
Topical anesthesia
  advantages of, 157–158, 158t
  agents for, 154t, 154–155
  application of, 145f
  delivery of, 158
  description of, 13, 157
  disadvantages of, 158, 158t
  patient selection for, 157
Toric reference marker, 103f
Toxic anterior segment syndrome, 195
Trabeculectomy, 232f
Tremor. See Hand tremor
Trendelenburg position, 67, 67f
Trephines, 104f
Triamcinolone acetonide, 194
Trypan blue, 195
Tying forceps, 92, 94f

U
Upper extremity pain, 46, 47t
Uveal wound healing, 236
Uveitis, 217

V
Vancomycin, 194
Van Lint block, 164f, 164–165
Vannas scissors, 92f
Vascular endothelial growth factor
  antagonists of, 195
  description of, 230, 239
Vasoconstriction, 173
Verhoeff–van Gieson stain, 253t
Versed. See Midazolam
Verteporfin, 123
Vertical mattress suture, 181f, 181–182
Vicryl sutures, 112, 113t, 237t
Virtual reality simulation training, 39–40
Viscodissection, 189, 191f
Viscoelastics
  cohesive
    advantages of, 187
    description of, 187–189

indications for, 189, 190f
    removing of, 190–191
    viscodissection use of, 189, 191f
composition of, 187
dispersive
    advantages of, 187–188
    description of, 187–188
    indications for, 189–190
injection of, 188, 189f
properties of, 187
removing of, 190–191
soft shell technique for, 188, 188f
Vitreous specimens, 260
Voluntariness, as informed consent precondition, 26–27
von Kossa stain, 253t
VR. *See* Virtual reality

W
Watzke sleeve spreading forceps, 95f
Wavelength of laser, 123f, 123–124
Westcott conjunctival scissors, 91f
Westcott tenotomy scissors, 91f
Williams lacrimal probe, 89f
Wire retractor, 86f
Working distance, 82
Work-related musculoskeletal disorders, 46, 47t, 58–59
Wound
    contraction of, 230, 234
    remodeling of, 231
Wound closure
    description of, 177
    primary, 231, 232f
    simple square knot for, 177–179, 178f
    sutures used in
        buried interrupted subcutaneous, 184, 184f
        horizontal mattress, 182f, 182–183
        near–far vertical mattress, 182, 182f
        running horizontal mattress, 183–184, 184f
        running subcuticular, 184–185, 185f
        simple continuous (running), 183, 183f
        simple interrupted, 181, 181f
        vertical mattress, 181f, 181–182

Wound healing
    anti-inflammatories' effect on, 238–239
    antiproliferative agents' effect on, 239
    corneal, 233–235
    description of, 225
    epithelial cell, 233
    by first intention, 225, 226f
    inflammatory phase of, 229
    length of time for, 226
    modification of, 237–240
    phases of, 226
    practical considerations, 231–232
    proliferative phase of
        angiogenesis, 230
        contraction, 230
        description of, 229–230
        epithelialization, 230
        granulation tissue formation, 229
    re-epithelialization, 231–232
    scleral, 235–236
    by second intention, 225, 226f, 231
    summary of, 227f–228f
    suture materials' effect on, 237, 237t
    by third intention, 225
    tissue maturation phase of
        characteristics of, 231
        description of, 231
    uveal, 236
Wrist, hand stabilization at, 74, 74f
Wrist rest, 72, 74f
Wrong-site surgery, 20, 199–201

X
Xylocaine. *See* Lidocaine

Z
Zenker acetic fixative, 252t
Ziegler cilia forceps, 93f
Ziegler knife, 107f
Ziegler lacrimal canal probe, 89f
Ziehl-Neelsen stain, 253t